# THE ENCYCLOPEDIA OF

# KIDNEY DISEASES AND DISORDERS

THE ENCYCLOPEDIA OF

# KIDNEY DISEASES
# AND DISORDERS

I. David Weiner, M.D.

Christine Adamec

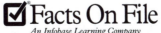

Facts On File

*An Infobase Learning Company*

**The Encyclopedia of Kidney Diseases and Disorders**

Copyright © 2012 by Christine Adamec

Facts On File
An imprint of Infobase Learning, Inc.
132 West 31st Street
New York NY 10001

**Library of Congress Cataloging-in-Publication Data**

Weiner, I. David.
The encyclopedia of kidney diseases and disorders / I. David Weiner, Christine Adamec.
p. ; cm.—(Library of health and living)
Includes bibliographical references and index.
ISBN-13: 978-0-8160-7544-7 (hardcover : alk. paper)
ISBN-10: 0-8160-7544-1 (hardcover : alk. paper) 1. Kidney—Diseases—Encyclopedias. I. Adamec, Christine A., 1949– II. Title. III. Series: Facts on File library of health and living.
[DNLM: 1. Kidney Diseases—Encyclopedias—English. WJ 13]
RC902.W397 2011
616.6'1003—dc22

Facts On File books are available at special discounts when purchased in bulk quantities for businesses, associations, institutions, or sales promotions. Please call our Special Sales Department in New York at (212) 967-8800 or (800) 322-8755.

You can find Facts On File on the World Wide Web at http://www.InfobaseLearning.com

Text design by Annie O'Donnell
Composition by Hermitage Publishing Services
Cover printed by Yurchak Printing, Landisville, Pa.
Book printed and bound by Yurchak Printing, Landisville, Pa.
Date printed: November 2011

Printed in the United States of America

10 9 8 7 6 5 4 3 2 1

This book is printed on acid-free paper.

# CONTENTS

# PREFACE

Kidney diseases and disorders are my particular passion and specialty: I am a practicing nephrologist and a medical school professor at the University of Florida in Gainesville. I take care of people with a wide variety of kidney diseases. I also teach future physicians what they need to know about nephrology, the branch of medicine concerned with the kidneys, so that they will be adept at treating future patients with kidney malfunction, from minor infections to the severity of kidney failure necessitating dialysis or a kidney transplantation. And I direct a research program aimed at better understanding how the kidney works in health and disease. I have coauthored this book, which discusses kidney illnesses at the layperson's level, to provide readers with a basic understanding of the key problems that may occur with the kidneys. These problems include chronic kidney disease, end-stage renal disease (kidney failure), kidney stones, and many other common diseases. Also discussed are some less common problems, such as Goodpasture syndrome or Alport syndrome. The book also covers common medical tests and procedures that nephrologists use to help them diagnose kidney disease and discusses how major kidney diseases can affect individuals in their daily lives. I also look at dietary changes that are needed by some individuals, such as patients who need to cut back on their consumption of certain foods or minerals to improve their health.

Many people with severe kidney disease have diabetes mellitus and/or hypertension, the top-two causes of kidney failure. I encourage anyone with these diseases to keep their blood sugar and their blood pressure as close to normal as possible in order to decrease the risk of developing serious kidney disease. It is also important for all adults to receive periodic blood testing of their kidney function; the majority of people with chronic kidney disease have no idea that their kidneys are deteriorating because they experience no symptoms until serious damage has occurred. If chronic kidney disease is identified and treated in the early stages, which it often can be with simple blood tests, then in many cases the kidneys can regain their health and the ravages of kidney disease may be altogether avoided. A simple blood test can provide this information.

The average person takes his or her kidneys for granted—until they malfunction or fail altogether—but as with most of the organs in the body, the kidneys require at least some routine maintenance. Simply seeing a physician at least on an annual basis and obtaining routine laboratory tests can ultimately mean the difference between kidney health and severe kidney disease. If a physician recommends a specialist, such as a nephrologist, then this recommendation should not be avoided or delayed.

If severe kidney disease does develop and the kidneys fail, many people can survive for years with dialysis or kidney transplantation. In fact, some transplantation procedures replace more than one failing organ at the same time, as with simultaneous kidney-liver transplants or kidney-pancreas transplants. Yet it is always best to try to keep the kidneys healthy and avoid the need for these survival procedures, which are emotionally and physically arduous for the patient as well as his or her family.

It is also important to take basic care of the body, which in turn will also help the kidneys. Overweight or obese people should lose weight and decrease the strain on their kidneys. Individuals with problems with too much sodium or potassium in their blood (or too little) should follow the recommendations of their physicians to resolve this issue and help to preserve their kidney function. People should avoid drinking to excess, and they should not smoke. If a physician recommends medications to treat diabetes, hypertension, or other illnesses that can impede or harm the kidneys' functioning, the doctor's recommendations should be followed closely. One example of a problem with compliance is that many people take their newly prescribed medications for a month or two and then decide that they do not really need them and stop taking them. Some individuals with gout, urinary and kidney infections, and many other diseases have done this. Often they have then ultimately found—to their consternation and severe pain—that the illness has returned in its full fury because the medication really *was* needed. Medication nonadherence is a major problem among many people, and this behavior is self-harming. If a medication causes distressing side effects, tell the doctor and do not just stop taking it. A lower dosage or a different medication might work more effectively.

This book offers entries with basic information on kidney diseases such as acute kidney injuries, polycystic kidney disease, and gout and on medications that could be harmful to the kidneys, as well as longer overview entries on topics such as the common medical tests used to diagnose kidney disease and how people with kidney prob-

lems live on a daily basis. Overview and lengthy discussions of dialysis and kidney transplantations and other topics are also included. The appendixes include important organizations that can help people with kidney disease, a quick-reference glossary, and other useful information.

Today, more than ever, there are many means to learn about kidney diseases and disorders, such as government Web sites on the Internet and self-help organizations throughout the country. There is also a plethora of medical journal articles written about kidney disease; far too many for the average person to access, read, and understand. This encyclopedia offers basic information as well as analysis of key studies selected to provide the most important and the most useful information for readers interested in learning about kidney diseases.

We are fortunate to be in an exciting medical era; I term this the third era of modern medicine. The first era was the development of the ability to predict the natural history of disease; the second entailed the development of techniques to treat the natural history of disease; and the third era, the most exciting to me, involves the ability to change the natural history.

I dedicate this book to my two uncles, who developed end-stage renal disease and required dialysis treatments for many years. While I treasure the time that I had with them while they received their dialysis treatments, I wish that their kidney disease had been identified and treated earlier so that their need for dialysis may have been prevented, which likely would have improved both the length and the quality of their lives.

I hope that you find this book very helpful and that it fulfills your information needs.

I. David Weiner, M.D.
C. Craig and Audrae Tisher Chair
in Nephrology, Co-holder
Professor of Medicine and Physiology
Division of Nephrology, Hypertension and
Transplantation
University of Florida College of Medicine

# ENTRIES A TO Z

**acquired cystic kidney disease (ACKD)** A disease that causes fluid-filled cysts to develop in the kidneys of children and adults with advanced CHRONIC KIDNEY DISEASE. Individuals receiving DIALYSIS are the most likely to develop acquired cystic kidney disease (ACKD) because of their kidney failure. An estimated 20 percent of individuals who initiate dialysis treatment already have ACKD, according to the National Institute of Diabetes and Digestive and Kidney Diseases (NIDDK). The longer that a person is on dialysis, the higher the probability that he or she will develop ACKD, and after eight years on dialysis, the broad majority (90 percent) of patients have ACKD.

These cysts may be caused by unknown substances that dialysis is unable to filter out. If tumors develop, they may become malignant in up to 20 percent of the cases. In contrast to autosomal dominant POLYCYSTIC KIDNEY DISEASE (ADPKD), ACKD is not genetically triggered nor are the kidneys enlarged. In addition, in ACKD, cyst formation occurs only in the kidneys, whereas with ADPKD, cysts may occur elsewhere in the body.

### Symptoms and Diagnostic Path

In most cases, there are no symptoms of ACKD; however, if INFECTION occurs, the individual may develop BACK PAIN and fever. Hematuria (blood in the urine) may occur if the cyst bleeds. Imaging tests such as ultrasound, a computerized tomography (CT) scan, or a magnetic resonance imaging (MRI) scan can detect the presence of ACKD. If cancer develops in a cyst, the person may develop progressive weight loss, anorexia, and weakness.

### Treatment Options and Outlook

Treatment is not necessary unless the patient experiences symptoms or the physician suspects that cancerous tumors may be present. Infections are treated with ANTIBIOTICS, and large cysts that are painful can be drained with a needle. Some physicians believe that all patients on dialysis should receive KIDNEY CANCER screening after several years on dialysis. If the patient receives a transplanted kidney, ACKD usually resolves in the remaining kidney. Patients with known ACKD should have regular imaging to screen for a possible transformation into cancer. Cancer, if it is present, generally requires the surgical removal of the cancer and the kidney.

### Risk Factors and Preventive Measures

Individuals on dialysis are at risk for ACKD. There are no known preventive measures, and if ACKD develops and causes symptoms, it should be treated.

**acute kidney injury (AKI)** Severe damage to and/or failure of one or both kidneys. Acute kidney injury (AKI) is also known as acute kidney failure or acute renal failure. In most cases, at least an overnight hospitalization will be needed to stabilize and treat the patient with this disorder.

AKI may be caused by an external trauma, such as an accident (for example, a car crash, fall, or other serious accident), a physical attack, a severe burn, or another external cause of the kidney injury. There are also many internal causes of AKI, such as severe dehydration,

1

disorders such as HEMOLYTIC UREMIC SYNDROME or SCLERODERMA, severe complications of pregnancy, or damage that is caused by medications, severe INFECTIONS, or from surgical procedures. Individuals in the intensive care unit (ICU) also have an elevated risk of AKI. Some research indicates that individuals who receive a liver transplantation are at risk for AKI.

According to Sushrut S. Waikar, M.D., and colleague Wolfgang C. Winkelmayer, M.D., in their editorial for the *Journal of the American Medical Association* in 2009, there are more than 1 million hospitalizations each year that are complicated by an acute kidney injury. An acute kidney injury is also a major marker for an extended hospital stay, as well as a cause for other morbidities (illnesses) and even death. The individual with an acute kidney injury often requires DIALYSIS in order to survive, although in many cases, the kidneys will recover sufficiently such that dialysis will no longer be required. However, this is not universally true, and many patients will be left with impaired renal function, also known as chronic kidney disease.

### Symptoms and Diagnostic Path

An acute kidney injury is diagnosed based on the patient's symptoms as well as the circumstances of the injury, such as an accident, an attack, or another cause of the AKI. Laboratory and imaging tests will also show damage to the kidneys.

Some symptoms and signs which may occur in individuals with an AKI include the following:

- nausea and/or vomiting
- shortness of breath
- bloody stools
- fatigue
- nosebleed
- prolonged bleeding
- swelling of the ankles, feet, and legs
- changes in urination such as decreased urination or no urination (anuria)

Laboratory tests will show abnormalities of the blood, such as abnormalities with tests of the blood urea nitrogen (BUN), serum creatinine, serum POTASSIUM, and the URINALYSIS. An abdominal ultrasound is generally the preferred imaging test for an AKI, but a magnetic resonance imaging (MRI) scan or a computerized tomography (CT) scan can also identify the problem.

### Treatment Options and Outlook

Treatment depends on the nature and severity of the injury. If the kidneys have failed, dialysis is needed. If dialysis appears to be needed on a permanent basis, then a KIDNEY TRANSPLANTATION may be considered. The outlook also depends on the presence of preexisting conditions; for example, individuals with prior CHRONIC KIDNEY DISEASE, DIABETES, or HYPERTENSION have a worse prognosis than those without these disorders before the kidney injury.

In some cases, the individual will need to make dietary changes, at least temporarily, such as adopting a diet that is high in carbohydrates and low in potassium, salt, and protein. The individual may receive intravenous supplementation of CALCIUM and glucose/insulin in order to treat a rise in the blood potassium levels. If an infection is present, ANTIBIOTICS will be administered.

### Risk Factors and Preventive Measures

Acute kidney injuries cannot be predicted; however, individuals who are elderly generally have a worse prognosis than younger individuals. Other risk factors include the development of severe infections, very low or very high blood pressure, the length of a surgery, the administration of medications or diagnostic agents that may damage the kidney, and the presence of underlying kidney or liver disease.

### Other Conditions Worsen the Outcome for the Acute Kidney Injury Patient

According to the United States Renal Data System (USRDS) in their 2009 data, chronic kidney disease (CKD) among acute kidney injury patients greatly escalates the risk for END-STAGE RENAL DISEASE (ESRD); for example, the ESRD rate for acute kidney injury patients with CKD was 32.8 per 1,000 patient years, compared to a rate of 4.4 for those with AKI only and 16.4 for those with CKD only. The term *patient years* is a statistical concept which takes into account the number of patients and the number of years they were studied. For example, if 100 patients were studied for 10 years, that would be equal to 1,000 patient years. To determine particular trends, the researchers look at how often a studied event, such as acute kidney injury, heart attack, or another medical event, occurred among the patients. Thus, as in the example, if there were 1,000 patient years and only one patient had the acute kidney injury, heart attack, or other event being studied, that would mean the rate would be one out of 1,000 patient years or .001 per patient year.

The USRDS also noted that the rate of AKI is apparently increasing in the United States, particularly among some populations such as the very elderly, although the reasons for this are unknown. (See Table 1.) The risk for AKI is slightly higher among older females than older males, as can be seen in Table 1. However, as can be seen from Table 2, most of the younger individuals with acute kidney injuries are males; for example, 59.7 percent of those ages 20–64 years with an acute kidney injury in 2007 were male.

Most older AKI patients are white (82.8 percent in 2007). This information was not provided for younger individuals with acute kidney injuries.

The rates of AKI vary considerably from state to state, although again, the reasons for this are yet unknown. In general, the rates for AKIs were about twice as high among individuals in Eastern states.

The USRDS also reports that the probability of ESRD or death after a hospital discharge for an acute kidney injury is significantly higher among AKI patients than among those discharged from the hospital for other reasons. The risk of death

is higher for older Medicare patients hospitalized for an AKI; for example, the death rate for elderly individuals ages 80 years and older who are hospitalized for an acute kidney injury is about 41 percent higher than the death rate for individuals ages 66–70 who are hospitalized for an AKI.

Patients with diabetes have an increased risk for ESRD after an acute kidney injury; according to the USRDS, they are 24 percent more likely to develop ESRD after a hospital discharge for an AKI than hospitalized AKI patients without diabetes. In addition, the risk of ESRD among those with both chronic kidney disease and an

**TABLE 1: DEMOGRAPHICS OF AMERICANS ON MEDICARE AGES 66 AND OLDER WITH ACUTE KIDNEY INJURY, 2002–2007 (DATA IN PERCENTS)**

|  | 2002 | 2005 | 2007 |
|---|---|---|---|
| Total Number | 8,924 | 14,863 | 19,369 |
| **Age** | | | |
| 66–69 | 12.3 | 11.9 | 12.2 |
| 70–74 | 19.8 | 17.9 | 17.2 |
| 75–79 | 23.3 | 22.8 | 21.0 |
| 80–84 | 21.8 | 22.7 | 22.7 |
| 85+ | 22.8 | 24.8 | 26.9 |
| **Gender** | | | |
| Male | 47.9 | 47.3 | 47.2 |
| Female | 52.1 | 52.7 | 52.8 |
| **Race** | | | |
| White | 82.1 | 81.3 | 82.8 |
| African American | 13.5 | 14.1 | 12.6 |
| Other | 4.4 | 4.6 | 4.5 |
| % Requiring Dialysis | 4.4 | 3.1 | 2.3 |
| Acute renal failure, unspecified | 18.3 | 23.5 | 23.2 |
| Pneumonia, organism unspecified | 3.8 | 4.1 | 3.5 |

Note: The data reported here have been supplied by the United States Renal Data System (USRDS). The interpretation and reporting of these data are the responsibility of the authors and in no way should be seen as an official policy or interpretation of the U.S. government.

Source: Adapted from United States Renal Data System. *USRDS 2009 Annual Data Report: Atlas of Chronic Kidney Disease and End-Stage Renal Disease in the United States.* Bethesda, Md.: National Institutes of Health, National Institute of Diabetes and Digestive and Kidney Diseases, 2009, p. 122.

TABLE 2: DEMOGRAPHICS OF PATIENTS WITH ACUTE KIDNEY INJURY IN THE UNITED STATES,
AGES 20–64 YEARS, 2002–2007

| | Market Scan (20–64 years) | | | Ingenix (20–64 Years) | | |
|---|---|---|---|---|---|---|
| | 2002 | 2005 | 2007 | 2002 | 2005 | 2007 |
| Total Number | 1,490 | 5,407 | 14,433 | 1,757 | 3,557 | 5,474 |
| **Age** | | | | | | |
| 20–44 | 12.3 | 11.9 | 12.2 | 9.2 | 13.6 | 15.2 |
| 45–54 | 19.8 | 17.9 | 17.2 | 26.4 | 26.5 | 26.3 |
| 55–64 | 23.3 | 22.8 | 21.0 | 64.4 | 59.9 | 58.5 |
| **Gender** | | | | | | |
| Male | 61.4 | 60.5 | 59.7 | 55.8 | 58.3 | 58.0 |
| Female | 38.6 | 39.5 | 40.3 | 44.2 | 41.7 | 42.0 |
| % Requiring Dialysis | 7.0 | 5.9 | 3.0 | 6.4 | 4.9 | 2.3 |
| Acute renal failure, unspecified | 20.5 | 22.1 | 19.7 | 19.2 | 21.8 | 20.4 |
| Pneumonia, organism unspecified | 2.6 | 2.1 | 2.0 | 1.9 | 1.8 | 2.2 |

Note: The data reported here have been supplied by the United States Renal Data System (USRDS). The interpretation and reporting of these data
   are the responsibility of the authors and in no way should be seen as an official policy or interpretation of the U.S. government.

Source: Adapted from United States Renal Data System. *USRDS 2009 Annual Data Report: Atlas of Chronic Kidney Disease and End-Stage Renal
Disease in the United States.* Bethesda, Md.: National Institutes of Health, National Institute of Diabetes and Digestive and Kidney Diseases, 2009,
p. 122.

acute kidney injury is almost four times higher than among AKI patients without chronic kidney disease. Individuals with hypertension also have a greater risk for ESRD after discharge for an acute kidney injury. (See Table 3.)

### Other Research on Acute Kidney Injury and Chronic Kidney Disease

Dr. Ron Wald and colleagues performed an analysis of 3,769 adult patients in Ontario, Canada, with acute kidney injury requiring dialysis and with an average age of 62 years. These subjects had survived at least 30 days after their discharge from the hospital. The researchers compared the acute kidney injury patients to 13,598 matched controls, and reported their findings in a 2009 issue of the *Journal of the American Medical Association*. About 25 percent of the acute kidney injury subjects had chronic kidney disease within the five years before they were hospitalized for an acute kidney injury.

The researchers found that an acute kidney injury that required an in-hospital dialysis was a risk factor for the need for chronic dialysis.

They also noted that individuals with severe kidney injuries necessitating dialysis have an in-hospital death rate of 45–70 percent. However, among those who do survive, research has indicated that up to 15 percent will continue to need dialysis. The researchers also found that in the case of patients with a prior history of acute kidney injury who then experienced a new kidney injury requiring dialysis before their hospital discharge but who recovered sufficiently and did not need dialysis anymore when they were discharged, such patients were *not* associated with a high risk for death. Rather, those with a prior kidney injury had a lower death risk. The researchers said:

Our findings expand on prior knowledge to provide clinicians with new information about the long-term effect of acute kidney injury that arises during a hospitalization. First, if affected patients survive to hospital discharge, then they remain at high risk of needing dialysis over the next 3 to 5 years. Patients who survive a hospitalization complicated by acute kidney injury requiring dialysis may benefit from specialized care to address complications of chronic kidney

## TABLE 3: RATES PER 1,000 PATIENT YEARS AND HAZARD RATES OF ESRD AFTER DISCHARGE FOR ACUTE KIDNEY INJURY, AGES 66 YEARS AND OLDER, 2005–2006

| | Medicare Rate[1] | Hospitalization Rate[2] |
|---|---|---|
| **Age** | | |
| 66–70 | 57.9 | 1.00 |
| 71–75 | 50.7 | 0.87 |
| 76–80 | 39.3 | 0.69 |
| 80+ | 25.2 | 0.45 |
| **Gender** | | |
| Male | 41.5 | 1.13 |
| Female | 34.7 | 1.00 |
| **Race** | | |
| White | 36.1 | 1.00 |
| African American | 46.8 | 1.10 |
| Other | 44.3 | 1.08 |
| **Baseline diabetes** | | |
| Yes | 51.8 | 1.24 |
| No | 28.2 | 1.00 |
| **Baseline hypertension** | | |
| Yes | 41.6 | 1.02 |
| No | 25.4 | 1.00 |
| **Baseline chronic kidney disease** | | |
| Yes | 92.1 | 2.85 |
| No | 21.4 | 1.00 |

[1] The Medicare Rate refers to patients in the Medicare database.
[2] The hospitalization rate refers to a database of hospitalized patients diagnosed with acute kidney injury discharge.
Note: The data reported here have been supplied by the United States Renal Data System (USRDS). The interpretation and reporting of these data are the responsibility of the authors and in no way should be seen as an official policy or interpretation of the U.S. government.
Source: Adapted from United States Renal Data System. *USRDS 2009 Annual Data Report: Atlas of Chronic Kidney Disease and End-Stage Renal Disease in the United States.* Bethesda, Md.: National Institutes of Health, National Institute of Diabetes and Digestive and Kidney Diseases, 2009, p. 128.

## TABLE 4: RATES PER 1,000 PATIENT YEARS AND HAZARD RATIOS OF DEATH AFTER DISCHARGE FOR ACUTE KIDNEY INJURY

| | Medicare Rate[1] | Hospitalization Rate[2] |
|---|---|---|
| **Age** | | |
| 66–70 | 312.0 | 1.00 |
| 71–75 | 350.9 | 1.09 |
| 76–80 | 417.9 | 1.32 |
| 80+ | 683.2 | 2.04 |
| **Gender** | | |
| Male | 522.5 | 1.09 |
| Female | 488.8 | 1.00 |
| **Race** | | |
| White | 512.2 | 1.00 |
| African American | 467.1 | 0.98 |
| Other | 478.8 | 0.95 |
| **Baseline diabetes** | | |
| Yes | 466.0 | 0.97 |
| No | 531.6 | 1.00 |
| **Baseline hypertension** | | |
| Yes | 487.2 | 0.86 |
| No | 531.6 | 1.00 |
| **Baseline chronic kidney disease** | | |
| Yes | 559.7 | 1.17 |
| No | 487.8 | 1.00 |

[1] The Medicare Rate refers to patients in the Medicare database.
[2] The hospitalization rate refers to a database of hospitalized patients diagnosed with acute kidney injury discharge.
Note: The data reported here have been supplied by the United States Renal Data System (USRDS). The interpretation and reporting of these data are the responsibility of the authors and in no way should be seen as an official policy or interpretation of the U.S. government.
Source: Adapted from United States Renal Data System. *USRDS 2009 Annual Data Report: Atlas of Chronic Kidney Disease and End-Stage Renal Disease in the United States.* Bethesda, Md.: National Institutes of Health, National Institute of Diabetes and Digestive and Kidney Diseases, 2009, p. 128.

disease, and also from concerted efforts to prevent progression to chronic dialysis. At the same time, their high mortality rate is similar to hospitalized patients without acute kidney injury or need for dialysis. Hence, an episode of acute kidney injury requiring in-hospital dialysis may not be an independent contributing factor to long-term survival.

See also MEDICATIONS THAT CAN HARM THE KIDNEYS.

*USRDS 2009 Annual Data Report: Atlas of Chronic Kidney Disease and End-Stage Renal Disease in the United States.* Bethesda, Md.: National Institutes of Health, National Institute of Diabetes and Digestive and Kidney Diseases, 2009.

Waikar, Sushrut S., M.D., and Wolfgang C. Winkelmayer, M.D. "Chronic on Acute Renal Failure: Long-Term Implications of Severe Acute Kidney Injury." *Journal of the American Medical Association* 302, no. 11 (2009): 1,227–1,228.

Wald, Ron, et al. "Chronic Dialysis and Death among Survivors of Acute Kidney Injury Requiring Dialysis." *Journal of the American Medical Association* 302, no. 11 (2009): 1,179–1,185.

**acute renal failure**   See ACUTE KIDNEY INJURY.

**acute tubular necrosis**   See MEDICATIONS THAT CAN HARM THE KIDNEY.

**African Americans**   See END-STAGE RENAL DISEASE; KIDNEYS AND KIDNEY DISEASE.

**albuminuria**   See PROTEINURIA.

**aldosterone and aldosteronism**   Aldosterone is a hormone that is produced by the adrenal glands. It allows for the absorption of SODIUM and is also involved in the movement of POTASSIUM to the kidney. Aldosteronism refers to excessively high levels of aldosterone within the body, a condition often directly associated with the presence of high blood pressure (HYPERTENSION). However, severe illness can lead to a dangerously *low* level of aldosterone, which is known as hypoaldosteronism.

When a person has low blood pressure (hypotension), is volume depleted, or loses significant amounts of both water and salts in the cells, then the level of aldosterone production will increase. This higher level of aldosterone both increases the blood pressure and stimulates the kidneys to retain salt and water, thereby helping to correct the volume depletion.

Primary hyperaldosteronism (also known as Conn's syndrome) occurs when the adrenal glands produce excessive amounts of aldosterone in the absence of volume depletion, hypotension, or other physiologically appropriate stimuli. It can be caused either by an excessive number of aldosterone-producing cells in the adrenal glands, which often involves both adrenal glands, or may be caused by a benign tumor in one of the adrenal glands.

Patients with primary hyperaldosteronism may have HYPOKALEMIA (abnormally low levels of potassium in the blood), which may lead to muscle weakness. However, the majority of patients who have primary hyperaldosteronism have either normal or low-normal levels of potassium. Secondary hyperaldosteronism refers to the presence of increased levels of aldosterone caused by an underlying existing disease, such as heart failure, liver cirrhosis, or NEPHROTIC SYNDROME.

### Symptoms and Diagnostic Path
Often there are no symptoms of either primary or secondary aldosteronism, other than the hypertension which is classically present with primary hyperaldosteronism. In this case, the hypertension is often very difficult to treat and may be resistant despite the use of as many as five or six antihypertensive medications. The disorder is diagnosed through the results of laboratory testing of the blood.

### Treatment Options and Outlook
The treatment of aldosteronism depends on whether it is a primary or secondary form. If it is a primary aldosteronism, the most serious cause is a tumor of the adrenal gland. In such cases, the tumor is usually removed along with the entire adrenal gland. For the patient whose adrenal tumor is removed, the expectation is for a 50 percent chance of cure of the hypertension and a 50 percent chance of a dramatic improvement in blood pressure control. For the patient with bilateral adrenal hyperplasia, treatment is based on medications; the adrenal glands produce compounds other than aldosterone, which precludes the removal of both adrenal glands. Mineralocorticoid receptor antagonists are used, and the dose is titrated to optimal improvement of the patient's blood pressure and hypokalemia.

Secondary aldosteronism is treated by addressing the underlying disease process. Mineralocorticoid receptor antagonists generally are not necessary.

### Risk Factors and Preventive Measures

The cause of primary hyperaldosteronism is unknown, and thus there are also no known preventive measures. If primary hyperaldosteronism develops, then it must be treated.

**alkalemia**    A condition in which the fluids in the body are excessively alkaline. (This is in contrast to the condition of being excessively acidic, another serious medical condition that is known as acidosis.) Hypokalemic alkalosis refers to the condition in which there is a lack of POTASSIUM in the patient's bloodstream along with excessive alkaline levels.

The primary fluids in the human body include blood, perspiration, saliva, and urine, and when their acidity/alkalinity deviates too far from the norm, this often indicates the presence of a disease or disorder. According to Sala Horowitz, Ph.D., in an article on acid-base balance, pH was originally known as "potential for hydrogen" because it was associated with hydrogen ions in fluid. For example, acids emit hydrogen ions, while bases (alkaline fluids) accept hydrogen ions. In general, on a scale of 0 (very acidic) to 14 (highly alkaline), an arterial blood pH of about 7.4 is normal. However, urinary pH can vary from 5 to 8 during a day, depending on the foods that the individual consumes. The kidneys work to maintain a normal pH level in the blood and urine. Alkalemia is generally defined as a blood pH greater than 7.45, according to Varon and Acosta in their chapter on renal and fluid electrolyte disorders in the *Handbook of Critical and Intensive Care Medicine*, published in 2010.

Causes of alkalemia include persistent vomiting or the use of DIURETICS, such as to treat hypertension or congestive heart failure. It may also result from taking high levels of some diuretic medications in an attempt to lose weight quickly. (This practice is not medically recommended; individuals seeking to lose a significant amount of weight should instead seek the assistance of their physicians to create a workable plan.) Other causes of alkalemia include any condition that causes a person to breathe excessively rapidly. This can result from anxiety, fear, or liver disease.

### Symptoms and Diagnostic Path

Alkalemia can worsen to a state of coma if the patient is not treated before that time. Other symptoms and signs of alkalemia may include

- muscle twitching
- nausea and vomiting
- prolonged muscle spasms
- light-headedness

Complications of alkalemia may include an ELECTROLYTE IMBALANCE and heart arrhythmias.

Alkalemia is diagnosed from the results of specific laboratory tests that measure the pH (levels of acidity or alkalinity) of the blood, also known as an arterial blood gas (ABG). Alkalemia can result either from breathing too rapidly or from loss of acids from the body; these causes can be differentiated from the levels of carbon dioxide ($CO_2$) and bicarbonate ($HCO_3$) in the blood, as measured in the ABG. Although the level of bicarbonate in the blood can also be measured in tests such as the basic metabolic panel, people with chronic lung disease may need altered $HCO_3$ levels to compensate for their lung problems, and thus they may not have alkalemia.

### Treatment Options and Outlook

The treatment for alkalemia in general is based on treating the underlying condition. In addition, potassium or chloride losses should be replaced. Potassium, if needed, should be given orally if the person is able to take oral medications, and intravenously, if not. In many cases, this treatment will resolve the problem entirely. If treated, the outlook for the patient is good.

### Risk Factors and Preventive Measures

Most people with healthy kidneys do not experience alkalosis; however, people with unhealthy kidneys are at risk for alkalosis, especially those with CHRONIC KIDNEY DISEASE. Among individuals with unhealthy kidneys, the prevention of alkalosis may include receiving regular laboratory tests of their alkalinity or acidity, and taking appropriate actions if the blood levels fall dangerously out of the normal range.

Horowitz, Sala. "Acid-Base Balance, Health, and Diet." *Alternative and Complementary Therapies* 15, no. 6 (2009): 292–297.

Varon, J., and P. Acosta. "Renal and Fluid-Electrolyte Disorders." *Handbook of Critical and Intensive Care Medicine.* New York: Springer, 2010.

**alpha blockers**   A category of medication used to treat HYPERTENSION, which is a common cause of kidney disease and kidney failure, and that works by reducing the nerve impulses which tighten the blood vessels. Alpha blockers are also known as peripherally acting alpha-adrenergic blockers. Examples of alpha blockers that are approved by the Food and Drug Administration (FDA) to treat hypertension in the United States include doxazosin (Cardura), dibenzyline (phenoxybenzamine), prazosin (Minipress), and terazosin (Hytrin).

Medications in this category are not generally considered the first line of defense in treating patients with high blood pressure, although they may be used as add-on drugs. According to an analysis of existing studies on alpha blockers by Bairaj S. Heran and colleagues in 2009 in *Cochrane Database of Systematic Reviews,* alpha blockers provide only a modest lowering of blood pressure, at best, and all alpha blockers seem to be about equally effective.

Alpha blockers can cause side effects of dizziness, fatigue, light-headedness, decreased sexual ability, and swelling of the hands, feet, ankles, or legs. Individuals using alpha blockers should contact their physicians if they have chest pain or irregular heartbeat. Men using alpha blockers should contact their doctors if they experience painful erection.

See also ANTIHYPERTENSIVE DRUGS; BETA BLOCKERS; CALCIUM CHANNEL BLOCKERS; DIURETICS.

Heran, Bairaj S., Brandon P. Galm, and James M. Wright. "Blood Pressure Lowering Efficacy of Alpha Blockers for Primary Hypertension." *Cochrane Database of Systematic Reviews* 4 (2009). Available online. URL: http://mrw.interscience.wiley.com/cochrane/clsystev/articles/CD00464. Accessed February 13, 2010.

**Alport syndrome**   A rare inherited disease that may cause kidney disease. In males, Alport syndrome is usually associated with severe disease, and almost all cases are genetically transmitted from females to males. This means that females are the carriers of the problem gene but usually do not develop the disease themselves. Males with Alport syndrome usually develop kidney disease that progresses to kidney failure. Females who carry the genetic defect that causes Alport syndrome are frequently asymptomatic, but may develop mild features of Alport syndrome. The disease generally develops in childhood. Alport syndrome may lead to kidney failure.

In 1927, Dr. Alport first identified the syndrome. However, the cause of the abnormality was unknown until 1966, when genetic links to collagen IV were first identified. Collagen type IV is one of the proteins that forms the glomerular basement membrane, i.e., the supporting structure for the glomerular loops.

Alport patients may have kidney disease, as well as ear cochlear abnormalities leading to high frequency deafness, and eye changes that are caused by abnormalities in the cornea and the lens of the eye. Rarely, children with Alport may also have mental retardation. It is estimated that Alport syndrome is present in one out of every 5,000 people in the population.

### Symptoms and Diagnostic Path

During the early stages of Alport syndrome, patients are generally asymptomatic; when symptoms occur, they are generally associated with the onset of the kidney disease. However, the following signs may be present in the early stages of the disease: sensorineural deafness, eye abnormalities, and tumors in the upper airways or the esophagus.

*Sensorineural deafness* Sensorineural deafness is a hearing abnormality detected only by audiometry (special tests of hearing). This test can confirm a hearing loss to high tones. Generally, the hearing loss is gradual, and eventually also involves lower frequencies, including those of conversational speech. Almost 90 percent of males with Alport syndrome develop a hearing loss by age 40.

*Eye abnormalities* Ophthalmologists will note a protrusion of the front portion of the eye lens in some patients with Alport syndrome. This eye abnormality develops in about 25 percent of males with Alport syndrome and worsens with age. Abnormalities in the retina may also occur to patients with Alport syndrome. Small white blotches develop in the retina at an early age among patients with Alport syndrome who later develop kidney disease caused by Alport syndrome. These abnormalities do not affect the individual's vision.

Corneal changes may also be present in the eye of the patient with Alport syndrome. Abnormalities in the cornea, referred to as corneal dystrophy, can present in the early stages of the syndrome. If this abnormality in the cornea is detected, it is highly suggestive of Alport syndrome.

*Tumors in the upper airways and esophagus* *Leiomyomatosis* is the term used to refer to tumors arising from the muscle cells. In patients with Alport syndrome, leiomyomatosis may develop in the esophagus (the food tube) and in the upper airways and can produce symptoms if the tumors grow and obstruct the esophagus and the upper airways.

*Other symptoms* Other symptoms that may occur in the patient with Alport syndrome are blood in the urine (hematuria) as well as coughing and swelling in the ankles. Blood in the urine is either noted by the physician during the physical examination for a visit to the doctor for other reasons or it may be noted by the patient himself or herself, since the urine is dark and large amounts of blood may be seen in the urine.

Hearing defects in both ears usually are noted in early adolescence. By about age 40, individuals with Alport syndrome will need hearing aids.

A protein leak in the urine (PROTEINURIA) may appear in childhood and it may worsen to NEPHROTIC SYNDROME in young adults.

Imaging studies are used to diagnose Alport syndrome. An ultrasound examination of the kidneys will rule out other causes of blood in the urine. In Alport syndrome, an ultrasound of the kidneys is often normal. However, in the later stages of the disease, the kidneys may appear shrunken.

A KIDNEY BIOPSY is the best means to diagnose Alport syndrome. However, a skin biopsy can also diagnose Alport syndrome. Genetic testing can make a definitive diagnosis.

### Treatment Options and Outlook

Patients with early kidney failure that is caused by Alport syndrome may be treated with medications for HYPERTENSION. KIDNEY TRANSPLANTATION is another important option for the treatment of kidney failure. However, first degree relatives of the patient should be screened very thoroughly to avoid taking the kidney from individual donors who may also be carriers of the disease.

### Risk Factors and Preventive Measures

The syndrome occurs in both males and females but it is more serious in males. As a result, according to the National Institutes of Health, young men with Alport syndrome who still retain their hearing should wear ear protection whenever they are in noisy environments, to decrease their risk for deafness.

Hudson, Billy G., et al. "Alport's Syndrome, Goodpasture's Syndrome, and Type IV Collagen," *New England Journal of Medicine* 348, no. 25 (June 19, 2003): 2,543–2,556.

**American Indians/Alaska Natives**  See KIDNEYS AND KIDNEY DISEASE.

**amyloidosis**  A rare disorder in which amyloid, which is a protein-like matter, amasses in one or more of the major organs of the body, such as in the KIDNEYS, heart, brain, gastrointestinal tract, or the skin. This condition occurs when the antibody-producing cells of the body fail to function normally, and instead they create these abnormal protein fibers of antibody fragments. The fragments may then deposit themselves in different organs of the body, including the kidneys. According to the National Institute of Arthritis and Musculoskeletal and Skin Diseases (NIAMS), about 1,200 to 3,200 new cases of amyloidosis are reported each year in the United States.

With amyloidosis, the body cannot break the deposited matter down, and as a result, this excess matter interferes with the normal functioning of the kidneys or the other organs in which these proteins deposit. Amyloidosis in the kidneys can cause PROTEINURIA, NEPHROTIC SYNDROME, and even kidney failure (see END-STAGE RENAL DISEASE).

There are several different types of amyloidosis. Primary amyloidosis is not associated with other diseases, while secondary amyloidosis results from another disease, such as rheumatoid arthritis or other inflammatory diseases. There is also a rare form of hereditary amyloidosis (familial amyloidosis) that affects the nerves and also some organs, which has been found primarily in individuals from Portugal, Japan, Sweden, and other countries. Another form of amyloidosis, associated with normal aging, primarily affects the heart. Each type of amyloidosis is caused by a different form of protein deposit.

### Symptoms and Diagnostic Path

Many people have few or no symptoms with amyloidosis. However, if symptoms are present, they may include fatigue, edema (especially of the ankles and legs), shortness of breath, diarrhea, weight loss, an enlarged tongue, numbness of the legs and arms, dizziness upon standing, and abnormal levels of protein in the urine (proteinuria).

If doctors suspect amyloidosis because the patient suffers from multiple organ failure for no apparent reason, they may test a sample of the patient's tissues for the abnormal proteins. Tissues that can be examined include tissues within abdominal fat and tissues of the skin, gums, kidney, liver, or rectum. Because the disease involves some but not all tissues, it is important to obtain the tissue from the affected organs when considering the diagnosis. When present, the amyloid proteins are detected under a microscope with special stains that are used by the laboratory technician.

### Treatment Options and Outlook

As of this writing, the treatment of amyloidosis is directed at treating the underlying cause. If the disease results from a chronic infectious or inflammatory condition, then treating the underlying disease may be helpful. If the disease is the result of a hereditary condition in which the liver is producing an abnormal amyloid precursor protein, then a liver transplantation may be helpful. Patients with advanced and possibly a life-threatening involvement of their heart and/or liver in addition to involvement of their kidneys may benefit from organ transplantation. If the disease results from the abnormal proliferation of certain blood cells, namely plasma cells, then chemotherapy that is directed at this condition may be beneficial.

If the accumulations of amyloid can be identified, in some cases, they can be surgically removed. The individual whose kidneys have failed because of amyloidosis can be treated with dialysis or a kidney transplant. However, a major problem is that the transplanted organs are also at risk for receiving deposits of amyloid and themselves becoming damaged. Thus, unless the root cause of the disorder can be identified and treated, the amyloidosis will continue to create amyloid fibrils that damage the organs of the body.

Some patients are treated with blood stem cells that are taken from their own blood and that are then used to replace their damaged bone marrow.

Because amyloidosis is rare and can be very damaging, it is best to see a physician who is an expert in the treatment of this disease; the few doctors with expertise in the treatment of amyloidosis are found at only a few major medical centers.

Some individuals with kidneys that have been damaged by amyloid deposits can no longer remove excess potassium or sodium from the body, and as a result, they must carefully restrict their dietary intake of these two minerals.

### Risk Factors and Preventive Measures

According to NIAMS, most patients (two-thirds) with amyloidosis are males, and 95 percent of all patients with this disorder are ages 40 years and older. The National Kidney and Urologic Diseases Information Clearinghouse (NKUDIC) reports that individuals who have been receiving HEMODIALYSIS for five or more years may subsequently develop amyloidosis because the amyloid cannot be filtered out in the process of dialysis. This form of amyloidosis is called dialysis-related amyloidosis, as opposed to primary amyloidosis. KIDNEY TRANSPLANTATION may be helpful in either slowing or altogether halting the progression of dialysis-related amyloidosis.

There are no known preventive measures for amyloidosis. If the disease develops, it should be treated.

See also DIALYSIS.

**analgesic nephropathy**  A form of kidney damage that is caused by the frequent use of painkillers. Chronic pain affects more than 50 million Americans, and physician visits for lower back pain alone result in more than 25 million physician visits each year. According to the National Institute of Diabetes and Digestive and Kidney Diseases (NIDDK), four of every 100,000 people in the United States develop analgesic nephropathy.

Analgesics are painkilling drugs, many of which can be obtained by patients over-the-counter (OTC) and without a prescription. An example of the excessive use of OTC medications is taking three or more pills per day every day for six years, according to the National Institutes of Health (NIH).

Examples of analgesics include acetaminophen (Tylenol), aspirin, and NONSTEROIDAL ANTI-INFLAMMATORY DRUGS (NSAIDs), such as ibuprofen and naproxen sodium. In some individuals, ingestion of large doses of analgesics for an extended period can harm the kidneys. In particular, the combination of medications that combine aspirin with phenacetin, paracetamol, or salicylamide, and with caffeine or codeine appears to result in the highest risk of analgesic nephropathy.

Phenacetin was a commonly used over-the-counter analgesic used many years ago, and at that time, prolonged, heavy use of phenacetin was a frequent cause of analgesic nephropathy. In some countries, analgesic nephropathy accounted for as much as 28 percent of all cases of END-STAGE RENAL DISEASE (renal failure). Accordingly, phenacetin was removed from the market, and it is no longer available in most countries. After phenacetin's removal, the number of people with analgesic nephropathy decreased worldwide. The finding that phenacetin can be converted by the body to acetaminophen has raised the question as to the safety of combination medications that include acetaminophen. Unfortunately, definitive proof as to whether or not long-term, regular use of acetaminophen causes kidney damage is not available at this time.

Long-term use of aspirin in therapeutic doses appears to be safe, but when used in combination with either phenacetin or acetaminophen, it may increase the risk of kidney damage from these medications. Long-term use of narcotic analgesics probably does not cause analgesic nephropathy.

The long-term use of NSAIDs appears to be safe, although it is possible that ingestion of large amounts of NSAIDs over a prolonged period of many years can lead to worsening renal function. Although they can cause papillary necrosis, this is a different condition from analgesic nephropathy. Because NSAIDs can have other effects on renal function, including reversible alterations in renal blood flow, their use should be discontinued in the patient with renal disease.

COX-2 inhibitors are newer forms of NSAIDs that have more specific effects, including a substantially lower risk of stomach-related complications compared to NSAIDs. Their short-term effects on the kidney appear to be similar to those of NSAIDs. Whether the long-term ingestion of large amounts of COX-2 inhibitors leads to kidney-related complications is not currently known.

Many people assume that over-the-counter medications are entirely safe, and that only prescribed medications could be harmful to them, but this is an erroneous assumption. (However, taking an occasional OTC painkiller for infrequent pain generally should not be harmful to most people.) The FDA warns consumers that all OTC pain medications should be used in strict accordance with the label directions. If the use of an OTC NSAID is needed for longer than 10 days, a physician should be consulted.

### Symptoms and Diagnostic Path

There may be no symptoms in individuals with analgesic nephropathy. If there are symptoms, they may be related to the nonspecific effects of decreased renal function, including such symptoms as:

- fatigue
- weakness
- increased urgency or frequency of urination
- decreased alertness, including drowsiness, confusion and lethargy
- nausea and vomiting
- easy bruising or bleeding
- hypertension

A physical examination of the patient may be completely normal or it may show that the patient's blood pressure is significantly elevated, with or without the accumulation of water, causing swelling of the ankles. The patient may also look pale, due to a combination of blood loss as well as abnormal kidney function. In addition, premature skin aging can be another sign of the overuse of analgesics.

Tests which may provide further information to the physician include a complete blood count (CBC), an examination of sediment in the urine, and a blood chemistry that includes the assessment of kidney function. In the past, a special X-ray study that included injecting dye and capturing the passage of dye via the kidneys with sequential X-ray images, termed an intravenous pyleogram (IVP), was used to diagnose NSAID toxicity. However, today a computed tomography (CT) scan can detect the kidney scars that develop as a consequence of long-term exposure to these drugs more effectively than the IVP. Sometimes a toxicology screen and urinalysis can also help in making the diagnosis.

Analgesic use can also result in the development of increased POTASSIUM levels as a consequence of the suppression of the hormone (renin) production from the kidney. Increased levels of potassium is called HYPERKALEMIA, and it can induce rhythm disorder of the heart. A combination of these types of kidney injury may occur when an individual is taking high dosages of nonsteroidal anti-inflammatory drugs.

### Treatment Options and Outlook

If analgesic nephropathy is suspected, then the patient is advised to stop taking all medications that may be contributing to the problem immediately. The physician should determine whether the damage to the kidney is temporary, chronic, or long-term. The physician will also decide whether a KIDNEY BIOPSY is needed to determine the exact cause of the kidney problem, and to eliminate other causes of kidney injury. If kidney failure has begun, this may require the replacement of kidney function through DIALYSIS or with a kidney transplant. If the kidney injury is not severe at the time of diagnosis, then the kidney may have a chance to heal itself with the complete elimination of the use of the problematic analgesics.

### Risk Factors and Preventive Measures

Analgesic nephropathy most commonly occurs among women older than age 30 years, according to the NIDDK. Patients receiving dialysis or who have had kidney transplants should seek to avoid daily or frequent use of OTC analgesics to prevent the development of kidney-related complications. Individuals who have not yet experienced analgesic nephropathy should seek to limit their use of analgesics, whenever possible.

See also ANTIBIOTICS; MEDICATIONS THAT CAN HARM THE KIDNEYS.


**anemia**   A medical problem in which the individual does not have sufficient red blood cells, which is a common problem among many individuals with kidney disease. According to the National Kidney Foundation, anemia is present when there is a hemoglobin concentration of less than 12 grams/deciliter (g/dl) for women and less than 13.5 g/dl for men.

Healthy kidneys produce erythropoietin (EPO), a hormone that stimulates the production of red blood cells, but diseased kidneys cannot produce sufficient amounts of EPO, thus leading to anemia. Almost everyone with END-STAGE RENAL DISEASE, the most severe stage of CHRONIC KIDNEY DISEASE, has anemia.

There are many different types of anemia; for example, some individuals with anemia have iron deficiency anemia, and they need to take iron supplements to counteract the effect of this disease.

Research has shown that the presence of anemia is a predictive factor for the development of CARDIOVASCULAR DISEASE. In addition, according to a study by Peter McCullough and colleagues in a 2007 issue of *Archives of Internal Medicine*, when anemia is combined with microalbuminuria and an abnormal estimated GLOMERULAR FILTRATION RATE (eGFR), then cardiovascular disease is common and the risk of death is increased. Unfortunately, research has shown that treating this anemia with erythropoietin-related medications does not reverse this increased risk of death.

### Symptoms and Diagnostic Path

Individuals with anemia may feel chronically fatigued and weak, and they may also appear paler than normal. The disease is readily diagnosed with a laboratory test of a complete blood count (CBC).

### Treatment Options and Outlook

The treatment of anemia depends upon the cause. If the patient is deficient in iron, then iron supplements are the basis of treatment. If the anemia is caused by a chronic disease, such as chronic kidney disease, that disease should be diagnosed and treated. If the problem is a lack of EPO, then the treatment involves the use of transdermal injections (through the outer skin layer only) of a genetically engineered form of the hormone. If DIALYSIS patients cannot tolerate EPO shots, then they may be given their EPO intravenously during their dialysis sessions. Nutritional deficiencies, such as of folate or B12, should be treated with appropriate medications. Blood loss from the gastrointestinal tract may need an evaluation and treatment by a gastroenterologist, a specialist in the gastrointestinal tract.

### Risk Factors and Preventive Measures

People with chronic kidney disease and those receiving dialysis often have anemia as a result of the lack of the production of EPO. Anemia is also common among people with chronic kidney disease. According to experts, when the anemia results from chronic kidney disease, it often is caused by a deficiency of erythropoietin.

See also HEMOLYTIC UREMIC SYNDROME.

Bahal O'Mara, Neeta. "Anemia in Patients with Chronic Kidney Disease." *Diabetes Spectrum* 21, no. 1 (2008): 12–18.

McCullough, Peter A., M.D., et al. "Independent Components of Chronic Kidney Disease as a Cardiovascular Risk State: Results from the Kidney Early Evaluation Program (KEEP)." *Archives of Internal Medicine* 167 (June 11, 2007): 1,122–1,129.

Singh, Ajay K., et al. "Correction of Anemia with Epoetin Alfa in Chronic Kidney Disease." *New England Journal of Medicine* 355, no. 20 (November 16, 2006): 2,085–2,098.

**angiotensin-converting enzyme inhibitors (ACEIs)**   One type of medication that is used to treat HYPERTENSION, a major cause of kidney disease and kidney failure, by blocking the effects of angiotensin II, a hormone that causes the blood vessels to constrict. As a result, the blood vessels relax. Examples of such medications are such drugs as captopril (Capoten), benazepril (Lotensin), enalapril (Vasotec), and ramipril (Altace). The cost of the ACEI varies with the medication, and prices can range from under about $10 to greater than $300. ACEIs are often used in conjunction with other ANTIHYPERTENSIVE DRUGS.

Sometimes ACEIs can be harmful to the kidneys, and consequently, individuals taking such medications should have their kidney function periodically monitored with blood tests on a schedule determined by the physician. According to the Agency for Healthcare Research and Quality in their 2007 report, ACEIs rarely cause side effects, and the main difference between the side effects of ACEIs and those of angiotensin II receptor blockers (ARBs) is that ACEIs are more likely to cause a dry cough. Neither ACEIs nor ARBs affect blood sugar levels or cholesterol levels.

An estimated 8 percent of individuals taking ACEIs stop taking the medication because of side effects. Some side effects are cough, dizziness, and headache. Very rarely, some individuals experience angioedema, which causes the tongue or lips to swell and means that an individual may be having a reaction to the drug. The individual should call the physician right away if this happens. Angioedema occurs in about one of every 10,000 individuals, so it is not at all common.

**TABLE 1: ACEIS**

| Generic Name | Brand Name | Generic Available? |
|---|---|---|
| Benazepril | Lotensin | Yes |
| Captopril | Capoten | Yes |
| Enalapril | Vasotec | Yes |
| Fosinopril | Monopril | Yes |
| Lisinopril | Prinivil, Zestril | Yes |
| Moexipril | Univasc | No |
| Perindopril | Aceon | No |
| Quinapril | Accupril | Yes |
| Ramipril | Altace | No |
| Trandolapril | Mavik | No |

ACEIs can cause birth defects, and individuals who are pregnant or even thinking about becoming pregnant should contact their physician before using ACEIs or if they are already using ACEIs.

See also ANGIOTENSIN II RECEPTOR BLOCKERS (ARBs); BETA BLOCKERS; CALCIUM CHANNEL BLOCKERS; DIURETICS.

Agency for Healthcare Research and Quality. *Comparing Two Kinds of Blood Pressure Pills: ACEIs and ARBs: A Guide for Adults.* October 2007. Available online. URL: http://www.effectivehealthcare.ahrq.gov/ehc/products/12/31/ACEI-ARBConsumer.pdf. Accessed February 15, 2010.

**angiotensin II receptor blockers (ARBs)**   Medications that are used to treat HYPERTENSION by blocking the effects of angiotensin II, a hormone that causes the blood vessels to constrict. ARBs are commonly used to treat high blood pressure. Hypertension is a major cause of kidney disease and kidney failure, which is why it is important to keep it under control. ARBs have been shown to help protect the kidneys from the effects of Type 2 DIABETES MELLITUS, particularly in patients who already have existing damage to their kidneys from their diabetes. Generic equivalents of ARBs are not currently approved for use in the United States as of this writing, and thus, patients must pay for the brand name drug.

| TABLE 1: ARBS | | |
|---|---|---|
| Generic Name | Brand Name | Generic Available? |
| Candesartan | Atacand | No |
| Eprosartan | Teveten | No |
| Irbesartan | Avapro | No |
| Losartan | Cozaar | No |
| Olmesartan | Benicar | No |
| Telmisartan | Micardis | No |
| Valsartan | Diovan | No |

ARBs can cause dizziness, headache, and cough, although ANGIOTENSIN-CONVERTING ENZYME INHIBITORS (ACEIs), another class of commonly used medications to treat hypertension, are more likely to cause cough. ARBs do not affect blood sugar levels or cholesterol levels directly.

According to the Agency for Healthcare Research and Quality, three of 100 people who take an ARB stop taking the medication because of side effects. There is also a very rare side effect called angioedema that occurs in one of 10,000 people taking ARBs or ACEIs. The primary symptom is swelling of the tongue or lips, and if this side effect occurs, the patient should call his or her doctor right away. Another common side effect is HYPERKALEMIA (increased serum POTASSIUM levels). Generally, this can be managed either with DIETARY CHANGES to decrease the intake of foods high in potassium, such as tomatoes and bananas, or with the addition of DIURETICS that increase the potassium mix creation by the kidneys.

See also ANTIHYPERTENSIVE DRUGS; BETA BLOCKERS; CALCIUM CHANNEL BLOCKERS.

Agency for Healthcare Research and Quality. *Comparing Two Kinds of Blood Pressure Pills: ACEIs and ARBs: A Guide for Adults.* October 2007. Available online. URL: http://www.effectivehealthcare.ahrq.gov/ehc/products/12/31/ACEI-ARBConsumer.pdf. Accessed February 15, 2010.

**antibiotics** Prescribed medications that are given to treat a bacterial infection in some part of the body, including the kidneys. (See PYELONEPHRITIS.) Antibiotics prevent an infection from worsening, and they are a lifesaver in the United States and around the globe. In many cases, the antibiotic is excreted by the kidneys, while in other cases, it is primarily metabolized by the liver. In patients who have CHRONIC KIDNEY DISEASE (CKD), appropriate adjustment of antibiotic dosing is important to avoid possible toxicity from elevated blood levels.

It is also important to try to avoid the unnecessary use of antibiotics, because the excessive use of the same medication (or sometimes of medications in the same class of drugs) can lead to antibiotic resistance, or the resistance of the bacteria to this particular type of antibiotic in the future. If this occurs, and if the patient becomes infected with the same bacteria again, then it could be possible that antibiotics to treat the infection effectively might not be available.

It is also important for patients who are prescribed antibiotics to take the entire course of the antibiotic (usually seven to 10 days, although sometimes a longer course is prescribed), unless the doctor tells the individual to stop taking the medication because of adverse side effects or for another reason. If an individual with an infection feels better after a day or two and stops taking the antibiotic, in most cases, the bacteria causing the infection are still present and the infection can recur shortly after stopping the antibiotic. It is also possible that stopping antibiotics early can increase the risk of developing antibiotic-resistant bacteria. As a result, medication adherence to the antibiotic regimen is very important.

Some antibiotics can be harmful to the kidneys, especially aminoglycoside antibiotics, and appropriate monitoring of blood levels of individuals taking these antibiotics is important in order to limit dose-related toxicities.

It is also important to tailor the dosage to the patient's age; for example, older individuals metabolize many medications at a slower rate than do younger individuals. Thus, a 70-year-old woman may need a lower dosage of a medication for an infection such as CYSTITIS than a 30-year-old woman would require with the same type of infection. Dosages of antibiotics should also be carefully tailored when prescribed for children or adolescents.

See also DIURETICS; INFECTIONS; LITHIUM AND BIPOLAR DISORDER; MEDICATIONS THAT CAN HARM THE KIDNEYS.

**antihypertensive drugs** Medications that are prescribed to treat high blood pressure (HYPERTENSION), including drugs in such categories as ALPHA BLOCKERS, ANGIOTENSIN-CONVERTING ENZYME INHIBITORS (ACEIs), ANGIOTENSIN II RECEPTOR BLOCKERS (ARBs), BETA BLOCKERS, CALCIUM CHANNEL BLOCKERS, and DIURETICS. Vasodilators and centrally-acting alpha adrenergics are also used to treat hypertension, as are renin inhibitors.

Many individuals with hypertension will need to take two or more medications to keep their hypertension under control adequately. There are also combination antihypertensive drugs as of this writing that combine two medications into one pill or capsule, thus increasing the patient's convenience as well as the likelihood of the patient remembering to take the medication. For example, Diovan HCT combines hydrochlorothiazide and valsartan, while Hyzaar combines hydrochlorothiazide and losartan. Caduet is a combination medication that combines amlodipine and atorvastatin, medications that are used to treat hypertension and high cholesterol.

Uncontrolled hypertension can lead to kidney disease and even kidney failure, and hypertension is the second leading cause of END-STAGE RENAL DISEASE (ESRD), after DIABETES MELLITUS. Untreated hypertension can also cause heart attacks, stroke, peripheral arterial disease, and even death. It is extremely important that individuals taking antihypertensive medications take them on the schedule recommended by the physician and report any side effects that may occur. Failure to adhere to the medication treatment plan generally decreases the likelihood of effective and adequate blood pressure control, and thus increases the risk of hypertension and other related complications.

The table provides information on both the brand and generic names of selected antihypertensive medications in each class of medications, as well as warnings, common side effects, and signs that indicate the patient should call his or her physician right away. Note that the table offers general information on various classes of medications; to obtain more detailed information on any particular medication, individuals should consult a physician or pharmacist.

### TABLE 1: ANTIHYPERTENSIVE MEDICATIONS

| Category of Medication | Brand Name | Generic Name | Warnings | Common Side Effects | Call Your Doctor If You Have These Signs |
|---|---|---|---|---|---|
| Angiotensin-Converting Enzyme (ACE) Inhibitors | Aceon | Perindopril | Pregnant women should consult with their doctor before using these drugs in pregnancy. Women attempting to become pregnant should, in general, not use these medications, as they can lead to severe fetal defects. | • Cough<br>• Hyperkalemia | • Chest pain<br>• Problems with breathing or swallowing<br>• Swelling in the face, eyes, lips, tongue, or legs<br>• Sudden or marked decrease in urine volume |
|  | Accupril | Quinapril |  |  |  |
|  | Altace | Ramipril |  |  |  |
|  | Capoten | Captopril |  |  |  |
|  | Lotensin | Benazepril |  |  |  |
|  | Mavik | Trandolapril |  |  |  |
|  | Monopril | Fosinopril |  |  |  |
|  | Prinivil | Lisinopril |  |  |  |
|  | Univasc | Moexipril |  |  |  |
|  | Vasotec | Enalapril |  |  |  |
|  | Zestril | Lisinopril |  |  |  |

| Category of Medication | Brand Name | Generic Name | Warnings | Common Side Effects | Call Your Doctor If You Have These Signs |
|---|---|---|---|---|---|
| Angiotensin Receptor Blockers (ARBs) | Atacand<br>Avapro<br>Benicar<br>Cozaar<br>Diovan<br>Micardis<br>Teveten | Candesartan<br>Irbesartan<br>Olmesartan<br>Losartan<br>Valsartan<br>Telmisartan<br>Eprosartan | Women who are pregnant or nursing should not use these drugs.<br>Women who are attempting to become pregnant should, in general, not use these medications, as they can lead to severe fetal defects. | • Low blood pressure<br>• Hyperkalemia | • Swelling of the face, throat, lips, eyes, hands, feet, ankles, or legs<br>• A sudden or marked decrease in urine volume |
| Beta Blockers | Bystolic<br>Coreg<br>Corgard<br>Inderal<br>Inderal LA<br>Kerlone<br>Levatol<br>Lopressor<br>Sectral<br>Tenormin<br>Toprol XL<br>Trandate<br>Visken<br>Zebeta | Nebivolol<br>Carvedilol<br>Nadolol<br>Propranolol<br>Propranolol<br>Betaxolol<br>Prebutol<br>Metoprolol<br>Acebutolol<br>Atenolol<br>Metoprolol<br>Labetalol<br>Pindolol<br>Bisoprolol | These medications should not be taken by patients with slow heart rate, heart block, or shock.<br>Women who are pregnant or nursing their babies should consult their physicians before starting beta blockers.<br>Elderly individuals and patients with kidney or liver problems, asthma, diabetes, or an overactive thyroid gland should talk to their doctors about specific risks with particular beta blockers. | • Fatigue<br>• Dizziness<br>• Feeling light-headed | • Chest pain<br>• Difficulty breathing<br>• Slow or irregular heartbeat<br>• Swelling in the hands, feet, or legs |
| Calcium Channel Blockers | Norvasc<br>Cleviprex<br>Cardizem<br>Dilacor XR<br>Tiazac<br>Plendil<br>DynaCire CR<br>Cardene<br>Adalar CC<br>Procardia<br>Nimotop<br>Sular<br>Calan<br>Covera HS<br>Isoptin<br>Verelan | Amlodipine<br>Clevidipine<br>Diltiazem<br>Diltiazem<br>Diltiazem<br>Felodipine<br>Isradipine<br>Nicardipine<br>Nifedipine<br>Nifedipine<br>Nimodipine<br>Nisoldipine<br>Verapamil<br>Verapamil<br>Verapamil<br>Verapamil | Patients with a heart condition or who are taking nitrates, quinidine, or fetanyl should avoid calcium channel blockers.<br>Individuals with liver or kidney problems should discuss the specific risks of any calcium channel blocker with their physician.<br>Women who are pregnant or nursing should talk to their doctor before starting any calcium channel blocker. | • Feeling drowsy<br>• Headache<br>• Upset stomach<br>• Ankle swelling<br>• Feeling flushed/warm | • Chest pain<br>• Serious rashes<br>• Swelling of the face, eyes, lips, tongue, arms, or legs<br>• Fainting<br>• Irregular heartbeat |

*(table continues)*

**TABLE 1** (continued)

| Category of Medication | Brand Name | Generic Name | Warnings | Common Side Effects | Call Your Doctor If You Have These Signs |
|---|---|---|---|---|---|
| Peripherally Acting Alpha-Adrenergic Blockers (Alpha Blockers) | Cardura<br>Dibenzyline<br>Minipress<br>Hytrin | Doxazosin<br>Phenoxybenzamine<br>Prazosin<br>Terazosin | The elderly or those with liver problems should talk to their doctor about the risks of these medications. | • Dizziness<br>• Feeling tired<br>• Feeling light-headed<br>• Vision problems<br>• Swelling of the hands, feet, ankles, or legs<br>• Decreased sexual ability | • Chest pain<br>• Irregular heart-beat<br>• Painful erec-tion in men |
| Centrally-Acting Alpha Adrenergics | Catapres<br>Tenex | Clonidine<br>Guanfacine | Women who are pregnant or nursing should talk to their doctor before using these drugs.<br>People with heart disease, recent heart attack, or kidney disease should talk to their doctor before using these drugs.<br>Drinking alcohol may make side effects worse. | • Dizziness<br>• Dry mouth<br>• Upset stomach<br>• Feeling drowsy or tired | • Fainting<br>• Slow or irregu-lar heartbeat<br>• Fever<br>• Swollen ankles or feet |
| Combination Medications for Hypertension | Diovan HCT<br><br>Exforge<br><br>Hyzaar<br><br>Lexxel<br><br>Lotrel<br><br>Tarka | Hydrochlorothiazide and Valsartan<br>Amlodipine and Valsartan<br>Hydrochlorothiazide and Losartan<br>Enalapril and Felodipine<br>Benzepril and Amlodipine<br>Verapamil and Trandoalpril | These medications are comprised of 2 different blood pressure medications. | The warnings and side effects of these drugs are the same as those listed earlier for both generic drugs. | See information on individual drugs. |
| Combination Medication for Hypertension and High Cholesterol | Caduet | Amlodipine and Atorvastatin | This combination medication is used to treat patients with both hypertension and high cholesterol.<br>The medication should be avoided by women who are pregnant or planning to become pregnant.<br>The medication should be avoided by women who are breastfeeding.<br>The medication should be avoided by patients with liver problems. | • Swelling of the legs or ankles (edema)<br>• Muscle or joint pain<br>• Headache<br>• Diarrhea or constipation<br>• Feeling dizzy<br>• Feeling tired or sleepy<br>• Gas<br>• Rash<br>• Nausea<br>• Stomach pain<br>• Fast or irregular heartbeat<br>• Face feels hot or warm (flushing) | • Muscle prob-lems such as weakness, tenderness, or pain that hap-pens without a good rea-son (such as exercise or an injury)<br>• Brown or dark-colored urine<br>• Skin or eyes looking yellow (jaundice)<br>• Feeling more tired than usual |

| Category of Medication | Brand Name | Generic Name | Warnings | Common Side Effects | Call Your Doctor If You Have These Signs |
|---|---|---|---|---|---|
| Diuretics (sometimes called "water pills") | Aldactazie Aldactone Demadex Diuril Enduron Microzide Oretic Lasix Saluron Thalitone Zaroxolyn | Spironolactone Torsemide Chlorothiazide Methyclothiazide Hydrochlorothiazide Furosemide Indapamide Hydroflumethiazide Chlorthalidone Metolazone | Patients who are breastfeeding should tell their doctors because these medications may pass into breast milk. These medications should be avoided by patients who have problems making urine. People with kidney or liver problems, pregnant women, and the elderly should consult with their doctor about the risks of using diuretics. | • Dizziness<br>• Frequent urination<br>• Headache<br>• Thirst<br>• Muscle cramps<br>• Upset stomach | • Severe rash<br>• Problems breathing or swallowing<br>• Hyperuricemia (Gout) |
| Renin Inhibitor | Tekturna | Aliskiren | Women who are pregnant or planning to become pregnant should talk to their doctor before using this drug. People with kidney problems should talk to their doctor before using this drug. People who are taking diuretics, other high blood pressure medications, heart medicines, or medicines to treat fungus should tell their doctor before using this medication. | • Diarrhea | • Low blood pressure<br>• Swelling of the face, throat, lips, eyes, or tongue |

Source: Adapted from Food and Drug Administration, "High Blood Pressure—Medicines to Help You." February 2009. Available online. URL: http://www.fda.gov/ForConsumers/ByAudience/ForWomen/ucm118594.htm. Accessed February 9, 2010.

**anti-rejection drugs** See IMMUNOSUPPRESSIVE DRUGS.

**Asians and Pacific Islanders** See KIDNEYS AND KIDNEY DISEASE.

**autosomal dominant polycystic kidney disease** See POLYCYSTIC KIDNEY DISEASE.

**autosomal recessive polycystic kidney disease** See POLYCYSTIC KIDNEY DISEASE.

**back pain and kidney disease**   Kidney disease can lead to a wide variety of types of back pain. Kidney infection (PYELONEPHRITIS) can lead to back pain which is typically in the flanks, and is associated with burning with urination (dysuria), frequency (need to urinate very often), and urgency (or an inability to delay when needing to urinate). The flank pain can typically be elicited by light taps, which will result in much more severe pain on one side than on the other. The area of increased tenderness is the likely site of pyelonephritis. CYSTITIS, a urinary tract infection involving only the bladder, is sometimes associated with a vague low back pain.

KIDNEY STONES that are in the process of passing may cause flank pain if it is in either the upper kidneys or the upper portion of the ureter. Once a kidney stone has passed approximately one-third of the way from the kidney to the bladder, the pain will classically be experienced in either the testicles in males or in the vulva in women. The pain with a kidney stone is frequently very severe, and it is associated with recurrent waves of pain. In very rare cases, an acute cessation of blood flow to the kidneys, such as with a blood clot to the kidneys, will result in severe flank pain.

Nevertheless, it is also important to recognize that the majority of cases of back pain have nothing to do with kidney disease or infection. Much more common causes include muscle strain, nerve disease, back disc disease, fibromyalgia, or many other possible causes. Back pain is an extremely common problem among adults, and it should be carefully evaluated by a physician, using the medical history of the patient and the current symptoms. Selected laboratory tests and imaging studies, such as X-rays, magnetic resonance imaging (MRI) scans, computerized tomography (CT) scans, and ultrasound studies are sometimes necessary to determine the cause of the back pain.

See also ANALGESIC NEPHROPATHY; MEDICATIONS THAT CAN HARM THE KIDNEYS; NONSTEROIDAL ANTI-INFLAMMATORY DRUGS (NSAIDs).

**Bartter's syndrome**   A salt-losing kidney disease that has been recognized since the mid-1900s. Its early recognition can prevent future metabolic and growth-related complications that are invariably associated with this disorder.

Bartter's syndrome was first noticed by Frederic Bartter in 1962, when he identified the syndrome in two African Americans, a 25-year-old man and a five-year-old boy. It was later discovered that it was kidney tubular defects in the patients that caused the disorder, and in addition, it was discovered that Bartter's syndrome was inherited if both parents carried at least one gene for the syndrome.

According to Lynda A. Frassetto in her article for eMedicine in 2008, Richard Lifton and his colleagues discovered that there were several forms of Bartter's syndrome with different genetic causes; for example, in the individual with Bartter I syndrome, the syndrome was caused by defects in the Na-K-2Cl transporter (Sodium-Potassium-2 Chloride transporter), which resulted from mutations in the SLC12A1 gene. Two other forms of Bartter's syndrome (Bartter syndrome II and III) were caused by other genetic mutations. To date, five different genes have been implicated in the development of Bartter's syndrome.

According to Salim K. Mujais and Adrian I. Katz, Bartter's syndrome is similar to GITELMAN SYNDROME in several key ways. In both conditions, the patient exhibits HYPOKALEMIA, metabolic alkalosis, low blood pressure (hypotension), salt wasting, and high blood levels of renin and ALDOSTERONE. However, patients with Bartter's syndrome usually come to medical attention in childhood or adolescence, while Gitelman syndrome is usually identified in adulthood. This is because the defects in renal sodium and potassium are worse with Bartter's syndrome than with Gitelman syndrome. In addition, Bartter's syndrome is characterized by hypercalciuria (high levels of calcium in the urine), while Gitelman syndrome is characterized by hypocalciuria (low levels of calcium in the urine).

### Symptoms and Diagnostic Path

Individuals with Bartter's syndrome have an enlargement of specific kidney cells termed the macula densa, as well as low blood pressure, hypokalemia that is usually severe, metabolic alkalosis, and elevated levels of the hormones aldosterone and renin. Untreated patients are usually below normal in height. The syndrome is characterized by the following symptoms:

- muscle cramping and weakness
- constipation
- increased frequency of urination
- growth failure

Bartter's syndrome is diagnosed by the finding of low levels of blood potassium in combination with elevated levels of potassium in the urine in a patient who is not taking DIURETICS. The absence of using diuretics is important to demonstrate, since many patients who were initially thought to have Bartter's syndrome were actually abusing diuretics (such as furo-semide or bumetanide) without their doctor's knowledge. (Diuretics can cause temporary weight loss and some people use them to excess.) Some patients are deficient in magnesium as well.

Other symptoms may include:

- elevated blood levels of the hormones renin and aldosterone
- elevated urine levels of potassium, calcium, and chloride
- low blood levels of chloride
- metabolic alkalosis

In addition, the increased excretion of calcium in the urine can result in stone formation in the kidneys. The blood pressure of the individual with Bartter's syndrome is generally low or low-normal.

If children with severe Bartter's syndrome survive, they may develop CHRONIC KIDNEY DISEASE in adulthood because of chronic scarring of the kidneys due to hypokalemia. Diuretic abuse should be excluded by the physician by screening the urine for the offending drugs.

### Treatment Options and Outlook

It is important for the patient with Bartter's syndrome to maintain a diet that is high in potassium. In addition, almost all patients with this diagnosis need to take supplemental potassium, often in very large doses.

Both Bartter's and Gitelman syndrome require lifelong therapy with potassium and magnesium supplements, as well as a liberal salt intake. High doses of medications such as spironolactone or amiloride can be used to treat the hypokalemia, alkalosis, and magnesium wasting.

NONSTEROIDAL ANTI-INFLAMMATORY DRUGS (NSAIDs) sometimes can be used to reduce the salt-wasting symptoms found with Bartter's syndrome. Prescribed ANGIOTENSIN-CONVERTING ENZYME (ACE) INHIBITORS may also be given, such as captropil (Capoten) or enalapril (Vasotec), which are drugs that work to lower the aldosterone levels and to prevent the loss of potassium. Spironolactone (Aldactone) may be given to increase the potassium blood levels. High doses of NSAIDs may be used, such as indomethacin (Indocin). While NSAIDs are occasionally effective, in the majority of patients, their use is limited by the gastrointestinal side effects that they can cause, and by only a minimal beneficial effect in most patients. If the patient is a child or the individual is someone in early adolescence, then growth hormone may be administered to treat short stature.

The outlook for patients with Bartter's syndrome is uncertain as of this writing. Some patients do well with treatment, while others will develop END-STAGE RENAL DISEASE (kidney failure). Some research has shown that in patients with Bartter's syndrome and kidney failure, a kidney transplant may cause an improvement or even a normalization of many of the abnormalities that are associated with Bartter's syndrome.

### Risk Factors and Preventive Measures

Because Bartter's syndrome is a genetic disorder, the major risk for developing this condition is having two parents that are carriers of the genetic mutation. Because carriers of this condition are asymptomatic, it is not possible to know whether the parents are carriers other than by genetic linkage analysis or if the parents have other children with Bartter's syndrome. In this case, all subsequent children will have a 25 percent chance of having it.

Patients with Bartter's syndrome should avoid all medications that can worsen the salt wasting and hypokalemia that are the major complications of this disorder. In particular, they should avoid using loop and thiazide diuretics. In conditions in which volume depletion of urine might occur to an individual, such as with a prolonged exposure to hot climates, strenuous physical exercise, or diarrhea, then patients should be aware that they are at an increased risk for worsening, and potentially serious, hypotension (low blood pressure) and hypokalemia.

Frassetto, Lynda A., M.D. "Bartter Syndrome." eMedicine, May 16, 2008. Available online. URL: http://www.emedicine.com/MED/topic213.htm. Downloaded May 24, 2008.

Mujais, Salim K., and Adrian I. Katz. "Potassium Deficiency." In *Seldin and Giebisch's The Kidney: Physiology and Pathophysiology. Volume 1,* edited by Robert J. Alpern and Steven C. Hebert. Burlington, Mass.: Academic Press, 2008: 1,349–1,385.

**Berger's disease**    See IGA NEPHROPATHY.

**beta blockers**    A category of medications that is used to treat hypertension, which is the second leading cause of kidney failure. These drugs reduce systolic-diastolic hypertension or systolic hypertension alone by slowing down the heart rate and causing the heart to beat with less force. They also decrease renin release, and thus improve blood pressure control by inhibiting the renin-angiotensin system. This category of medications has been used to reduce hypertension since the 1970s. The cost of beta blockers can vary from only about $10 per month to greater than $200 per month. Many beta blockers are available in generic forms, which are much less costly than brand name prescriptions. As of this writing, nebivolol (Bystolic) is the only beta blocker not available in a generic form. Note that sometimes physicians prefer to prescribe brand name drugs even when generics are available, and this issue should be discussed with the doctor.

Beta blockers are not considered the first line of therapy for patients with uncomplicated hypertension but may be added on to other medications, such as diuretics. However, if an individual has hypertension and other compelling indications, such as congestive heart failure, diabetes mellitus, post-myocardial infarction (heart attack), or high coronary artery disease risk, treatment including a beta blocker may be beneficial.

According to *Consumer Reports Best Buys Report* in 2009, beta blockers were the fifth most prescribed medication in the United States in 2008; nearly 131 million prescriptions were filled for this drug. Note that beta blockers are also used to treat other conditions besides hypertension, such as angina, heart failure, and treatment after a heart attack (myocardial infarction).

According to authors Qi Che, M.D., and colleagues in their 2009 article on beta blockers in *Current Drug Therapy*, there are three primary types of beta blockers, including nonselective beta blockers, selective beta blockers, and beta blockers with peripheral vasodilatation effects. Nonselective beta blockers are drugs that block both the beta-1 and beta-2 adrenergic receptors, and include nadolol (Corgard), pindolol (Visken), propranolol (Inderal), and timolol (Blocadren).

Selective beta blockers primarily block beta-1 receptors and they include such drugs as atenolol (Tenormin), betaxolol (Kerlone), bisoprolol (Zebeta), exmolol (Brevibloc), and metoprolol (Lopressor and Toprol). Because inhibiting the beta-2 receptor can cause worsening of asthma control in susceptible patients, the beta-1–selective beta blockers may be preferred to nonselective beta blockers in susceptible individuals. Beta blockers with peripheral vasodilatation effects act through antagonism of the alpha 1 receptor, such as with labetolol (Normadyne) or carvidilol (Coreg), or they increase the release of nitric oxide, such as with the medication nebivolol (Bystolic). These medications may be beneficial in patients whose hypertension is not responding optimally to either nonselective or selective beta blockers because they have the ability to improve blood pressure control through multiple mechanisms.

Some beta blockers, such as atenolol and nadolol, are excreted by the kidney, and the dosage of these medications must be adjusted in individuals with chronic kidney disease or whose kidneys are impaired by other illnesses.

Che and colleagues question whether beta blockers are as useful as believed, pointing out that in some clinical trials, the outcomes for individuals who took beta blockers were worse than the outcomes for hypertensive subjects who used other antihypertensive medications. Say the authors, "Until these drugs are proved beneficial, they should be used as antihypertensive therapy only in patients with compelling cardiac indications for them or as add-on agents in those with uncontrolled or resistant hypertension."

Beta blockers have side effects, as do all medications, and may cause fatigue and sleepiness as well as constipation, headache, erectile dysfunction, cold feet and hands, and a mild depression. In general, the beta blockers used to treat hypertension are atenolol, metoprolol tartrate, nadolol, and propranolol. Individuals taking beta blockers should call their physicians if they experience chest pain, difficulty breathing, a slowed or irregular heartbeat, or swelling in the hands, feet, or legs.

Individuals who are elderly or who have kidney or liver problems or diabetes should talk to their doctor about the risks of using beta blockers. Pregnant women or women who are nursing should consult with their doctor before taking beta blockers.

See also ALPHA BLOCKERS; ANGIOTENSIN-CONVERTING ENZYME INHIBITORS; ANGIOTENSIN II RECEPTOR BLOCKERS; ANTIHYPERTENSIVE DRUGS; CALCIUM CHANNEL BLOCKERS; DIURETICS.

### TABLE 1: BRAND AND GENERIC NAME OF BETA BLOCKERS

| Brand Name | Generic Name |
| --- | --- |
| Blocadren | Timolol |
| Bystolic | Nebivolol |
| Brevibloc | Exmolol |
| Coreg | Carvedilol |
| Corgard | Nadolol |
| Inderal, Inderal LA | Propranolol |
| Kerlone | Betaxolol |
| Levatol | Penbutolol |
| Lopressor | Metoprolol |
| Sectral | Acebutolol |
| Tenormin | Atenolol |
| Toprol XL | Metoprolol |
| Trandate | Labetalol |
| Visken | Pindolol |
| Zebeta | Bisoprolol |

Che, Qi, Martin J. Schreiber, Jr., M.D., and Mohammed A. Rafey, M.D. "Beta-Blockers for Hypertension: Are They Going Out of Style?" *Cleveland Clinic
Journal of Medicine* 76, no. 9 (2009): 533–542.

Consumers Union. *Treating High Blood Pressure and Heart
Disease: The Beta-Blockers. Comparing Effectiveness,
Safety, and Price.* June 2009. Available online. URL:
http://www.consumerreports.org/health/resources/
pdf/best-buy-drugs/CU-Betablockers-FIN060109.
pdf. Accessed February 15, 2010.

**biopsy**  See KIDNEY BIOPSY.

**bipolar disorder**  See LITHIUM AND BIPOLAR
DISORDER.

**bisphosphonates**  Medications that are used
to treat patients with osteoporosis as well as
patients with diseases such as Paget's disease,
HYPERCALCEMIA of malignancy, and several
other diseases and disorders. Some examples of
bisphosphonate drugs include such medications
as etidronate (Didronel), ibandronate (Boniva),
alendronate (Fosamax), risedronate (Actonel),
zoledronate (Zometa), tiludronate (Skelid), and
pamidronate (Aredia). Individuals with kidney
disease must be carefully monitored while on
these medications. In addition, these drugs have
a risk for leading to the development of kidney
disease.

These medications must usually be taken on
an empty stomach and consumed with water,
and then the individual must stand up for about
an hour afterwards because these drugs can
irritate the esophagus (the food tube leading to
the stomach) and may also cause esophagitis
(inflammation of the esophagus, making it hard
to swallow foods) or even ulceration in the stomach. Women with postmenopausal osteoporosis
generally take the oral form of a bisphosphonate. However, intravenous bisphosphonates
are apparently less likely to cause esophagitis
because they bypass the digestive system.

Nephrotoxicity (harm to the kidneys) that
may be caused by bisphosphonates has been seen
in the form of toxic acute tubular necrosis and
FOCAL SEGMENTAL GLOMERULOSCLEROSIS. According to Mark A. Perazella and Glenn S. Markowitz
in their article on bisphosphonate nephrotoxicity
in *Kidney International* in 2008, when stringent
compliance and care is used by physicians, the
risk for kidney damage is decreased. The authors
say with regard to zoledronate and pamidronate,
"With both of these agents, severe nephrotoxicity can be largely avoided by stringent adherence
to guidelines for monitoring serum creatinine
prior to each treatment, temporarily withhold-
ing therapy in the setting of renal insufficiency,
and adjusting doses in patients with pre-existing
chronic kidney disease."

In treating other than postmenopausal osteoporosis, generally higher dosages of bisphosphonates are used, often administered intravenously.
In these cases, the risk for nephrotoxicity is
elevated.

In their 2009 article published in the *Clinical
Journal of the American Society of Nephrology,* Nigel
D. Toussaint and colleagues discussed the pros
and cons of using bisphosphonates with patients
who have CHRONIC KIDNEY DISEASE (CKD) but
who still need protection for their bones in order
to avoid bone fractures because of their high risk
for such fractures. According to these authors,
low bone mass is common among individuals with CKD. Some research has shown that
among patients with CKD 1–3 (there are five
stages of CKD, from Stage 1, the least severe,
to Stage 5, which is the stage at which the kidneys fail), with secondary causes of their low
bone density and with normal blood levels of
CALCIUM, phosphate, vitamin D, parathyroid,
and alkaline phosphatase (ALP), bisphosphonate
use is generally safe and it effectively reduces
the risks for fractures. The value of the use of
bisphosphonates in individuals with more severe
levels of CKD (4–5), however, is unknown
because this circumstance has rarely been studied. The authors concluded that:

> Although there is a paucity [very limited
> amount] of evidence, bisphosphonates may be

used for osteoporosis in CKD 1 to 3. A number of other bone pathologies result in low BMD [bone mineral density] in CKD 4 and 5, which should warn against the common perception that these agents may provide bone protection in all stages of CKD. In severe CKD, bisphosphonates should only be used with caution in carefully selected patients and after consideration of bone biopsy, because of the possibility of worsening low bone turnover, osteomalacia, and mixed uraemic osteodystrophy, and exacerbating hyperparathyroidism.

See also MEDICATIONS THAT CAN HARM THE KIDNEYS.

Perazella, Mark A., and Glen S. Markowitz. "Bisphosphonate Nephrotoxicity." *Kidney International* 74 (2008): 1,385–1,393.

Petit, William A., Jr., M.D., and Christine Adamec. *The Encyclopedia of Endocrine Diseases and Disorders.* New York: Facts On File, 2005.

Toussaint, Nigel D., Grahame J. Elder, and Peter G. Kerr. "Bisphosphonates in Chronic Kidney Disease; Balancing Potential Benefits and Adverse Effects on Bone and Soft Tissue." *Clinical Journal of the American Society of Nephrology* 4 (2009): 221–233.

**bladder cancer**   A malignant tumor of the bladder which may damage other parts of the body, such as the kidneys. According to the National Cancer Institute (NCI), there were an estimated 70,980 new cases of bladder cancer in 2009 in the United States, and 14,330 people died from bladder cancer in that year. Cancer can also occur in the small thin tubes (ureters) that connect the bladder to the kidneys, but bladder cancer occurs far more commonly than ureteral cancer. Bladder cancer is the fourth most common type of cancer in males, and it is the eighth most common form of cancer in females. The incidence of bladder cancer has stayed about the same for 20 years, as of this writing, according to Konety, Joyce, and Wise in *Urologic Diseases in America*, published in 2007.

There are five stages of bladder cancer, ranging from Stage 0, in which noninvasive tumors are located within the bladder lining, to Stage IV, when the cancer has spread to regional lymph nodes or has spread (metastasized) to distant parts of the body. With Stage I, the tumor extends through the bladder lining but not into the muscle layer. With Stage II, the tumor has invaded the muscle layer. With Stage III, the tumor has gone into the tissue that surrounds the bladder.

### Symptoms and Diagnostic Path
Bladder cancer may include the symptoms that follow. Note that these symptoms may also indicate the presence of other noncancerous disorders, such as a bladder infection (CYSTITIS) or a kidney infection (PYELONEPHRITIS); however, individuals with these symptoms should see a physician for a diagnosis. The symptoms include microscopic blood in the urine (hematuria) or visible blood (macrohematuria).

Other possible symptoms that may occur with bladder cancer include

- abdominal pain
- urinary incontinence
- anemia
- weight loss
- fatigue
- bone pain

If the physician suspects that bladder cancer may be present, he or she will usually order an ultrasound and also a computer tomography (CT) scan of the bladder. In some cases, a microscopic analysis of the urine, which is called cytology, can identify the presence of cancer cells. The doctor may also perform a CYSTOSCOPY to visualize the interior bladder and obtain a biopsy of abnormal tissue in order to definitively diagnose the cancer. The doctor may also order a urinalysis.

### Treatment Options and Outlook
The treatment depends upon the stage of the cancer. If it is Stage 0 or 1, according to Konety, Joyce, and Wise, a transurethral resection of the

tumor is the most often used approach to treat early bladder cancer.

If the tumor is at either Stage II or III, then either part or all of the bladder may be removed (a radical cystectomy). However, about 30 percent of individuals experience complications from a cystectomy, and unless deemed necessary, the physician will avoid this procedure.

In men who have a cystectomy for bladder cancer, in addition to the bladder being removed, the prostate and seminal vesicles are also taken out by the surgeon because of their closeness in proximity to the bladder and the risk that the cancer could have spread to these areas. If the patient with bladder cancer is a woman, then the urethra, uterus, and the front of the vagina are also surgically extracted for the same reasons: the risk that the bladder cancer could have spread to adjacent areas.

After a cystectomy, the urine that is created by the kidneys will be channeled into a special bag that is periodically changed and which will have to be managed by the patient or other caregivers.

If the tumor is a Stage IV, surgery is usually not performed because the cancer is not curable.

When the tumor has extended into the renal pelvis, a nephroureterectomy is performed. In some cases, both the kidney and ureter may be surgically removed.

Chemotherapy may also be used to treat bladder cancer and to shrink the tumor and reduce pain. The most frequently used chemotherapy drugs for bladder cancer as of this writing include Mitomycin, Doxorubicin, and Epirubicin.

Immunotherapy (also known as biological therapy) is another treatment for bladder cancer, using bacteria known as Bacille Calmette-Guerin (BCG). This is a genetically modified form of bacteria. The majority of people who are treated with BCG (up to 90 percent) will experience some initial side effects, such as urinary frequency, urinary urgency, and painful urination, but these symptoms usually subside within days.

### Risk Factors and Preventive Measures

Males have a greater risk for bladder cancer than females, according to the National Cancer Institute (NCI), and over the 2002–06 period, the incidence rate of bladder cancer in the United States per 100,000 people was 37.1 for men and 9.3 for women. White male non-Hispanics had the highest rate, or 40.3 per 100,000 men, and American Indian/Alaska Natives had the lowest rate among males, or 12.4 per 100,000 men. (See Table 1.)

Among females, white females had the highest incidence rate (9.9 per 100,000 females) and American Indian/Alaska Native had the lowest rate (3.4 per 100,000 women). Note that *incidence* refers to the number of newly diagnosed cases of bladder cancer in a year. In contrast, the world *prevalence* refers to everyone alive who has been diagnosed with the disease. For example, on July 1, 2006, according to the NCI, the prevalence of bladder cancer was 527,496, which included 388,965 living men and 138,531 women who had ever been diagnosed with bladder cancer.

| TABLE 1: INCIDENCE OF BLADDER CANCER BY RACE AND ETHNICITY, 2002–2006 | | |
|---|---|---|
| Race/Ethnicity | Male | Female |
| All Races | 37.1 per 100,000 men | 9.3 per 100,000 women |
| White | 40.3 per 100,000 men | 9.9 per 100,000 women |
| Black | 20.0 per 100,000 men | 7.9 per 100,000 women |
| Asian/Pacific Islander | 16.5 per 100,000 men | 4.0 per 100,000 women |
| American Indian/Alaska Native | 12.4 per 100,000 men | 3.4 per 100,000 women |
| Hispanic | 19.8 per 100,000 men | 5.3 per 100,000 women |

**TABLE 2: DEATH RATES FROM BLADDER CANCER BY RACE AND ETHNICITY, 2002–2006**

| Race/Ethnicity | Male | Female |
|---|---|---|
| All Races | 7.5 per 100,000 men | 2.2 per 100,000 women |
| White | 7.9 per 100,000 men | 2.2 per 100,000 women |
| Black | 5.5 per 100,000 men | 2.8 per 100,000 women |
| Asian/Pacific Islander | 2.7 per 100,000 men | 1.0 per 100,000 women |
| American Indian/Alaska Native | 2.7 per 100,000 men | 1.1 per 100,000 women |
| Hispanic | 3.9 per 100,000 men | 1.3 per 100,000 women |

Males also have a higher death rate from bladder cancer than females; according to the NCI the death rate for 2002–06 per 100,000 people was 7.5 for men and 2.2 for women. In considering race, white males have a death rate of 7.9 per 100,000 individuals, compared to a much lower death rate of 2.7 per 100,000 people for both American Indian/Alaska Native males and Asian/Pacific Islander males.

In contrast, the incidence rate for black females was somewhat higher than it was among white females, or 2.8 per 100,000 black females, compared to 2.2 per 100,000 white females. Again, however, the lowest death rates from bladder cancer were seen among Asian/ Pacific Islander females or 1.0 per 100,000 women, followed by an almost identical rate of 1.1 per 100,000 American Indian/Alaska Native women. The death rate was also low among Hispanic females, or 1.3 per 100,000 women. The reasons for these discrepancies are unknown. (See Table 2.)

The cause of bladder cancer is unknown; however, it is known that smokers have five times the risk of developing bladder cancer compared to nonsmokers. As a result, individuals who smoke should stop SMOKING immediately to decrease their risk of developing bladder cancer or of causing a recurrence of the cancer. Quitting smoking will also decrease the risk for many other forms of cancer, as well as many diseases that are directly caused by or associated with smoking.

According to Konety, Joyce, and Wise, other factors that are linked to bladder cancer are a past exposure to the dyes that are used in the printing and rubber industries. In addition, a past history of radiation therapy or cyclophosphamide chemotherapy may increase the risk for the development of bladder cancer.

Chronic irritation, such as seen with recurrent bladder infections, the frequent use of urethral catheters or the presence of bladder or kidney stones, increases the risk of the development of squamous cell carcinoma of the bladder.

See also KIDNEY CANCER; MYELOMA KIDNEY.

Konety, Adrinath R., M.D. Geoffrey F. Joyce, and Matthew Wise. "Bladder and Upper Tract Urothelial Cancer." In *Urologic Diseases in America*, edited by Litwin M. S. and C. S. Saigal, 223–280. Bethesda, Md.: National Institute of Diabetes and Digestive and Kidney Diseases (NIDDK), 2007.

**bladder infection**    See CYSTITIS.

**bone disease, renal**    See CHRONIC KIDNEY DISEASE—MINERAL BONE DISORDER (CKD-MBD).

**calcium**    An essential mineral that is vital to the maintenance of healthy bones, teeth, and blood, as well as to life itself. Calcium is processed by the kidneys and excreted in the urine and feces. Individuals who are hypocalcemic (deficient in calcium) need to take supplemental calcium in the form of calcitriol in order to create and maintain normal blood levels of calcium. HYPOCALCEMIA may be caused by an issue with the parathyroid glands, such as by their damage or removal. In contrast, some individuals have excessively high levels of calcium, which is a condition that is known as HYPERCALCEMIA.

Hypocalcemia may also be caused by vitamin D deficiency. Vitamin D deficiency is an increasing problem in many countries, and probably related to both decreased dairy intake, particularly milk, and by decreased sun exposure (skin exposure to the sun is necessary in the activation process of vitamin D). Patients with advanced kidney disease, particularly those requiring DIALYSIS, may develop hypocalcemia because of kidney disease–related defects in vitamin D metabolism.

Many vegetables and some grains contain naturally occurring calcium. Some beverages are calcium-fortified, such as orange juice and soy milk, as well as mineral water. According to Deborah A. Straub in her article on calcium for *Nutrition in Clinical Practice* in 2007, most people in the United States do not consume sufficient daily amounts of calcium in their diet. Some factors increase the loss of calcium in the urine in females, such as a high intake of caffeine (greater than 300 mg per day) and low estrogen levels. About 11 percent of adults in the United States take calcium supplements.

Hypocalcemia can have important side effects in patients with kidney disease. The major issue is that hypocalcemia will cause the parathyroid glands to secrete more parathyroid hormone, and parathyroid hormone has adverse effects on many body tissues. Abnormal calcium levels are seen with individuals with severe CHRONIC KIDNEY DISEASE. For example, according to the United States Renal Data System (USRDS), based on data from 1999–2006, abnormal calcium levels equal to or less than 8.9 mg/dl are found in about 7 percent of individuals who do not have chronic kidney disease. These levels stay about the same until Stages 4–5 (the last stages) of chronic kidney disease, when about 22 percent of individuals have abnormal calcium levels.

Calcium interacts with some medications that are commonly used by many patients, such as thyroid medication, BISPHOSPHONATES, corticosteroids, and other drugs. See Table 1 for further information. In addition, some types of medications contain calcium, particularly antacids.

### Daily Requirements for Calcium

The needed daily milligrams of calcium vary by the individual's age and gender, as well as by whether a woman is pregnant or lactating (breastfeeding). See Table 2 for the adequate daily intakes of calcium according to the Office of Dietary Supplements in the National Institutes of Health.

Sometimes a calcium deficiency is inadvertently self-induced; for example, some severely

## TABLE 1: CALCIUM SUPPLEMENT–DRUG INTERACTIONS

| | |
|---|---|
| Levothyroxine | Administrations of calcium and levothyroxine should be separated by 4 hours; calcium reduces levothyroxine absorption by forming insoluble complexes. |
| Histamine 2 blockers and proton pump inhibitors | H2 blockers and proton pump inhibitors decrease the absorption of calcium carbonate, which requires an acidic environment. |
| Tetracyclines | Tetracyclines should be taken 4–6 hours before or after calcium supplements; calcium decreases the absorption of tetracycline by forming insoluble complexes. |
| Bisphosphonates | Bisphosphonates should be taken at least 30 minutes before calcium supplementation. Ideally, calcium should be taken at another time of day. |
| Quinolone antibiotics | Quinolone antibiotics should be taken at least 2 hours before or 4–6 hours after calcium supplementation; calcium decreases absorption of the drug by forming insoluble complexes. |
| Digoxin | Hypercalcemia increases the risk of fatal cardiac arhythmmia [when patients take digoxin]. |
| Thiazide diuretics | Thiazide diuretics decrease the excretion of calcium. Calcium supplementation in moderate doses increases the risk of milk-alkali syndrome. Serum calcium and parathyroid levels should be monitored regularly. |
| Corticosteroids | Corticosteroids in doses of 7.5 mg/day or more can cause significant bone loss, as they decrease calcium absorption, increase calcium excretion, and inhibit bone formation. Patients using these drugs should take calcium and vitamin D supplements. |
| Anticonvulsants, phenytoin, fosphenytoin, carbamazepine, phenobarbital | These anticonvulsants decrease calcium absorption by increasing the metabolism of vitamin D. Hypercalcemia and osteomalacia have been identified in patients receiving chronic therapy. Patients receiving these drugs should take calcium and vitamin D supplements. |

Source: Straub, Deborah A. "Calcium Supplementation in Clinical Practice: A Review of Forms, Doses, and Indications." *Nutrition in Clinical Practice* 22 (2007), p. 294.
NUTRITION IN CLINICAL PRACTICE ONLINE by Deborah A. Straub. Copyright 2007 by SAGE PUBLICATIONS INC. JOURNALS. Reproduced with permission of SAGE PUBLICATIONS INC. JOURNALS in the format Tradebook via Copyright Clearance Center.

obese individuals undergo bariatric surgery in order to reduce their weight significantly after all other weight loss efforts have failed. If they have a gastric bypass procedure, most of the stomach and duodenum as well as the upper small intestine is bypassed. This leads to an absorption deficiency of such minerals as calcium, and consequently, the individuals who have this surgery will need to take calcium supplements for the rest of their lives.

## TABLE 2: ADEQUATE INTAKES FOR CALCIUM

| Age | Male | Female | Pregnant | Lactating |
|---|---|---|---|---|
| Birth to 6 months | 210 mg | 210 mg | | |
| 7–12 months | 270 mg | 270 mg | | |
| 1–3 years | 500 mg | 500 mg | | |
| 4–8 years | 800 mg | 800 mg | | |
| 9–13 years | 1,300 mg | 1,300 mg | | |
| 14–18 years | 1,300 mg | 1,300 mg | 1,300 mg | 1,300 mg |
| 19–50 years | 1,300 mg | 1,300 mg | 1,000 mg | 1,000 mg |
| 50+ years | 1,200 mg | 1,200 mg | | |

Source: Office of Dietary Supplements. Dietary Supplement Fact Sheet: Calcium. National Institutes of Health. Updated October 7, 2009. Available online. URL: http://ods.nih.gov/factsheets/Calcium_pf.asp. Accessed December 29, 2009.

## Types of Calcium Supplements

Calcium citrate is one form of an over-the-counter (OTC) supplement that is given to treat a calcium deficiency. Another supplemental option is calcium carbonate. Both these forms of calcium may cause stomach upset. Calcium lactate is also a form of a calcium supplement, although this form of calcium is difficult to obtain other than by mail order. Calcium gluconate is yet another form of calcium supplement. These OTC calcium supplements may also be given with calcitriol, a prescribed form of vitamin D that boosts the blood calcium levels in those who need it.

See also MAGNESIUM; POTASSIUM; SODIUM.

Office of Dietary Supplements. *Dietary Supplement Fact Sheet: Calcium.* National Institutes of Health. Updated October 7, 2009. Available online. URL: http://ods.nih.gov/factsheets/Calcium_pf.asp. Accessed December 29, 2009.

Straub, Deborah A. "Calcium Supplementation in Clinical Practice: A Review of Forms, Doses, and Indications." *Nutrition in Clinical Practice* 22 (2007): 286–296.

**calcium channel blockers**   A class of medications that is used to treat heart disease, HYPERTENSION, and a variety of other diseases and disorders, such as migraine headaches, an irregular heartbeat, or chest pain. Hypertension is a leading cause of kidney disease and kidney failure. Calcium channel blockers are also sometimes used to treat Raynaud's phenomenon, a medical problem that causes a decreased circulation to the extremities.

Calcium channel blockers are also called calcium blockers or calcium antagonists. Drugs in this category impact the movement of calcium into the heart and blood vessel cells, thus relaxing the blood vessels and thereby increasing the level of oxygen and the blood supply to the heart.

Some examples of calcium channel blocker medications include amlodipine (Norvasc), bepridil (Vascor), nimodipine (Nimotop), and verapamil (Calan, Calan Sustained Release, and Isoptin). (See Table 1 for more examples of calcium channel blocker medications.)

### TABLE 1: CALCIUM CHANNEL BLOCKERS

| Brand Name | Generic Name |
| --- | --- |
| Norvasc | Amlodipine |
| Cardizem | Diltiazem |
| Dilacor XR | Diltiazem |
| Tiazac | Diltiazem |
| Plendil | Felodipine |
| DynaCirc CR | Isradipine |
| Cardene | Nicardipine |
| Adalat CC | Nifedipine |
| Procardia | Nifedipine |
| Nimotop | Nimodipine |
| Sular | Nisoldipine |
| Calan | Verapamil |
| Coversa HS | Verapamil |
| Isoptin | Verapamil |
| Verelan | Verapamil |

Source: FDA Office of Women's Health, Medicines to Help You: High Blood Pressure. 2007. Available online. URL: http://www.fda.gov/womens/medicinecharts/highbloodpressure.html. Downloaded May 20, 2007.

### Precautions with Calcium Channel Blockers

Individuals with some diseases and disorders should be carefully monitored when they take calcium channel blockers. Patients who are taking specific medications, particularly nitrate medications (drugs that are given to treat heart disease), quinidine (a medication for the treatment of abnormal heart rhythms), or fentanyl (a medication that is given to treat pain) should avoid taking calcium channel blockers.

Individuals who take calcium channel blockers should either limit or avoid their consumption of both grapefruit juice and grape juice, because these juices will significantly increase the absorption of the medication.

Although each calcium channel blocker medication has its own particular side effects, in general, the possible side effects of calcium channel blockers are:

- swelling of ankles or feet
- irregular or speeded up heartbeat
- constipation
- slowed heart rate
- worsening shortness of breath

In addition, some patients who begin taking a calcium channel blocker may experience headaches; however, in many cases, the patient's body eventually adjusts to the medication and these headaches disappear.

Anyone taking calcium channel blockers who exhibits any of the following signs should immediately contact their physician:

- severe rash
- fainting
- irregular heartbeat
- increased chest pain
- difficulty breathing

See also ANGIOTENSIN-CONVERTING ENZYME INHIBITORS; ANTIHYPERTENSIVE DRUGS; BETA BLOCKERS; DIURETICS; MEDICATIONS THAT CAN HARM THE KIDNEYS.

FDA Office of Women's Health. Medicines to Help You: High Blood Pressure. 2007. Available online. URL: http://www.fda.gov/womens/medicinecharts/highbloodpressure.html. Downloaded May 20, 2007.

**cancer**  See BLADDER CANCER; KIDNEY CANCER; MYELOMA KIDNEY.

**cancer, bladder**  See BLADDER CANCER.

**cancer, kidney**  See KIDNEY CANCER.

**cardiovascular disease (CVD)**  Refers to the presence of either heart disease (heart attack or heart failure), peripheral arterial disease, or stroke. Cardiovascular disease increases the risk for both kidney disease and kidney failure. Alternatively, kidney disease itself also elevates the risk for the development of cardiovascular disease. Most individuals with cardiovascular disease have HYPERTENSION, and it may be controlled insufficiently.

According to Stein Hallan, M.D., and colleagues, their research has showed that both a reduced kidney function and the presence of microalbuminuria (a type of protein sometimes found in the urine) were risk factors for cardiovascular death, independent of other risk factors. This research was based on nearly 10,000 participants in Norway who were followed for more than eight years. The estimated glomerular filtration rate (eGFR) and the albumin-creatinine ratio (ACR) were especially significant risk factors among those individuals ages 70 years and older.

In another study by Nisha I. Parikh, M.D., and colleagues, cardiovascular disease risk factors among those with CHRONIC KIDNEY DISEASE (CKD) were evaluated based on more than 3,000 subjects, in whom 8.6 percent had CKD. The researchers found that individuals with CKD were more likely to be older, obese, and with high triglyceride levels and low levels of high-density lipoprotein (HDL), the good CHOLESTEROL. The researchers noted that a diagnosis of CKD should trigger an analysis of potentially modifiable risk factors for cardiovascular disease in patients. The researchers said:

> There is a significant burden of CVD risk factors among participants with CKD in the community. Participants with CKD are more likely to be treated for hypertension, elevated LDL-C levels, and diabetes, but rates of control are uniformly low in those with and without CKD. In general, when we stratified our analysis using an age cutoff of 65 years, older individuals demonstrated more significant differences in hypertension prevalence, treatment, and control.

In another study by Essam F. Elsayed, M.D., and colleagues of more than 13,000 subjects, the researchers found that cardiovascular disease was associated with an increased likelihood of kidney disease and kidney function decline. The researchers provided possible explanations for this unidirectional cause:

> First, the presence of baseline CVD may identify individuals with greater duration and severity of shared CVD and kidney risk factors, particularly DM [diabetes mellitus] and hypertension. Second, atherosclerotic disease may also affect the renal vasculature, causing disease of small or large vessels and resulting in CKD. Third, the presence of baseline CVD may identify individuals who will eventually develop heart failure, and these individuals may develop kidney function decline due to decreased kidney perfusion. Fourth, CVD predisposes individuals to cardiac procedures, including cardiac catheterization, which may result in kidney damage from intravenous contrast or atheroemboli.

See also DIABETES MELLITUS; END-STAGE RENAL DISEASE.

Elsayed, Essam F., M.D., et al. "Cardiovascular Disease and Subsequent Kidney Disease." *Archives of Internal Medicine* 167 (2007): 1,130–1,136.

Hallan, Stein, M.D., et al. "Association of Kidney Function and Albuminuria with Cardiovascular Mortality in Older vs. Younger Individuals: The HUNT II Study." *Archives of Internal Medicine* 167, no. 22 (2007): 2,490–2,496.

Parikh, Nisha I., M.D., et al. "Cardiovascular Disease Risk Factors in Chronic Kidney Disease: Overall Burden and Rates of Treatment and Control." *Archives of Internal Medicine* 166 (2006): 1,884–1,891.

**Caucasians/whites** See KIDNEYS AND KIDNEY DISEASE.

**causes of kidney diseases** There are many possible causes of serious kidney diseases such as CHRONIC KIDNEY DISEASE, recurrent KIDNEY STONES, and other disorders, but there are some diseases that bring the greatest risk for the development of kidney disease. These diseases include DIABETES MELLITUS, HYPERTENSION, and GLOMERULONEPHRITIS, as well as some urologic diseases and other causes. Diabetes is the primary cause of chronic kidney disease, followed by hypertension as the second leading cause.

If chronic kidney disease progresses, it leads to END-STAGE RENAL DISEASE (ESRD), at which point the kidneys have either failed or they will fail imminently. With the failure of the kidneys comes the need for either DIALYSIS or a KIDNEY TRANSPLANTATION in order for the individual to survive. Researchers have also found that the presence of CARDIOVASCULAR DISEASE is a risk factor for kidney disease, just as kidney disease is itself a risk factor for the development of cardiovascular disease.

ACUTE KIDNEY INJURY may cause kidney disease leading to kidney failure. Acute kidney injury refers to a sudden and severe harm to the kidney, either from external forces (such as a reaction to nephrotoxic medications, such as radiocontrast dye) or from internal forces (such as severe low blood pressure caused by sepsis). Acute kidney injury (AKI) is also known as acute renal failure or acute kidney failure. It is also a cause of kidney failure, although not everyone with AKI needs to receive permanent dialysis, and some patients will regain their kidney function. AKI itself may be caused by severe infections, surgery, some medications that can harm the kidneys, or by complications that can occur in the intensive care unit (ICU) of the hospital.

### Diabetes Mellitus and Kidney Disease

According to the United States Renal Data System (USRDS) as well as many other sources, diabetes mellitus was the major cause of end-stage renal disease in 2007, and it continues to be the major risk factor for ESRD in 2010, as of this writing.

Diabetes is an increasing problem in the United States, and according to the Centers for Disease Control and Prevention (CDC), an estimated 23.6 million people in the United States had diabetes in 2007; however, of this number, 5.7 million had not been diagnosed. The largest single percentage of those with diabetes were individuals who were ages 60 years and older, among whom 23.1 percent had diabetes. In general, men are slightly more likely to have diabetes than women; 11.2 percent of all men ages 20 years and older and 10.2 percent of all women ages 20 and older have diabetes.

Among non-Hispanic blacks, 14.7 percent ages 20 years and older have diabetes, compared to 9.8 percent of non-Hispanic whites. Other groups have high rates of diabetes, such as American Indians and Alaska Natives.

According to the CDC, 46,739 people with diabetes began treatment for end-stage kidney disease in the United States and Puerto Rico in 2005, and 178,698 diabetics with ESRD were either on dialysis or had had a kidney transplant.

### Hypertension and Kidney Disease

The United States Renal Data System reports that hypertension is the second leading cause of kidney failure in the United States. According to the National Kidney and Urologic Diseases Information Clearinghouse, in 2007, there were nearly 31,000 new cases of patients with kidney failure in the United States that were caused by hypertension. Even if hypertension is not considered the cause of kidney failure, by the time patients are in Stages 4–5 of the five stages of kidney failure in chronic kidney disease, 84.1 percent of them have hypertension, according to data analyzed over the period 1999 to 2006 by the United States Renal Data System.

Control of high blood pressure with medications, weight loss, and stress reduction can significantly reduce the risk of kidney disease as well as the risk for cardiovascular disease.

### Severe Infections

In the United States, most people recover from the broad variety of infections. Rarely, however, infections can severely damage the kidneys, particularly if these infections are not diagnosed and treated and especially if they are recurrent. Chronic incidents of PYELONEPHRITIS (kidney infection) may be harmful to the kidneys. In very rare cases, infection with an organism such as *Streptococcus* can lead to POSTSTREPTOCOCCAL GLOMERULONEPHRITIS, particularly if the individual resides in a less developed country or in a very poor part of a developed country.

An infection with HEPATITIS C can harm the kidneys as well as the liver. Other sexually transmitted diseases can lead to kidney disease or failure, such as infection with the human immunodeficiency virus (HIV), which can lead to HUMAN IMMUNODEFICIENCY VIRUS ASSOCIATED NEPHROPATHY (HIVAN).

HEMOLYTIC UREMIC SYNDROME–THROMBOTIC THROMBOCYTOPENIA PURPURA (HUS-TTP) is caused by an infection with specific forms of the bacteria *Escherichia coli (E. coli)* in the digestive system, often caused by consumption of contaminated food. In the most severe case, it can lead to kidney failure.

### Endocrine Disorders

Some endocrine disorders can lead to kidney disease, especially HYPERPARATHYROIDISM, excessive levels of parathyroid hormone produced by the parathyroid glands. This disorder may also result from the presence of kidney disease. Hyperparathyroidism can lead to the development of kidney stones.

Diabetes mellitus is also an endocrine disorder and is the leading cause of kidney disease and kidney failure. Good control of blood sugar levels significantly decreases the risk for both kidney disease and kidney failure.

### Cancer

Cancer may be the cause of kidney disease, as with multiple myeloma causing MYELOMA KIDNEY. KIDNEY CANCER is another form of cancer. The risk for kidney cancer (as well as other forms of cancers) can be estimated by answering questions at the Stetman Cancer Center site at http://www.yourdiseaserisk.siteman.wustl.edu/hccpquiz.pl?lang=english&func=prev&quiz=kidney&page=&prev=0. Individuals with some risk factors, such as smoking, can learn that they should stop smoking immediately to decrease their risk for kidney cancer. Smoking does not directly cause kidney cancer but does increase the risk for the development of this form of cancer. Other risk factors for kidney cancer include high blood pressure, obesity, and long-term dialysis. Males have a greater risk for kidney cancer than females. Individuals with a rare genetic disease known as Von-Hippel-Lindau syndrome have an elevated risk for developing kidney cancer. Individuals who are exposed to some substances also have an increased risk for kidney cancer, such as those who are exposed to cadmium or asbestos.

BLADDER CANCER can also metastasize (spread) into the kidneys. Other cancers that do not directly involve the kidney can also lead to a specific form of glomerular disease, membranous glomerulonephritis. If the cancer is cured, then the membranous glomerulonephritis will typically resolve.

### Genetic Causes of Some Kidney Diseases

Some kidney diseases largely stem from genetic issues; for example, POLYCYSTIC KIDNEY DISEASE is an inherited disease that causes multiple kidney cysts to form—as many as thousands of cysts per kidney. The most frequently seen form of this disease is autosomal dominant polycystic kidney disease (ADPKD), which stems from a genetic mutation in either the PKD1 or PKD2 gene.

**Polycystic kidney disease**   According to Peter C. Harris and Vicente F. Torres in their 2009 article for the *Annual Review of Medicine,* ADPKD is usually not diagnosed until adulthood, and it has an incidence of one in every 400–1,000 individuals. However, patients may have an onset of their symptoms as early as the teenage years. Alternatively, there may be no clinically apparent disease until the patient is in the 70s, 80s, or even later. Because of its high incidence, ADPKD is one of the most common autosomal dominant genetic conditions.

In many cases, this disease leads to ESRD. Harris and Torres report that 4.4 percent of all patients needing dialysis or a kidney transplantation have ADPKD. The authors say that typical symptoms are hematuria (blood in the urine), renal colic (pain emanating from the kidneys), urinary tract infections, flank pain, and hypertension. Adults who are at risk for ADPKD can be diagnosed with ultrasound, computerized tomography (CT), or magnetic resonance imaging (MRI).

A less common form of polycystic kidney disease is autosomal recessive polycystic kidney disease (ARPKD), which is believed to occur in one in 20,000 individuals. It may present in utero or in newborns with grossly enlarged kidneys, as well as with limb and spine abnormalities. Of those who survive the neonatal period, about a third will need renal replacement therapy. ARPKD stems from a genetic mutation in PKHD1.

**Alport syndrome**   Another disease that harms the kidneys and which is genetically based is ALPORT SYNDROME. Females are the carriers of the problem gene but they usually do not develop the disease themselves. Males with Alport syndrome typically develop kidney disease that progresses to kidney failure.

**Rare genetic diseases**   Another kidney disease with a genetic link, albeit a very rare condition, is BARTTER'S SYNDROME, a syndrome linked to five different genes in its development. The first syndrome typically presents at a young age with hypotension, hypokalemia, and evidence of volume depletion.

DENYS-DRASH SYNDROME is another rare and genetically linked disease that causes harm to the kidneys. It is usually identified in children and it leads to kidney failure. FABRY'S DISEASE is a genetically based disorder which is more serious in males than females. Affected individuals typically have symptoms that begin during their childhood or adolescence. AMYLOIDOSIS is an inherited disease that causes a protein-like material known as amyloid to accumulate in different parts of the body, including the kidneys, causing damage to the organs to which it attaches. (Alzheimer's disease is characterized by plaques of amyloid in the brain.) SICKLE CELL DISEASE (also known as sickle cell anemia) is another hereditary disease that harms the kidneys.

Some forms of kidney stones are genetically linked; for example, individuals with stones comprised of cystine usually have inherited a genetic predisposition for the formation of these types of stones.

CRYSTAL NEPHROPATHY is a form of kidney disease that is caused by the development of crystals that dam up the urine flow and can cause acute renal failure. It may be caused by the administration of high dosages of intravenous acyclovir.

### Autoimmune Disorders

An autoimmune disorder refers to a circumstance in which the immune system mistakes an individual's own tissue as a foreign invader and attacks that tissue. There are many types of autoimmune disorders that can be harmful to the kidney; for example, SJÖGREN'S SYNDROME and LUPUS NEPHRITIS are both autoimmune disorders. Some autoimmune disorders are rare but they can be very lethal; for example, GOODPASTURE SYNDROME may lead to kidney failure within days. MEMBRANOPROLIFERATIVE GLOMERULONEPHRITIS (MPGN) is a rare autoimmune disorder that primarily attacks children and young adults.

WEGENER'S GRANULOMATOSIS is a rare autoimmune disease that can be harmful to the kidneys because it damages the blood vessels of the kidneys and other organs. SCLERODERMA is an autoimmune dermatologic disease that can cause harm to the kidneys and sometimes lead to kidney failure.

### Physical Abnormalities

Some individuals are born with physical abnormalities of the kidneys that may cause no problems for years and then be discovered at a later date when kidney function is impaired. For example, some individuals are born with one kidney rather than the usual two kidneys. As long as the individual remains healthy, the one kidney may be able to manage the task of filtering out impurities. Often the abnormality is not discovered until imaging scans or other procedures are performed.

Another type of physical abnormality is the ECTOPIC KIDNEY, which occurs when the kidney is in an unusual position in the body. This condition may lead to recurrent infections as well as the development of bladder stones and kidney stones.

REFLUX NEPHROPATHY is a condition in which the urine flows backward up into the kidney. This may lead to the development of recurrent infections, which can lead to damage to the kidneys and chronic kidney disease.

### Combined Risk Factors for Kidney Disease

Many people have a combination of risk factors for kidney disease, such as having both diabetes and hypertension, which together further escalate the risk of kidney failure. Some medications can increase the risk for (or cause) kidney diseases, particularly among individuals who are ELDERLY and who have diabetes and/or hypertension. (See MEDICATIONS THAT CAN HARM THE KIDNEYS.)

Some kidney diseases are caused or exacerbated by an individual's diet and lifestyle choices; for example, some individuals develop kidney stones because of a genetic risk to react to a diet that is high in a substance known as calcium oxalate. Decreasing the oxalates in the blood will then decrease the risk for the development of kidney stones. Although this propensity may be caused by rare genetic diseases causing HYPEROXALURIA, it may also be caused by a diet replete with foods that are very high in oxalates, such as berries and some fruits and vegetables.

Another tendency that may increase the risk for kidney stones that can be altered by DIETARY CHANGES is a predisposition to excessive urinary uric acid excretion. Individuals with this predisposition need to restrict their dietary intake of purines, which can involve limiting their consumption of organ meats, fish, and shellfish, to name just a few common foods that are high in purines. In addition, individuals who form uric acid stones need to limit their overall consumption of meats.

It should also be noted that kidney disease can occur with *no* family history and in a seemingly healthy person who is of normal weight and who does not smoke or drink alcohol and who exercises on a regular basis. Genetic and environmental factors can increase or decrease risks for diseases but even the most favorable sustained conditions cannot altogether eliminate the risk for kidney disease and other diseases.

### Lifestyle Choices That Increase the Risk for Kidney Disease

Some lifestyle choices increase the risk for kidney disease, either directly or indirectly. For example, OBESITY increases the risk for diabetes, which then in turn increases the risk for kidney disease. Severe obesity can also cause the development of certain types of glomerular disease, most commonly focal segmental glomerulosclerosis (FSGS).

SMOKING is a lifestyle choice that is also a risk factor for kidney disease. Heavy drinking also increases the risk for kidney disease. In one important study, researchers studied the association between smoking, heavy drinking, and the subsequent development of chronic kidney disease (CKD), based on data from 4,898 individuals including 324 subjects with CKD. The subjects were studied over the period 1988 to 1995. The researchers found a strong correlation between heavy drinking and/or smoking and the later development of CKD.

In this study, published in 2006 in the *American Journal of Epidemiology,* heavy drinking was defined as the consumption of four or more alcohol servings per day. The rate of CKD among individuals who consumed from zero to three servings of alcohol per day was about 6 percent but rose dramatically to nearly 16 percent among those who drank four or more servings of alcohol per day.

Among smokers, 3.6 percent of those who never smoked had CKD, while the rate was 5.8 percent among those who were former smokers. The prevalence of CKD among current smokers was 15.1 percent.

The researchers found that current smokers had about twice the odds of developing CKD as never-smokers, and heavy drinkers also had about twice the odds of developing CKD compared to non-heavy drinkers. The highest odds ratio for the development of CKD was seen among those who were *both* heavy drinkers and current smokers: These subjects faced nearly a five-fold increased risk for developing CKD. Clearly, giving up smoking and heavy drinking is important for those who wish to decrease their risk for chronic kidney disease. Since chronic kidney disease further increases the risk for cardiovascular disease and kidney failure, these are yet further reasons for giving up tobacco and moderating or giving up alcohol.

A lack of exercise and a general sedentary life may lead to obesity and then to an elevated risk for the development of kidney disease. Obesity itself is a risk factor for kidney disease, including kidney failure. In study results from more than 320,000 adults studied between 1964 and 1985, published in *Annals of Internal Medicine* in 2006, the researchers found that a higher body mass index was significantly associated with a risk for end-stage renal disease (kidney failure). The relative risk for the development of ESRD was nearly twice as high for overweight individuals compared to normal-weight individuals. The relative risk increased with increasing body mass index (BMI) and was more than seven times greater for those with extreme obesity or a body mass index equal to or greater than 40. The researchers noted that a high BMI was an independent risk factor for the development of kidney failure.

### Unknown Causes

Sometimes the reason for kidney disease and/or kidney failure is unknown, even if the diagnosis of the cause is made. For example, Henoch-Schönlein purpura (HSP) is one disorder that causes kidney disease but whose cause is unknown. When the cause of a disease is not known, the physician seeks to treat the symptoms and reduce the risks of kidney disease or kidney failure as well as any other medical problems associated with the disease.

Harris, Peter C., and Vicente E. Torres. "Polycystic Kidney Disease." *Annual Review of Medicine* 60 (2009): 321–337.

Hsu, Chi-yan, et al. "Body Mass Index and Risk for End-Stage Renal Disease." *Annals of Internal Medicine* 144 (2006): 21–28.

MedicineNet. "Kidney Cancer: Who's at Risk?" Available online. URL: http://www.medicinenet.com/kidney_cancer/page2.htm. Accessed November 8, 2010.

Shankar, Anoop, Ronald Klein, and Barbara E. K. Klein. "The Association among Smoking, Heavy Drinking, and Chronic Kidney Disease." *American Journal of Epidemiology* 164, no. 3 (2006): 263–271.

Tryggvason, Karl, M.D., Jaakko Patrakka, M.D., and Jorma Wartiovaara, M.D. "Hereditary Proteinuria Syndromes and Mechanisms of Proteinuria." *New England Journal of Medicine* 354, no. 13 (2006): 1,387–1,401.

**childhood nephrotic syndrome**  Signs of damage in childhood to the glomeruli, the tiny blood-filtering units of the kidney. Nephrotic syndrome in children or adults results from diseases that affect the glomeruli. When diagnosed, childhood nephrotic syndrome is most commonly found among children between the ages of 18 months and five years, and it is also found more often among boys. The most frequently occurring cause of childhood nephrotic syndrome is MINIMAL CHANGE DISEASE, which has this name because when examined with conventional light microscopes, the kidney appears relatively normal. Children with minimal change disease are treated with corticosteroid medications such as prednisone.

Often childhood nephrotic syndrome abates when children reach late adolescence, and usually the kidneys have not been permanently damaged.

### Symptoms and Diagnostic Path

The most common symptoms and signs of childhood nephrotic syndrome are:

- high levels of urinary protein (PROTEINURIA)
- low levels of blood protein
- swelling of body tissue (edema) due to a buildup of water and salt, particularly in the tissues surrounding the eyes (in adults, the swelling is more likely to occur in the ankles and feet)
- high levels of lipids and CHOLESTEROL in the blood (hyperlipidemia, hypercholesterolemia)

If childhood nephrotic syndrome is suspected, the doctor may order a urine sample to check for the protein levels in the child's urine. This typically is found with a routine URINALYSIS, for screening purposes; if positive, formal measurement of the urine protein-to-creatinine ratio in a random sample is performed for accurate quantification of the degree of proteinuria. Although the physician may also request a 24-hour urine collection, this test is less frequently performed because of the difficulty and inconvenience of collecting urine for 24 hours.

### Treatment Options and Outlook

Treatment is based upon the cause of the nephrotic syndrome. Screening tests for systemic lupus erythematosus (SLE) and other systemic diseases should be performed. Because minimal change disease is the most common cause of idiopathic childhood nephrotic syndrome, treatment is generally directed at this diagnosis with the use of glucocorticoids, such as prednisone, if the screening serologic tests do not identify an underlying etiology. In most cases, idiopathic nephrotic syndrome will resolve and the prednisone can be gradually discontinued. In cases where either the proteinuria does not resolve or where it returns after discontinuing the prednisone, a KIDNEY BIOPSY may be needed to identify whether another condition is the cause of the childhood nephrotic syndrome.

DIURETICS are often prescribed to decrease tissue swelling. ANGIOTENSIN-CONVERTING ENZYME INHIBITORS may be prescribed to decrease proteinuria.

### Risk Factors and Preventive Measures

The disorder is most common in children ages 18 months to 5 years with kidney disease and is more common among boys than girls.

See also CHILDREN AND KIDNEY DISEASE; NEPHROTIC SYNDROME.

**children and kidney disease** Disorders and diseases of the kidneys that are experienced by children and adolescents, such as CHILDHOOD NEPHROTIC SYNDROME, MINIMAL CHANGE DISEASE, and others. Some non-kidney diseases that children may have, such as Type 1 or Type 2 DIABETES MELLITUS or HYPERTENSION, can directly affect and harm the kidneys. Children may also suffer from CHRONIC KIDNEY DISEASE (CKD), and sometimes they experience kidney failure that is caused by either chronic kidney disease in its final stage END-STAGE RENAL DISEASE [ESRD], or by ACUTE KIDNEY INJURY (AKI). Some kidney diseases are genetically linked.

### Genetic Disorders

Some kidney diseases are directly caused by genetic mutations; for example, DENYS-DRASH SYNDROME is a rare disease that is identified in some children and which ultimately leads to kidney failure. Other hereditary diseases that can lead to kidney failure are POLYCYSTIC KIDNEY DISEASE and ALPORT SYNDROME. Once identified, these diseases should be treated as soon as possible to reduce the risk for kidney failure.

### Systemic Diseases

Some children suffer from systemic diseases than can lead to kidney failure, such as lupus or diabetes mellitus. With lupus, an overactive immune system attacks body tissues, including the kidneys, a condition known as LUPUS NEPHRITIS. Among adults, diabetes is the leading cause of kidney failure; however, it is not the leader among children. Despite this, many experts are concerned about the increasing number of children and adolescents with Type 2 diabetes, which portends ill for these children in terms of their risk for developing chronic kidney disease and kidney failure. As with adults, when both diabetes and hypertension are present, the risk for chronic kidney disease is elevated in children.

### Chronic Kidney Disease

According to Valerie L. Johnson, M.D., most chronic kidney disease in children is caused by either a urologic disease or a medical issue that they inherited. She also noted that the most frequently seen causes of childhood CKD include a urinary tract blockage; an unusual growth of the kidneys; or the presence of either REFLUX NEPHROPATHY or FOCAL SEGMENTAL GLOMERULOSCLEROSIS. Johnson said that some children with CKD experience growth failure, while others do not; generally it is younger children whose growth is the most affected by CKD.

Some children with kidney disease have a greater probability of receiving treatment from a nephrologist while others have a lower rate, depending on age. According to the United States Renal Data System (USRDS), the odds of a child with chronic kidney disease ages 14 years old or younger being under the care of a nephrologist prior to the development of end-stage renal disease, which is kidney failure, is up to 72 percent higher than an adult with CKD. However, the situation reverses itself for adolescents ages 15–19, who are 6 percent *less* likely to be seeing a nephrologist prior to ESRD than an adult with CKD. The reasons for these findings are unknown.

### Acute Kidney Injury

According to Zappitelli, acute kidney injury (AKI) may be caused by INFECTIONS, medications, and other causes, such as a urinary tract obstruction, an obstruction of a SOLITARY KIDNEY, or GLOMERULONEPHRITIS. It may also be caused by postoperative trauma and severe dehydration.

Exposure to some toxic materials or to snake or animal venom can also cause AKI.

***Nephrotoxic medications causing acute kidney injury in children***   Some medications can cause kidney damage in children, leading to AKI, and according to Ludwig Patzer, these reactions represent 16 percent of all the cause of acute kidney injury in children, particularly drugs that fit the following categories:

- nonsteroidal anti-inflammatory medications (NSAIDs)
- antibiotics
- antiviral agents
- calcineurin inhibitors
- radiocontrast media
- cytostatics

***Toxic animal venom***   Some animal bites can cause a nephrotoxic reaction, such as bites from snakes, spiders, bees, wasps, and some marine animals, such as jellyfish, carp, and sea anemones.

***Infections***   Some children develop serious kidney diseases because of infections; for example, an infection of the digestive system with *E. coli (Escherichia coli)* can lead to gastroenteritis. This infection stems from contaminated foods, as with contaminated meat, juice, or dairy products. It can also occur from swimming in lakes or pools that are contaminated with fecal matter. Most children recover within several days but some children develop HEMOLYTIC UREMIC SYNDROME, where, as a result of the reaction to infection, the body begins to strike the root cells, causing severe ANEMIA and the development of rapidly progressive acute renal failure. According to the National Institute of Diabetes and Digestive and Kidney Diseases (NIDDK), this is a rare occurrence.

The symptoms may occur within a week of infection, and they may include bleeding from the mouth or nose, unexplained bruises, and decreased urination. The child may also experience high blood pressure and swelling of the face, hands, or feet or even swelling of the entire body. Extreme fatigue is another symptom. In the most extreme case, the child will need DIALYSIS; some children develop permanent kidney damage, and they will need either continued dialysis or kidney transplantation. According to the National Kidney and Urologic Diseases Information Clearinghouse, some parents feel very guilty when their children develop hemolytic uremic syndrome; however, the course of the disease cannot be predicted, and most children will recover completely. Of those children who do develop kidney disease, there are no known risk factors.

Another microbe that can lead to kidney failure is streptococcus, and this form of bacterium may lead to POSTSTREPTOCOCCAL GLOMERULONEPHRITIS. The source of this infection may be contact with other children or adults with streptococcus. Most children recover with treatment; however, in some cases, the immunologic reaction to the streptococcus infection leads to kidney damage.

### Kidney Failure

Kidney failure may be caused by acute kidney injury (formerly known as acute renal failure) or by end-stage renal disease (ESRD), the fifth and final stage of chronic kidney disease.

According to the National Institute of Diabetes and Digestive and Kidney Diseases (NIDDK), about 30 in every 100,000 people in the general population develop kidney failure every year; however, the rate of kidney failure is much lower among children ages 19 and younger, or about one to two cases per 100,000 children. Thus, adults have a 20 times greater risk for kidney failure than children. Some children have a greater risk for kidney failure than others; for example, African Americans in their late teens with kidney disease have three times greater risk of developing kidney failure than white teenagers with kidney disease. In addition, boys are more likely to develop kidney failure than girls. The reasons for these disparities are frequently debated by experts but the actual causes are unknown.

If the child's kidneys fail, in addition to the problems that adults experience, such as severe fatigue, weak bones, SLEEP PROBLEMS, DEPRESSION, and nerve damage, children with kidney failure may also experience problems with their growth and development. Children with kidney failure may receive dialysis or a KIDNEY TRANSPLANTA-TION; sometimes they will receive a preemptive transplantation when it is anticipated that the kidneys will fail imminently, in order that they may avoid dialysis altogether. They may receive a donation from a living donor or a deceased donor. If the parent donates the kidney, then there is a greater likelihood of a good match.

The U.S. Renal Data System (USRDS) noted that 7,209 pediatric patients received treatment for ESRD in 2007, or a rate of 84.6 per million population. They also noted that the rate of ESRD caused by cystic kidney disease has increased by 27 percent since 2000 to the 2007 rate of 36.4 per million population.

The USRDS also noted in their 2009 report that there is a high rate of death caused by both infections and cardiovascular complications among children with ESRD, with the emphasis on cardiovascular problems.

*Treatment for kidney failure: dialysis*   Children who receive HEMODIALYSIS at a clinic may receive dialysis three times a week but sometimes small children will need more frequent dialysis treatments. The child may experience some initial problems with hemodialysis because of the rapid changes that occur during the treatments; for example, the child may experience muscle cramps, hypotension (below-normal blood pressure), weakness, dizziness, and nausea. In most cases, children need several months to adjust to dialysis. Dialysis may be very distressing for the child (and parents) but it can mean the difference between life and death.

*Treatment: kidney transplantation*   Many children with kidney failure are treated with kidney transplantation. As with adults, children who receive a kidney transplant must take IMMUNO-SUPPRESSIVE DRUGS, which increase their risk for infections and for cancer.

According to the National Kidney and Urologic Diseases Information Clearinghouse, children have more active immune systems than adults, which means that they need proportionately higher dosages of immunosuppressants. However, these drugs can cause weight gain, acne, unusual hair growth, and the development of malignant tumors. They may also affect growth and development.

Another limitation of kidney transplantation in children is a smaller size of the body, particularly in young children. This can limit the use of an adult kidney in a small child. Nevertheless, despite its limitations, kidney transplantation in children with end-stage renal disease is generally associated with a much better long-term outcome than either hemodialysis or peritoneal dialysis.

### Special Issues with Children with Kidney Disease

There are some special issues to consider for children with severe kidney disease, particularly those children with kidney failure, including such issues as bone problems, growth failure, hypertension, CARDIOVASCULAR DISEASE, high CHOLESTEROL levels, and a VITAMIN D deficiency.

*Bone problems and growth failure*   Bone problems and decreased growth are common complications in children with chronic kidney disease. These problems result from a combination of a number of factors. In particular, the growth and development of bones are affected, which are critical in the development of the child. Many of the complications of chronic kidney disease interfere with normal bone growth and development.

PHOSPHORUS blood levels may become high when a child has failed kidneys, and this development can impede the child's normal growth. The doctor may wish the child to limit the consumption of foods that are high in phosphorus, such as cheese, milk, cola drinks, nuts, and other items. Parents generally need to work with a dietitian to help create a diet that is low in phosphorus and that also meets the child's need for calories. Children may also need to take phosphate binder medications in order to lower their phosphorus levels and avoid HYPERPHOSPHATEMIA.

CALCIUM and a synthetic form of vitamin D may be prescribed to children with chronic kidney disease, and according to the NIDDK, these supplements help with the growth process. They may be given by pill or by injection, depending on the physician's recommendation. Systemic acid accumulation, termed metabolic acidosis, is common in chronic kidney disease and directly interferes with bone formation. Treatment with alkalizing agents such as sodium bicarbonate is necessary and important for normal bone growth and development and for skeletal muscle development.

Because of problems with growth failure in childhood, children with chronic kidney disease may become short adults. According to the USRDS, growth failure continues to be a problem for children with chronic kidney disease in the United States; for example, two-thirds of children and adolescents with pediatric end-stage renal disease are in the lowest height quintile and 50 percent are in the lowest weight quintile. This means that they are in the bottom 20 percent of children of their age for both height and weight. The USRDS says that there is relatively low use of growth hormone to treat growth failure among children who have kidney disease.

It should be noted that short stature can be a significant problem for children when they grow into adults. Says Johnson, "Studies of short stature in adulthood have demonstrated a significant negative impact on quality of life. Increases in final adult height are associated with increased likelihood of being married or living outside the parent's home. There is also a relationship with being employed full time. Short stature is, in addition, associated with an increased risk of morbidity and mortality."

To avoid such problems, children with chronic kidney disease are often treated with recombinant human growth hormone (rHGH), which is safe to use in children with kidney disease, even when they are receiving dialysis or have had a kidney transplant.

*Hypertension*  Some children with chronic kidney disease have abnormalities of their blood pressure, according to Janis M. Dionne and colleagues. These researchers reported on 42 children ages 2–19 years old with chronic kidney disease from Stage 2–5. They found that less than 10 percent had problems with hypertension in the daytime, but during the night, 14 percent had systolic hypertension and 24 percent experienced diastolic hypertension. The experts recommended a 24-hour ambulatory blood pressure monitoring to detect hypertension in children with CKD as early as Stage 2 CKD. The researchers also found that PROTEINURIA (protein in the urine) was associated with a failure to have a nocturnal (night-time) dipping in the children's blood pressure, as was a worsening GLOMERULAR FILTRATION RATE.

According to Joseph T. Flynn and colleagues in their 2008 article on children with CKD and hypertension, data from the Chronic Kidney Disease in children (CKiD) Study reveals that factors that have been found to be associated with an elevated blood pressure are African American race, a shorter time frame of having CKD, not taking ANTIHYPERTENSIVE DRUGS, and HYPERKALEMIA (an elevated rate of POTASSIUM in the blood). Of those children who *were* taking antihypertensive medications and had high blood pressure, hypertension correlated with being male, having a shorter duration of CKD, and an absence of taking either an ANGIOTENSIN-CONVERTING ENZYME (ACE) INHIBITOR or an ANGIOTENSIN II RECEPTOR BLOCKER (ARB).

The researchers noted that children with CKD and hypertension often can be undertreated or even untreated. The researchers said, "Our finding that patients receiving ACE inhibitors or ARBs were less likely to have uncontrolled hypertension points the way for development of strategies to improve the treatment of hypertension in children and adolescents with CKD, which in turn offers the potential to reduce cardiovascular risk and possibly ameliorate the progression of CKD in this vulnerable patient population."

*Cardiovascular disease* Children with CKD have an increased risk for cardiovascular disease (CVD). Greenbaum et al. point out that among children, adolescents have a greater risk for cardiovascular disease than younger children and female children have a greater risk than male children for CVD. As with adults, African-American children have an elevated risk for CVD compared to individuals of other races.

*Cholesterol levels* According to the USRDS, among children who have ESRD, African-American children have an elevated risk of a cholesterol level above 170 mg/dl at the beginning of their therapy, while white children have a lowered risk of having a high cholesterol level compared to children in other racial and ethnic groups. Children with secondary glomerulonephritis are the most likely to have elevated lipid levels. In contrast, children with cystic kidney disease, inherited kidney disorders or congenital kidney diseases (*congenital* means that they are born with the disease) have a much lower risk of having hyperlipidemia (an elevated lipid level).

*Vitamin D deficiency* Greenbaum and colleagues reported that although experts have known for many years that many adults with CKD are deficient in vitamin D, the same deficiency has only recently been noted among children and adolescents with kidney disease. In fact, some studies have shown that the majority of the child subjects were deficient in vitamin D. Vitamin D is important in controlling inflammation, decreasing levels of the hormone renin, and managing other important functions, and thus, children with CKD need to be monitored for their vitamin D levels and treated for any identified deficiencies.

The development of vitamin D deficiency is related to multiple factors. Children with chronic kidney disease often have to restrict their milk intake because of the high phosphorus load that is present in milk, yet milk is an important source of vitamin D. Many children with chronic kidney disease spend less time outdoors in the sun, and sun exposure is necessary for normal intrinsic vitamin D production. Finally, the kidneys play an essential role in the activation of vitamin D; with chronic kidney disease, there is impaired activation of vitamin D and subsequent decreased levels of the active forms of vitamin D.

### Lifestyle Issues

Children with CKD or kidney failure and their parents need to consider issues important to all children but they may loom larger for those with children with kidney disease; for example, children with kidney transplants must have their immunizations carefully monitored and must avoid some types of immunizations. Children with kidney failure may have a poor appetite and nutritional considerations are very important in this group.

*Immunizations* Children who have had kidney transplants are receiving immunosuppressive drugs to avoid the rejection of the kidney, and thus, they should not receive any immunizations that contain live viruses, such as the oral polio vaccine, the measles, mumps and rubella (MMR) vaccine, or the varicella (chickenpox) vaccine. If possible, these immunizations should be given before the transplant occurs. Other standard vaccinations are given to children with kidney failure.

*Nutrition and nutritional supplements* Children with advanced kidney disease may have a poor appetite or may even fail to have sufficient energy to eat. They may need to take nutritional supplements and sometimes tube feedings are needed. Children with kidney disease should not be given over-the-counter (OTC) vitamins because these vitamins may be high in phosphorus and other elements that are problematic for the child with kidney disease. Instead, the physician will prescribe vitamins and minerals as needed.

Children with chronic kidney disease need an intake of a certain number of calories per day per pound. (See Table 1.) For example, as seen from the table, an infant in the age range of

## TABLE 1: ENERGY NEEDS FOR CHILDREN WITH KIDNEY DISEASE

| | Age Range | Calories/Pound/Day | |
|---|---|---|---|
| Infant | 0–6 months | 49 | |
| | 7–12 months | 45 | |
| Toddler | 1–3 years | 46 | |
| Child | 4–6 years | 41 | |
| Adolescents | | **Girls** | **Boys** |
| | 11–14 years | 21 | 25 |
| | 15–18 years | 18 | 20 |

Source: National Institute of Diabetes and Digestive and Kidney Diseases. "Nutrition in Children with Chronic Kidney Disease." National Institutes of Health. March 2006.

0–6 months needs 49 calories per pound. Thus, a 10-pound infant needs 490 calories per day. When children reach adolescence, the caloric needs of boys exceed those of girls, as shown in the table.

The protein needs of children with kidney disease also need to be taken into account, depending on whether they are pre-dialysis or are on dialysis, as shown in Table 2; for example, the child age 4–6 years needs 0.5 grams per pound per day if he or she is pre-dialysis; however, the protein need increases to 0.7 grams per pound per day if the child is receiving hemodialysis and is even greater (0.9) if the child is receiving PERITONEAL DIALYSIS. Thus, a 10-year-old child weighing 60 pounds would need 27 grams of protein per day before dialysis. This may mean that the child needs to eat a half sandwich or smaller portions because many foods are high in protein. The same child would need to eat 36 grams of protein per day if on hemodialysis and 48 g per day if on peritoneal dialysis.

*Issues in school* Children with CKD or ESRD may miss many days of school, and the school needs to be advised of the health problem. These absences may make it difficult for the child to keep up at grade level. Children with serious kidney diseases are eligible for special services as needed under the Individuals with Disabilities Education Act (IDEA), the Americans with Disabilities Act, and other state and federal laws. The child may also need to receive tutoring and vocational rehabilitation.

### Children and Kidney Disease Worldwide

Kidney disease is a major problem in the United States as compared to other countries; for example, as far as diagnosed incidence (new cases of kidney disease in a year) and prevalence (all diagnosed cases), children in the United States lead children in many other countries in terms of incidence and they are third in terms of prevalence, according to researchers Bradley A. Warady and Vimal Chadha in their 2007

## TABLE 2: PROTEIN NEEDS FOR CHILDREN WITH KIDNEY DISEASE

| | Age Range | Grams/Pound/Day | | | |
|---|---|---|---|---|---|
| | | **Pre-Dialysis** | **Hemodialysis** | | **Peritoneal Dialysis** |
| Infant | 0–6 months | 1 | 1.2 | | 1.3–1.4 |
| | 7–12 months | 0.71 | 1.1 | | 1.0–1.1 |
| Toddler | 1–3 years | 0.5 | 0.7 | | 0.9 |
| Child | 4–6 years | 0.5 | 0.7 | | 0.9 |
| | 7–10 years | 0.45 | 0.6 | | 0.8 |
| Adolescents | 11–14 years | 0.45 | 0.6 | | 0.8 |
| | | | **Girls** | **Boys** | |
| | 15–18 years | 0.4 | 0.5 | 0.6 | 0.6–0.7 |

Source: National Institute of Diabetes and Digestive and Kidney Diseases. "Nutrition in Children with Chronic Kidney Disease." National Institutes of Health. March 2006.

INCIDENCE AND PREVALENCE OF KIDNEY FAILURE IN CHILDREN WORLDWIDE

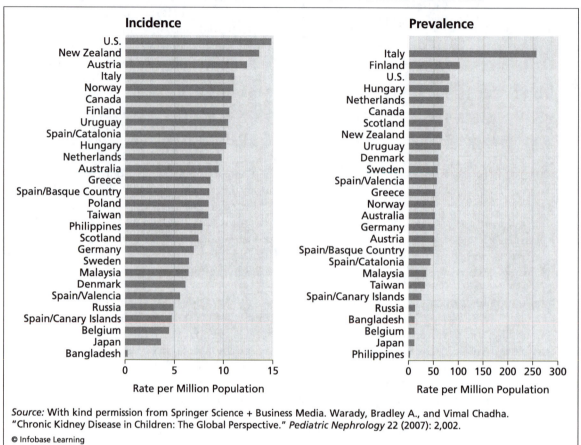

Source: With kind permission from Springer Science + Business Media. Warady, Bradley A., and Vimal Chadha. "Chronic Kidney Disease in Children: The Global Perspective." *Pediatric Nephrology* 22 (2007): 2,002.

© Infobase Learning

article in *Pediatric Nephrology*. As can be seen from the graphs, with regard to the incidence of ESRD, after the United States, the following countries are in the lead: New Zealand, Austria, Italy, and Norway. In terms of prevalence, Italy has the greatest number of cases, followed by Finland, the United States, Hungary, and the Netherlands.

### Parents and Children Dealing with Children's Kidney Disease

Quite understandably, it is very difficult for the parents of children with a serious kidney disease to deal with this problem. They may feel as if it is their fault, even when physicians are certain

that the kidney disease could not have been caused in any way by the parent and they tell the parents this. If it is a genetic disease that the child has, some parents feel guilty about passing on their "bad genes," yet in most cases, the parents did not know they had a genetic risk that could be passed on to their children.

In a meta-analysis of 16 articles on the issues of parents of children with chronic kidney disease, authored by Allison Tong and colleagues for *Pediatrics* in 2008, the analysts found 10 themes and 3 clusters of issues. These clusters included intrapersonal living, which included the parents living with ongoing stress and uncertainty and also maintaining watchfulness despite their own fatigue; interpersonal living, which involved the medicalizing of the parental role, a dependence on and sometimes conflict with medical professionals, as well as disruptions of their relationships with peers; and external issues, such as seeking information, managing the child's medical regimen, following the child's nutritional needs and restrictions, managing financial issues, and balancing the medical care that the child needs with the parents' other domestic responsibilities.

Of the role of parents of children with chronic kidney disease, Tong et al. reported, "They monitor their child's health and recognize symptoms that warrant more specialized assessment and intervention. Many of these are requirements for all parents of children with chronic disease, but the demands on parents of children with kidney disease are greater because of the complexity of the care, especially for children who are on home dialysis." As a result, parents need considerable support from experts as well as families and friends.

Of course it is difficult for children themselves to have chronic kidney disease. They may see that their friends and others their own age do not have the same health and dietary restrictions and limitations. It may not seem fair to them that they have this illness, and parents or guardians can explain that sometimes life does present challenges that seem unfair to most people, but you deal with them as best you can.

See also HUMAN IMMUNODEFICIENCY VIRUS ASSOCIATED NEPHROPATHY (HIVAN); MEDICATIONS THAT CAN HARM THE KIDNEYS.

Cerdá, Jorge, et al. "The Contrasting Characteristics of Acute Kidney Injury in Developed and Developing Countries." *Nature Clinical Practice Nephrology* 4, no. 3 (2008): 138–153.

Chadha, Vimal, and Bradley A. Warady. "Epidemiology of Pediatric Chronic Kidney Disease." *Advances in Chronic Kidney Disease* 12, no. 4 (2005): 345–352.

Dionne, Janis M., Margaret M. Turik, and Robert M. Hurley. "Blood Pressure Abnormalities in Children with Chronic Kidney Disease." *Blood Pressure Monitoring* 13 (2008): 205–209.

Flynn, Joseph T., et al. "Blood Pressure in Children with Chronic Kidney Disease: A Report from the Chronic Kidney Disease in Children Study." *Hypertension* 52 (2008): 631–637.

Greenbaum, Larry A., M.D., Warady, Bradley A., M.D., and Susan L. Furth, M.D. "Current Advances in Chronic Kidney Disease in Children: Growth, Cardiovascular, and Neurocognitive Risk Factors." *Seminars in Nephrology* 29, no. 4 (2009): 425–434.

Johnson, Valerie L., M.D. "Growth Failure in Children with Chronic Kidney Disease." *aakpRENAL LIFE* 26, no. 5 (2010). Available online. URL: http://www.aakp.org/aakp-library/Growth-Failure-Children/. Accessed March 2, 2011.

National Kidney and Urologic Diseases Information Clearinghouse. "Growth Failure in Children with Kidney Disease." National Institute of Diabetes and Digestive and Kidney Diseases. Washington, D.C., 2009.

Patzer, Ludwig. "Nephrotoxicity as a Cause of Acute Kidney Injury in Children." *Pediatric Nephrology* 23 (2008): 2,159–2,173.

Phillips Andreoli, Sharon. "Acute Kidney Injury in Children." *Pediatric Nephrology* 24 (2009): 253–263.

Tong, Allison, et al. "Experiences of Parents Who Have Children with Chronic Kidney Disease: A Systematic Review of Qualitative Studies." *Pediatrics* 121 (2008): 349–360.

United States Renal Data System. *USRDS 2009 Annual Data Report.* Vol. 3: *Reference Tables on ESRD in the United States,* "Chapter Eight: Pediatric ESRD." Bethesda, Md.: National Institutes of Health, National Institute of Diabetes and Digestive and Kidney Diseases, 2009.

Warady, Bradley A., and Vimal Chadha. "Chronic Kidney Disease in Children: The Global Perspective." *Pediatric Nephrology* 22 (2007): 1,999–2,009.

Zappitelli, Michael, M.D. "Epidemiology and Diagnosis of Acute Kidney Injury." *Seminars in Nephrology* 28, no. 5 (2008): 436–446.

**cholesterol**    A general term that refers to both high-density lipoproteins (HDL), otherwise known as "good" cholesterol, and low-density lipoproteins (LDL), often called "bad" cholesterol. (Elevated HDL levels predict decreased risk of cardiovascular complications, whereas elevated LDL cholesterol predicts an increased

**TABLE 1: DESIRABLE CHOLESTEROL LEVELS**

| | |
|---|---|
| Total cholesterol | Less than 200 mg/dL |
| LDL ("bad" cholesterol) | Less than 100 mg/dL* |
| HDL ("good" cholesterol) | 60 mg/dL or higher |
| Triglycerides | Less than 150 mg/dL |

*Optimal for people at risk for heart disease.

Source: Centers for Disease Control and Prevention. *Cholesterol Fact Sheet.* Atlanta, Ga.: CDC, September 2009.

risk.) Total cholesterol refers to the sum of all cholesterol in a person's blood, which includes HDL and LDL cholesterol together as well as triglycerides and other cholesterol components. An excessive buildup of LDL can lead to hyperlipidemia and may also cause atherosclerosis, a buildup of plaque in the arteries. In turn, atherosclerosis can then lead to RENAL ARTERY STENOSIS, a dangerous narrowing of the arteries leading to the kidneys.

Triglycerides are another form of fat that affects cholesterol levels, and triglycerides should be kept to a reasonably low level, as shown in Table 1. Treatment may be needed if triglycerides are borderline high (150–199 mg/dL) or high (200 mg/dL or more). Studies have shown that individuals with CHRONIC KIDNEY DISEASE (CKD) are likely to have low levels of high-density lipoprotein (HDL) and elevated LDL levels, as are individuals with END-STAGE RENAL DISEASE (ESRD), or kidney failure.

According to the Centers for Disease Control and Prevention (CDC), about 16 percent of all adults in the United States have an elevated total cholesterol level: 240 mg/dL and greater. Women in the United States are more likely than men to have high cholesterol levels. Some racial and ethnic groups have a greater risk for high cholesterol levels; for example, according to the CDC, Mexican-American males have the highest percentage of high levels among men (17.7 percent) and white females have the highest percentage of high cholesterol levels among females, or 17.9 percent.

The rate of high cholesterol also varies by age. Men ages 45–54 have the highest rates for males (20.8 percent), and women ages 55–64 years

have the highest rates of high cholesterol for females (30.5 percent).

The percentage of people who have had their cholesterol checked varies from state to state, as shown in Table 2. For example, individuals with the worst records for having their cholesterol checked live in Alaska, Arkansas, Arizona, Idaho, Kansas, Montana, Nevada, New Mexico, Oklahoma, Oregon, Texas, and Utah, while individuals residing in Connecticut, Delaware, and other states and the District of Columbia have the highest rates for having their cholesterol checked. (See Table 2.)

High cholesterol levels are often treated with medications that are known as HMG-CoA inhibitors, referred to as "statins" because statin is part of the generic name of the medication, as with atorvastatin (Lipitor) and lovastatin (Altoprev and Mevacor). Other statin medications are rosuvastatin, fluvastatin, pitavastatin, pravastatin, and simvastatin. High cholesterol is also treated with medications that are called bile acid sequestrants, such as colestipol (Colestid) and colesevelam (Welchol) and other medications in this category of drugs. In addition, fibrates are used to treat high cholesterol, including fenofibrate (Antara,

**TABLE 2: PERCENTAGE OF ADULTS AGED 20 YEARS AND OLDER WHO HAD THEIR CHOLESTEROL CHECKED WITHIN THE PAST FIVE YEARS, 2007**

| | |
|---|---|
| 65.9%–72.3%: Alaska, Arkansas, Arizona, Idaho, Kansas, Montana, Nevada, New Mexico, Oklahoma, Oregon, Texas, Utah | 74.8%–79.4%: Alabama, Florida, Hawaii, Kentucky, Louisiana, Michigan, Minnesota, North Carolina, Pennsylvania, South Carolina, Vermont, West Virginia, Wisconsin |
| 72.7%–74.7%: California, Colorado, Illinois, Indiana, Iowa, Mississippi, Missouri, Nebraska, North Dakota, Ohio, South Dakota, Washington, Wyoming | >79.5%: Connecticut, Delaware, District of Columbia, Georgia, Maine, Maryland, Massachusetts, New Hampshire, New Jersey, New York, Puerto Rico, Rhode Island, Tennessee, Virginia |

Source: Centers for Disease Control and Prevention. *Cholesterol Fact Sheet.* Atlanta, Ga.: CDC, September 2009. Available online. URL: http://www.cdc.gov/dhdsp/data_statistics/fact_sheets/docs/fs_cholesterol.pdf. Accessed March 2, 2011.

Fenoglide, Lipofen, Tricor, and Triglide) as well as gemfibrozil (Lopid). Another medication used to treat high cholesterol is niacin and nicotinic acid (Niaspan). Sometimes cholesterol absorption inhibitors are used to treat high cholesterol levels, such as ezetimibe (Zetia). Omega-3 fatty acids may be used, such as Lovaza.

Combination medications are sometimes used to treat high cholesterol levels, such as Advicor (a combination of niacin and lovastatin), Simcor (a combination of niacin and simvastatin), and Vytorin (a combination of ezetimibe and simvastatin). If the individual has both hypertension and high cholesterol levels, he or she may be treated with Caduet, a combination medication that includes amlodipine and atorvastatin.

Dietary changes are also recommended for people with high cholesterol levels, with fewer carbohydrates and more fruits and vegetables. It is very important for smokers to give up SMOKING in order to get their cholesterol levels down. Regular exercise is also an important feature of gaining mastery over high cholesterol levels.

The desired goal for LDL depends on the cardiovascular risk of the individual. Patients at low risk should have medications added to lower their cholesterol if above 130 mg/dl; those at intermediate risk should use medications to keep their LDL cholesterol below 100 mg/dl, and those at highest risk, such as with a known history of a myocardial infarction (heart attack) may need to target LDL cholesterol to less than 70 mg/dl.

See also HYPERURICEMIA; IgA NEPHROPATHY; MINIMAL CHANGE DISEASE; NEPHROTIC SYNDROME; VITAMIN D.

Food and Drug Administration Office of Women's Health. *Medicines to Help You: Cholesterol.* August 2009.

**chronic kidney disease (CKD)**  The presence of kidney disease that lasts for three or more months, associated with either decreased GLOMERULAR FILTRATION RATE (GFR) or with the leakage of blood proteins through the kidneys into the urine, is termed chronic kidney disease. Chronic kidney disease (CKD) progresses from Stage 1, which is a very mild form of kidney disease, and Stage 2, also a mild stage, to the moderate and increasingly severe phases of Stages 3–5 kidney disease. In Stage 5, the patient is either receiving DIALYSIS or will imminently or now needs a KIDNEY TRANSPLANTATION. At that point, the kidney has failed, a condition also known as END-STAGE RENAL DISEASE (ESRD). Not everyone with chronic kidney disease progresses to the final stage of kidney disease, and many remain at the earlier stages. Some also die of other diseases before their kidneys deteriorate to the level of Stage 5.

Chronic kidney disease is pervasive in the United States, affecting approximately one in every 11 adults, or more than 20 million people in 2009. There are usually no symptoms or only minor symptoms of chronic kidney disease until the disease is advanced and the kidneys are failing, although some people may have signs. As a result, anyone who is at high risk for chronic kidney disease, such as someone with diabetes or HYPERTENSION, should be evaluated regularly for chronic kidney disease. Note that individuals with either diabetes mellitus or hypertension together represent more than two-thirds of all cases of ESRD.

The National Kidney and Urologic Diseases Information Clearinghouse reports that between 1990 and 2000 the numbers of people needing dialysis or transplantation doubled to 380,000. At this rate of increase, if new interventions do not decrease the rate at which people develop ESRD, the numbers of individuals whose kidneys will fail may reach 700,000 by 2010.

### The Glomeruli and Their Filtration of Toxins

The glomeruli are tiny balls of capillaries that lie within the kidney, and blood is filtered through them. (One of these units is a glomerulus.) Each kidney has about 1 million glomeruli actively working to process the blood and protect the body. When the kidney is healthy, an astonishing 170 liters of fluid per day are successfully processed and filtered. Among women who are pregnant, the kidneys process more than 200 liters per day, and the failure to do so could lead to increased complications during the pregnancy.

When the kidneys are not healthy, the glomerular filtration rate (GFR) is much less efficient, and toxins start to build up in the body. While the kidneys have many functions, in general these functions work in parallel with glomerular function. As such, the GFR is an excellent global measure of overall kidney function.

Kidney function is typically assessed by assessing GFR. The most common way to do so is through blood tests that measure the amount of a substance named creatinine in the blood. Laboratories will then use the level of blood creatinine, in conjunction with the patient's age, gender, and race, to calculate the estimated GFR (eGFR). At present, this is the best routinely available measure of actual GFR. In the past, measurement of the blood creatinine level, without performing calculations that take into account the effect of age, gender, and race on the serum creatinine level, was the most common method to assess kidney function. However, this is now known to be less accurate. Other measurements are either not as accurate or are so difficult to perform that they are not available.

Research published in 2009 by Stein Hallan and colleagues in the *Journal of the American Society of Nephrology* revealed that by using two measures, the glomerular filtration rate and the urinary albumin levels, physicians can predict which patients are the most at risk for developing kidney failure.

Table 1 provides a description as well as a glomerular filtration rate for each of the five stages of chronic kidney disease. For example, as can be seen from Table 1, at Stage 1 of chronic kidney disease, there is some kidney damage, but the glomerular filtration rate is either normal or elevated. The GFR steadily decreases with each worsening stage. By Stage 5, the kidney has failed, and the glomerular filtration rate is less than 15 ml min$^{-1}$ (1.73m$^2$)$^{-1}$, and most individuals will require treatment with either dialysis or a renal transplant. The presence of protein in the urine (PROTEINURIA) is another indicator of kidney disease, and two positive proteinuria tests over several weeks indicates that there is persistent protein in the urine and indicates a positive diagnosis of CKD.

### Early Detection of Chronic Kidney Disease with Routine Screening

Many kidney experts believe that more patients with unidentified chronic kidney disease could be detected earlier if more patients were routinely screened for CKD. In a study by Ayub Akbari, M.D., and colleagues and reported in *Archives of Internal Medicine* in 2004, the researchers studied 324 patients ages 65 years and older and had the laboratory analyze their GFRs.

#### TABLE 1: THE STAGES OF CHRONIC KIDNEY DISEASE

| Stage | Description | Glomerular Filtration Rate, ml/min/1.73m |
|---|---|---|
| 1 | Kidney damage with normal or increased glomerular filtration rate, and with an albumin creatinine ratio of ≥ 30 mg | ≥ 90 and albumin creatinine ratio of ≥ 30 mg/g |
| 2 | Kidney damage with mild decreased glomerular filtration rate | 60–89 and albumin creatinine ratio of ≥ 30 mg/g |
| 3 | Moderately decreased glomerular filtration rate | 30–59 |
| 4 | Severely decreased glomerular filtration rate | 15–29 |
| 5 | Kidney failure | < 15 (or on dialysis) |

Source: Adapted from U.S. Renal Data System. *USRDS 2008 Annual Data Report: Atlas of Chronic Kidney Disease and End-Stage Renal Disease in the United States*. Bethesda, Md.: National Institutes of Health, National Institute of Diabetes and Digestive and Kidney Diseases, 2008, Chapter One, p. 27.
Note: The data reported here have been supplied by the United States Renal Data System (USRDS). The interpretation and reporting of these data are the responsibility of the authors and in no way should be seen as an official policy or interpretation of the U.S. government.

Before the study, 22.4 percent of patients with CKD had already been diagnosed; however, the recognition of CKD increased to a much higher rate of 85.1 percent after the intervention. Prior to the study, recognition of CKD was more likely to occur among patients with diabetes and male subjects. (This may be because these individuals were more likely to be screened for kidney disease.) After the study, there were no differences between gender and the presence or absence of diabetes and the detection of CKD.

The researchers said, "These data demonstrate that when serum creatinine concentrations are measured in elderly patients, the laboratory reporting of calculated GFR along with a targeted educational intervention can vastly improve detection of CKD by primary care physicians. In addition, our intervention eliminated the effects of 2 factors, sex and presence or absence of diabetes, both of which previously influenced the detection of CKD."

They also added, "Our findings become increasingly important when the population health implications of CKD are examined. The dialysis population in the United States and Canada is expanding at an alarming rate."

### Risk Factors for CKD

Chronic kidney disease is a major problem, particularly among African Americans and American Indians, as well as among individuals of all other races and ethnicities. Whites have the lowest risk for kidney disease compared to other races and ethnicities, but the risk is still high for whites, and kidney disease is the ninth leading cause of death in the United States.

African Americans have a four times greater risk for chronic kidney disease compared to white Americans, and American Indians have about three times the risk of whites. Further, Hispanic Americans have almost twice the risk of chronic kidney disease than that experienced by non-Hispanic whites. The high rate in African Americans probably reflects a combination of genetic factors, a higher rate of hypertension and diabetes mellitus, increased renal sensitivity to

the effects of hypertension and diabetes mellitus, and, in some cases, decreased access to medical care. It may also include other factors as yet unknown. However, identifying the reasons for the high rate of kidney disease among individuals of some races and ethnicities is important, so that they can be resolved and the health consequences that are associated with CKD and/or ESRD minimized or avoided.

In one interesting study by Thomas A. LaVeist and colleagues, published in the *Journal of General Internal Medicine* in 2009, the researchers looked at the prevalence of diabetes based on race, which is significant in that diabetes is the primary cause of kidney failure. The researchers found that when African Americans and whites resided in similar risk environments, their health outcomes were also more similar. In their study, blacks and whites lived in the same urban and low-income community. It is unknown if the same finding is true for individuals with kidney disease but this provocative finding gives pause to the possibility that it may be true.

Elderly individuals also have an elevated risk for the development of chronic kidney disease, as do other individuals with hypertension and diabetes. Other diseases that may lead to the development of chronic kidney disease are ALPORT SYNDROME, GLOMERULONEPHRITIS, KIDNEY STONES and recurring kidney infections (PYELONEPHRITIS), POLYCYSTIC KIDNEY DISEASE, and REFLUX NEPHROPATHY.

SMOKING, a modifiable risk factor, is another risk factor for the development of chronic kidney disease.

In addition, inherited kidney diseases may lead to CKD, as may disease of the kidney tissue, vascular (blood vessel) disease, chronic obstruction of the bladder, and the poorly controlled use of some medications. For example, lithium, a medication that is used to treat bipolar disorder (also known as manic depression), can be toxic to the kidneys. In addition, the use of some illegal drugs may damage the kidneys, such as the abuse of or dependence on heroin.

In a study published in 2007 in *Archives of Internal Medicine* by Heejung Bang and colleagues, the researchers described their prediction model for the development of chronic kidney disease, which they called SCreening for Occult REnal Disease (SCORED). Based on their analysis of more than 8,500 individuals nationwide in the United States, the researchers found that the following factors increased the individual's risk for the development of chronic kidney disease:

- anemia
- female sex
- hypertension
- diabetes
- peripheral vascular disease
- a history of cardiovascular disease
- a history of congestive heart failure
- the presence of proteinuria

### Signs and Symptoms of CKD

When signs and symptoms of chronic kidney disease are present (which often they are not, in the early stages of the disease), they may include the following:

- itching and dry skin
- swollen feet and ankles
- persistent fatigue
- SLEEP PROBLEMS
- puffiness around the eyes, particularly in the morning
- poor appetite
- the need to urinate more frequently, especially at night
- difficult to control hypertension

Later symptoms that may occur after the disease progresses further may include the following:

- confusion and decreased alertness
- nausea and vomiting, particularly in the morning

- decreased sensation in the hands and feet
- easy bruising or bleeding
- decreased urinary output
- seizures
- white crystals either in or on the skin (uremic frost)

### Considering Diabetic Nephropathy

It is essential for people who have diabetes to maintain as close to normal a level of blood sugar as possible, both to avoid chronic kidney disease and to limit its progression in those who have already developed it.

In a study by Lori D. Bash and colleagues and published in the *Archives of Internal Medicine* in 2008, the researchers studied 1,871 adults with DIABETES MELLITUS (DM) who were followed up for 11 years in the Atherosclerosis Risk in Communities (ARIC) study. The researchers found that hyperglycemia (excessive levels of blood glucose) was an important risk factor for the development of diabetic nephropathy. In some cases, the patient also had diabetic retinopathy (a serious eye disease that is common among people with diabetes) or diabetic nephropathy with albuminuria (albumin in the urine, a measure of disease). In other cases, the chronic kidney disease was in a less specific form.

The researchers said:

> In this population-based setting, approximately one-third of CKD incidence occurred in the presence of both albuminuria and retinopathy and one-third occurred in the absence of both conditions. These data suggest that glycemia control is an important modifiable risk factor in the pathology of kidney disease in individuals with DM [diabetes mellitus], both in the presence and absence of other microvascular damage. These results also suggest that urinary albumin screening alone may not be adequate for CKD detection in individuals with type 2 DM.

In another study of patients with diabetes in England, reported in *Diabetic Medicine* in 2007, researchers J. P. New and colleagues found that

31 percent of more than 5,000 diabetic patients had clinically significant CKD, rates that were similar to what studies have found in the United States, according to the researchers. However, the researchers also found that the currently used measures of renal function were inadequate and that 63 percent of patients with diabetes with a significant reduction in their kidney function had been recorded as having normal albumin levels in the urine. The researchers recommended using an estimated glomerular filtration rate (eGFR) as a superior way to ascertain the presence of kidney disease. (Many laboratories in the United States use the eGFR.)

### Lower Rates of CKD in Europeans

In a study by Hallan et al. published in the *Journal of the American Society of Nephrology* in 2006, Hallan and his colleagues reported that the incidence (new cases) of ESRD is three times higher in the United States than in Europe. The researchers sought to find reasons for this discrepancy by analyzing data from more than 65,000 adults in Norway who were diagnosed with chronic kidney disease.

The researchers found a similar prevalence (the total number of people in the general population with the disease, including old and new cases) of chronic kidney disease in the Norwegian patients as compared to American patients; however, they also found that the patients in the United States were referred significantly later in the course of their disease to nephrologists and also that the Americans also had a higher prevalence of having both diabetes and OBESITY. The researchers further determined that the lower rate of progression to ESRD in the Norwegian patients with chronic kidney disease caused them to be at a lower risk than the U.S. patients.

### Treatment of CKD and Hyperparathyroidism with Vitamin D (Calcitriol)

Patients with CKD need their underlying diseases to be under as effective control as possible, whether these diseases are diabetes, hypertension, ANEMIA, or other disorders. In addition,

other treatments may be recommended. For example, according to Csaba P. Kovesdy, M.D., and colleagues in their 2008 report in the *Archives of Internal Medicine*, treatment of the development of secondary HYPERPARATHYROID-ISM (the excessive production of parathyroid hormone, produced by the parathyroid glands which are embedded in the thyroid gland) with vitamin D (calcitriol) can be effective at increasing the survival of patients with CKD prior to dialysis. Secondary hyperparathyroidism is a common problem among individuals with chronic kidney disease.

In this study of 520 male military veterans, 258 of the subjects received treatment with calcitriol for about two years, during which time they were followed. The researchers said:

> It is remarkable that the beneficial outcomes seen in patients treated with calcitriol in our study were present despite the following characteristics that should have worsened their prognosis compared with the patients who were not treated with this agent: older age, lower diastolic blood pressure (associated with higher mortality in CKD), higher PTH [parathyroid hormone] level (associated with higher mortality in patients receiving dialysis), lower eGFR (associated with higher mortality in CKD), and a rise in serum phosphorus level (associated with higher mortality in dialysis patients and possibly in patients with CKD).

### Worsening Levels of Disease with Progressive Stages of CKD

With worsening kidney disease, other chronic health problems become more common. As can be seen from the end of Table 2, based on data from the National Health and Nutrition Examination Survey (NHANES), about 19.8 percent of all individuals in Stage 1 have diabetes, but by Stages 4–5 of chronic kidney disease, 36.0 percent have developed diabetes. The proportion of patients with hypertension also increases with worsening kidney function: 35.8 percent of the subjects had hypertension at Stage 1, while the majority (84.1 percent) had hypertension at Stage 5. Another health problem that is more

**TABLE 2: PREVALENCE OF COMORBIDITIES IN THE NHANES POPULATION (PERCENT) NHANES 1999–2006, PARTICIPANTS AGES 20 AND OLDER**

| | Diabetes | Hyper-tension | Cardio-vascular Disease | Obesity | Smoking |
|---|---|---|---|---|---|
| **Age 20–39** | | | | | |
| Stage 1 | 8.4 | 16.2 | 0.2 | 36.3 | 36.3 |
| Stage 2 | 9.0 | 19.6 | 2.3 | 36.9 | 44.5 |
| Stage 3 | 10.6 | 23.0 | 7.6 | 20.3 | 18.1 |
| Stage 4–5 | 0.0 | 67.0 | 16.8 | 51.9 | 32.6 |
| Non-CKD | 1.3 | 9.9 | 1.0 | 30.3 | 27.3 |
| **Age 40–59** | | | | | |
| Stage 1 | 25.6 | 46.2 | 7.6 | 32.5 | 45.1 |
| Stage 2 | 25.8 | 48.8 | 10.8 | 24.3 | 55.8 |
| Stage 3 | 13.8 | 49.9 | 15.7 | 18.9 | 40.5 |
| Stage 4–5 | 39.5 | 96.7 | 45.3 | 37.1 | 50.3 |
| Non-CKD | 5.6 | 27.3 | 6.0 | 25.3 | 34.8 |
| **Age 60+** | | | | | |
| Stage 1 | 36.2 | 62.9 | 28.3 | 28.3 | 34.6 |
| Stage 2 | 24.1 | 57.8 | 30.6 | 14.9 | 35.8 |
| Stage 3 | 19.2 | 63.9 | 36.6 | 9.0 | 32.8 |
| Stage 4–5 | 39.8 | 83.6 | 72.3 | 15.2 | 36.9 |
| Non-CKD | 11.6 | 48.7 | 18.5 | 13.0 | 31.9 |
| **Male** | | | | | |
| Stage 1 | 26.8 | 38.3 | 10.8 | 40.1 | 44.0 |
| Stage 2 | 27.1 | 49.7 | 23.0 | 21.1 | 48.3 |
| Stage 3 | 18.9 | 59.1 | 38.0 | 11.4 | 29.8 |
| Stage 4–5 | 33.7 | 83.3 | 59.8 | 25.1 | 32.1 |
| Non-CKD | 4.6 | 22.6 | 6.5 | 29.0 | 28.7 |
| **Female** | | | | | |
| Stage 1 | 14.9 | 34.1 | 5.5 | 28.9 | 36.6 |
| Stage 2 | 17.7 | 46.8 | 14.3 | 22.9 | 41.4 |
| Stage 3 | 17.2 | 60.3 | 27.4 | 11.3 | 36.7 |
| Stage 4–5 | 38.1 | 84.8 | 65.6 | 19.3 | 44.4 |
| Non-CKD | 4.9 | 24.0 | 5.2 | 22.0 | 33.4 |
| **Non-Hispanic white** | | | | | |
| Stage 1 | 19.0 | 35.3 | 9.6 | 38.1 | 35.3 |
| Stage 2 | 18.7 | 46.0 | 20.0 | 21.7 | 43.3 |
| Stage 3 | 15.8 | 58.6 | 31.7 | 11.2 | 33.9 |
| Stage 4–5 | 34.2 | 81.4 | 68.8 | 22.1 | 33.3 |
| Non-CKD | 4.3 | 24.1 | 6.4 | 26.0 | 30.3 |
| **Non-Hispanic African American** | | | | | |
| Stage 1 | 23.6 | 46.7 | 10.4 | 31.0 | 50.5 |
| Stage 2 | 36.2 | 62.3 | 19.6 | 26.9 | 58.4 |
| Stage 3 | 34.6 | 81.1 | 36.3 | 14.6 | 45.0 |
| Stage 4–5 | 34.5 | 92.1 | 51.7 | 27.7 | 36.0 |
| Non-CKD | 6.5 | 29.5 | 5.3 | 26.8 | 41.9 |
| **Other race** | | | | | |
| Stage 1 | 18.7 | 30.2 | 3.0 | 27.9 | 39.4 |
| Stage 2 | 28.7 | 48.8 | 10.1 | 20.6 | 41.6 |
| Stage 3 | 26.6 | 55.6 | 22.9 | 9.8 | 26.8 |
| Stage 4–5 | 46.8 | 84.2 | 52.4 | 13.5 | 66.8 |
| Non-CKD | 5.7 | 16.0 | 3.7 | 22.3 | 27.5 |
| **All** | | | | | |
| Stage 1 | 19.8 | 35.8 | 7.7 | 33.5 | 39.5 |
| Stage 2 | 22.2 | 48.1 | 18.4 | 22.1 | 44.7 |
| Stage 3 | 17.8 | 59.9 | 31.4 | 11.4 | 34.1 |
| Stage 4–5 | 36.0 | 84.1 | 62.8 | 22.1 | 38.7 |
| Non-CKD | 4.7 | 23.3 | 5.8 | 25.4 | 31.1 |

Source: Adapted from U.S. Renal Data System. *USRDS 2008 Annual Data Report: Atlas of Chronic Kidney Disease and End-Stage Renal Disease in the United States.* Bethesda, Md.: National Institutes of Health, National Institute of Diabetes and Digestive and Kidney Diseases, 2008, Chapter One, p. 30.

Note: The data reported here have been supplied by the United States Renal Data System (USRDS). The interpretation and reporting of these data are the responsibility of the authors and in no way should be seen as an official policy or interpretation of the U.S. government.

common with decreased kidney function is cardiovascular disease. In particular, patients with CKD have higher risk of cardiac disease and stroke than people with normal kidney function, and this effect persists even after taking into account the hypertension and diabetes that they may have.

Table 2 also compares individuals in terms of their age, gender, race, and ethnicity in the presence of chronic kidney disease at various stages.

### Clinical and Biochemical Abnormalities in CKD

As individuals develop worsening chronic kidney disease, their laboratory levels of potassium, uric acid, calcium, phosphorus, bicarbonate, and parathyroid hormone become significantly more abnormal as well. In addition, their blood pressure and their levels of elevated triglycerides, reduced high density lipoproteins (HDL), their

**TABLE 3: AWARENESS AND CONTROL OF HYPERTENSION AND HYPERLIPIDEMIA, BY CKD STAGE (PERCENT)**

|  | Non-CKD | CKD Stage 1–2 | CKD stage 3–4 |
|---|---|---|---|
| **Hypertension control among hypertensive patients** | | | |
| Unaware of need for | 29 | 40 | 25 |
| Aware, but not treated | 11 | 13 | 7 |
| Aware, treated, uncontrolled | 24 | 36 | 48 |
| Aware, treated, controlled | 36 | 11 | 20 |
| **Control of hyperlipedemia among hyperlipedemic patients** | | | |
| Unaware of need for | 34 | 36 | 44 |
| Aware, but not treated | 9 | 7 | 8 |
| Aware, treated, uncontrolled | 22 | 28 | 30 |
| Aware, treated, controlled | 35 | 29 | 18 |

Source: Adapted from U.S. Renal Data System. *USRDS 2008 Annual Data Report: Atlas of Chronic Kidney Disease and End-Stage Renal Disease in the United States.* Bethesda, Md.: National Institutes of Health, National Institute of Diabetes and Digestive and Kidney Diseases, 2008, Chapter One, p. 34.
Note: The data reported here have been supplied by the United States Renal Data System (USRDS). The interpretation and reporting of these data are the responsibility of the authors and in no way should be seen as an official policy or interpretation of the U.S. government.

elevated fasting glucose, and their elevated waist circumference also tend to deviate much further from the norm than in the early stages of the disease. For example, at Stage 1, only 5.9 percent had abnormal levels of potassium. By Stage 3, that percentage had increased to 20.7 percent and then further increased to more than half (52.0 percent) at Stages 4 and 5. Levels of uric acid, calcium, and phosphorus were also increasingly elevated at each successively higher level of chronic kidney disease.

### Patients' Lack of Awareness of the Need to Control Hypertension and Hyperlipidemia

Keeping their blood pressure and high cholesterol levels under good control is essential to avoid worsening kidney disease among patients with chronic kidney disease, yet many people with chronic kidney disease are unaware of this need, as illustrated in Table 3. As can be seen from the table, 40 percent of patients with chronic kidney disease and hypertension in Stages 1 and 2 are unaware of the importance of getting their high blood pressure under control. Only 11 percent of the subjects in this category were aware of the need for control, had their hypertension treated, and had their hypertension under control.

Similarly, 36 percent of individuals with stage 1 or stage 2 CKD with hyperlipidemia were unaware of the need to control their hyperlipidemia. Even more disturbingly, 44 percent of patients in the advanced stages of CKD Stage 3–4 were *still* unaware of the importance of controlling their cholesterol problems. It is unclear if they failed to listen to their physicians, if the physicians did not stress the importance to them sufficiently, or if other causes are at work.

See also CHILDREN AND KIDNEY DISEASE; CHOLESTEROL; DIABETIC NEPHROPATHY; ELDERLY AND CHRONIC KIDNEY DISEASE; MEDICATIONS THAT CAN HARM THE KIDNEYS; NEPHROLOGISTS.

Akbari, Ayub, M.D., et al. "Detection of Chronic Kidney Disease with Laboratory Reporting of Estimated Glomerular Filtration Rate and an Educational Program." *Archives of Internal Medicine* 164 (2004): 1,788–1,792.

Bang, Heejung, et al. "SCreening for Occult Renal Disease (SCORED): A Simple Prediction Model for Chronic Kidney Disease." *Archives of Internal Medicine* 167 (February 26, 2007): 374–381.

Bash, Lori D., et al. "Poor Glycemic Control in Diabetes and the Risk of Incident Chronic Kidney Disease Even in the Absence of Albuminuria and Retinopathy: Atherosclerosis Risk in Communities

(ARIC) Study." *Archives of Internal Medicine* 168, no. 22 (December 8/22, 2008): 2,440–2,447.

Coresh, Josef, M.D., et al. "Prevalence of Chronic Kidney Disease in the United States." *Journal of the American Medical Association* 298, no. 17 (2007): 2,038–2,047.

Hallan, Stein I., et al. "International Comparison of the Relationship of Chronic Kidney Disease Prevalence and ESRD Risk." *Journal of the American Society of Nephrology* 17, no. 8 (2006): 2,275–2,284.

Kovesdy, Csaba P., M.D., et al. "Association of Activated Vitamin D Treatment and Mortality in Chronic Kidney Disease." *Archives of Internal Medicine* 168, no. 4 (February 25, 2008): 397–403.

LaVeist, Thomas A., et al. "Environmental and Socio-Economic Factors as Contributors to Racial Disparities in Diabetes Prevalence." *Journal of General Internal Medicine* 24, no. 10 (2009): 1,144–1,148.

Levin, Adeera, M.D., et al. "Guidelines for the Management of Chronic Kidney Disease." *Canadian Medical Association Journal* 179, no. 11 (November 18, 2008): 1,154–1,162.

New, J. P., et al. "Assessing the Prevalence, Monitoring and Management of Chronic Kidney Disease in Patients with Diabetes Compared with Those without Diabetes in General Practice." *Diabetic Medicine* 24 (2007): 364–369.

Saydah, S., et al. "Prevalence of Chronic Kidney Disease and Associated Risk Factors—United States, 1999–2004." *Morbidity & Mortality Weekly Report* 56 (2007): 161–165.

**chronic kidney disease–mineral bone disorder (CKD-MBD)**  Harm to the bones that is caused by malfunction of the kidneys, a common complication of individuals with CHRONIC KIDNEY DISEASE (CKD) and found among the majority of patients receiving DIALYSIS. This disorder was formerly known as renal osteodystrophy.

There are four main types of bone disease seen in CKD-MBD, and many patients can have more than one type. The latter is called mixed uremic osteodystrophy. The different types include:

1. osteitis fibrosa cystica, which is generally due to secondary hyperparathyroidism

2. adynamic bone disease, in which bone turnover is low, and generally results from excessive suppression of the parathyroid glands

3. osteomalacia, a problem which is relatively uncommon at present and previously was due primarily to bone aluminum deposition resulting from the use of aluminum-containing medicines as phosphate binders

4. mixed uremic osteodystrophy, which has elements of both high and low bone turnover

Another type, which is different from the other types of CKD-MBD, presents as bone cysts that result from beta2-microglobulin–associated amyloid deposits; this is seen almost exclusively in patients who are on hemodialysis for prolonged periods.

According to the organization Kidney Disease Improving Global Outcome (KDIGO), CKD-MBD is characterized by one or more of the following signs:

- abnormal metabolism of CALCIUM, PHOSPHORUS, parathyroid hormone, and/or VITAMIN D
- abnormalities in bone turnover, mineralization, volume, strength, and other factors
- calcification of vascular tissue or other soft tissue

According to Priscilla P. How and colleagues in their 2008 article for the *Journal of Pharmacy Practice*, chronic kidney disease–mineral bone disorder (CKD-MBD) is caused by a reduction in the activation of Vitamin D and an impeded excretion of phosphorus in association with abnormal levels of parathyroid hormone (PTH).

Some individuals with CKD may have a secondary HYPERPARATHYROIDISM, which leads to hormonal changes and in turn to mineral and bone disorders. CKD-MBD is important to identify and treat, because it is also a risk factor for the development of CARDIOVASCULAR DISEASE. Many of the medications that are used to treat osteoporosis in adults, such as BISPHOSPHONATES, need to be avoided in patients diagnosed with chronic kidney disease. Children with kidney failure may develop growth failure because their level of blood phosphorus becomes high and interferes with the formation of healthy bone and growth.

### Symptoms and Diagnostic Path

There are often few or no symptoms of CKD-MBD, although bone and joint pain may be present. The disorder is diagnosed with a blood test that measures the levels of calcium, phosphorus, parathyroid hormone, and calcitriol. In some cases, an elevated level of alkaline phosphatase in the blood can point to CKD-MBD. However, as reported, it is important to recognize that there are other causes of alkaline phosphatase, including the liver. A bone biopsy may also be done to determine the bone density. Patients who are in CKD Stages 3–5 and not receiving dialysis should be checked for HYPERPHOSPHATE-MIA, HYPOCALCEMIA and a deficiency of vitamin D as well as for elevated levels of parathyroid hormone.

### Treatment Options and Outlook

The treatment depends on the cause of the disease. If overactive parathyroid glands are producing too much parathyroid hormone, then the patient is treated with dietary changes, medication, and sometimes with dialysis. If the levels remain high despite this treatment, then the parathyroid glands (which are embedded in the thyroid gland) may need to be surgically removed.

If the individual has hyperphosphatemia, then the goal is to lower the blood levels of phosphorus while maintaining steady levels of calcium.

In the case of calcitriol, if the blood levels are too low, the patient can take an oral dose of synthetic calcitriol and calcium supplements as needed. In addition, if the blood levels of parathyroid hormone are markedly elevated and continue to rise, then treatment with calcitriol or other active vitamin D analogues is recommended.

Careful monitoring of PTH levels during treatment is important. High levels of PTH can be associated with causing CKD-MBD, specifically causing a high turnover form. On the other hand, excessive lowering of the PTH level can lead to other types of CKD-MBD, particularly adynamic bone disease.

Dietary changes to reduce the dietary levels of phosphorus are another form of treatment for CKD-MBD. Most foods contain phosphorus but phosphorus levels are particularly high in some foods, such as milk, cheese, peas, nuts, peanut butter, and dried beans. The patient is also advised to limit the intake of cocoa, cola drinks, and other dark soft drinks as well as beer. Sometimes medications are given to increase the binding of phosphorus in the bowel, including such over-the-counter (OTC) drugs as calcium carbonate (available in many brands) or prescribed drugs such as sevelamer bicarbonate (Renvelal) or lanthanum carbonate (Fosrenol).

Exercise can improve bone strength in some patients but it is important to consult with the physician to determine what types of exercise are recommended and how often they should be performed.

### Risk Factors and Preventive Measures

According to the National Institute for Diabetes and Digestive and Kidney Diseases (NIDDK), about 90 percent of all dialysis patients have CKD-MBD. Patients with CKD are also at risk for this disorder. If the disorder is identified, it should be treated. According to the KDIGO, patients with CKD should have their blood levels of calcium, phosphorus, parathyroid hormone, and alkaline phosphatase measured starting at Stage 3 of the five stages of chronic kidney disease. As abnormalities worsen, the frequency of the monitoring should increase accordingly.

Patients with CKD-MBD should exercise as recommended by their physicians. SMOKING should be avoided.

See also CHILDREN AND KIDNEY DISEASE; HEMO-DIALYSIS; KIDNEY TRANSPLANTATION; PERITONEAL DIALYSIS.

Cibulka, R., and J. Racek. "Metabolic Disorders in Patients with Chronic Kidney Failure." *Physiological Research* 56 (2007): 697–705.

How, Priscilla P., Darius L. Mason, and Alan H. Lau. "Current Approaches in the Treatment of Chronic Kidney Disease Mineral and Bone Disorder." *Journal of Pharmacy Practice* 21, no. 3 (2008): 196–213.

Kidney Disease Improving Global Outcomes (KDIGO). *Best Practices in CKD-MBD: A Focus on Phosphorus.* 2009. Available online. URL: http://www.kidney. org/professionals/tools/pdf/BestPracticesInCKD_ MBD.pdf. Accessed February 13, 2010.

Martin, Kevin J., and Esther A. González. "Metabolic Bone Disease in Chronic Kidney Disease." *Journal of the American Society of Nephrology* 18 (2007): 875–885.

Moe, Sharon M., and Tilman Drueke. "Improving Global Outcomes in Mineral and Bone Disorders." *Clinical Journal of the American Society of Nephrology* 3 (2008): S127–S130.

**common medical tests and procedures**  Key laboratory tests, imaging procedures, and other procedures that are the most useful in detecting the presence of serious kidney disease, as well as its improvement or worsening, are often ordered by physicians. Often laboratory screens of kidney disease are ordered as part of a panel of laboratory tests by physicians, and thus one visit to the phlebotomist (blood test taker) can yield sufficient blood to test for kidney function, glucose levels (to check for DIABETES MELLITUS), and other major functions. If the chemistry panel yields abnormal results, then further testing can be performed.

### Vital Signs

One of the most common medical tests is the measurement of blood pressure, a routine test that is nearly always performed at each patient encounter. A normal blood pressure is less than 120/80. People with known kidney disease should seek to keep their blood pressure below 130/80.

Elevated blood pressure may indicate undiagnosed kidney disease. If the individual has already been diagnosed with HYPERTENSION, it is important to try to keep the blood pressure as close to normal as possible. If a blood pressure check reveals a high blood pressure, then the patient will need to take action to bring the blood pressure down, through medication and through lifestyle advice, such as using a low salt diet, losing weight if overweight, and stopping SMOKING if a smoker.

The temperature and pulse are also taken during nearly every patient encounter. An elevated pulse may go along with an elevated blood pressure, although it is possible to have a normal blood pressure and a heightened pulse. A fever may indicate the presence of an INFECTION, such as CYSTITIS or PYELONEPHRITIS, requiring ANTIBIOTICS. Of course fever could indicate infection with a virus.

### Laboratory Tests of Blood and Urine

Common tests of the blood and urine can detect indicators of kidney disease, enabling both diagnosis and treatment, often well before serious damage occurs to the kidneys.

***Blood tests***  A complete blood count (CBC) is often taken, and this test can show if there are insufficient red blood cells, which may occur when the kidneys fail to make erythropoietin, a hormone controlling production of red blood cells. Tests of creatinine or blood urea nitrogen (BUN) help determine whether waste products are being eliminated. If they are not, this may indicate a kidney problem. Normal blood levels of creatinine are 0.5–1.3 mg/dl and for BUN are 20 mg/dL or less. Elevated creatinine or BUN levels may indicate kidney disease, dehydration, or heart failure.

A formerly common test for kidney function is creatinine clearance performed using a 24-hour urine collection. More recently, the estimated GLOMERULAR FILTRATION RATE (eGFR) is used to estimate the kidney function level based on the person's serum creatinine, by gender, race and age. This is a blood test that requires no injection or urine collection and provides the same important data.

Physicians may also order a test for Cystatin C, which is a blood test to help detect and monitor kidney function in individuals with extreme OBESITY, those with liver cirrhosis, and patients with malnourishment. The blood may also be tested for levels of calcium and parathyroid hormone. Abnormal levels may indicate kidney disease and should be followed up with further testing. Levels of albumin in the blood may also be tested for the possibility of either NEPHRITIC SYNDROME or NEPHROTIC SYNDROME, two serious kidney disorders. Electrolyte levels in the blood may also be tested for imbalances, which could indicate kidney dysfunction. Testing for alkaline phosphatase can indicate whether the patient has chronic kidney failure.

Other blood tests may include tests for iron levels, such as the serum ferritin test. An iron deficiency may indicate a lowered level of red blood cells and the presence of kidney disease.

**Urine tests** Physicians can order screens of the urine for blood in the urine (hematuria) or for the presence of white blood cells that indicate infection. If the urine is cultured and it is infected, the culture can show the type of bacteria, and thus the doctor will know which medication is most effective in killing this form of bacterium. Blood in the urine may indicate infection or it may indicate the presence of a KIDNEY STONE, bladder stone, cancer in the kidneys, ureter, or bladder, or trauma to the urinary tract system.

Doctors also test for protein in the urine (PRO-TEINURIA), which indicates kidney disease. Tests can also check for albumin in the urine (albuminuria). Albumin is a form of protein and may indicate kidney disease.

The urine may also be checked for the sediment level. The urine is spun in a centrifuge and the sediment in the bottom is examined microscopically for bacteria, white blood cells, red blood cells, yeast, and crystals that may indicate the development of kidney stones.

Sometimes a 24-hour screen of the urine can be used to check kidney function over the course of a day. It is also sometimes used subsequent to the finding of kidney stones to help the physician determine the type of stones that are present, which may indicate the need to change the diet. Some doctors do not order such a screen because the broad majority of kidney stones are comprised of calcium or oxalate.

*Imaging Tests*

Nephrologists and other physicians may order imaging tests to determine the cause of pain or other symptoms of kidney disease. The three primary types of imaging tests are computerized tomography (CT) scans, magnetic resonance imaging (MRI) tests, and ultrasound. Sometimes a nuclear scan is also needed. The results of imaging tests are interpreted by a radiologist, who provides a diagnosis and related information to the prescribing physician.

***Computerized tomography scans and magnetic resonance imaging scans*** Renal imaging with a CT scan or an MRI can show kidney enlargements and other types of kidney damage. These tests can show the presence of tumors, kidney stones, and other solid masses. The Food and Drug Administration (FDA) advises that patients with moderate to END-STAGE RENAL DISEASE (ESRD) should avoid imaging studies that use contrast agents (dyes) that contain gadolinium, because some patients with kidney disease who receive gadolinium have an increased risk of developing nephrogenic systemic fibrosis, a potentially fatal disease. If gadolinium must be used for some good reason, then the patient may need to receive DIALYSIS after a magnetic resonance imaging (MRI) scan or after a magnetic resonance angiography (MRA) scan.

***Positron emission tomography (PET) scan*** A positron emission tomography (PET) scan shows the rate at which the tissues use an artificial form of glucose; for example, cancer cells use increased amounts of glucose for nutrition, and a PET scan may be helpful in selected cases at determining whether cancer involving the kidneys is present.

***Radioactive nuclear scans*** Sometimes a renal scan is performed using the injection of a radioisotope that is injected into the vein and goes into the bloodstream. This scan takes from 30 minutes to an hour and provides images of the kidneys and their functioning. This scan shows the position, size, and shape of the kidneys. It may be used for patients who are allergic to the contrast dye that is used in the intravenous pyelogram. Patients are asked to drink extra fluids before the examination to increase the volume of urine.

An abnormal result on this test may indicate chronic kidney disease or ACUTE KIDNEY INJURY. It may also indicate abnormalities in blood flow to the kidneys, hydronephrosis (blockage of the urine exit from one or both kidneys), and other conditions.

The renal perfusion scintiscan is another nuclear medicine test that is specific to the kidneys and also uses a radioactive tracer to provide information about the kidneys. The bladder fills up with urine during the course of the test and may feel uncomfortable for the patient who feels urgency to urinate. Abnormal results with this test may indicate renal artery stenosis.

*Renal ultrasounds*   A renal ultrasound uses ultrasonic waves to image the kidneys and bladder. It can show the presence of kidney stones and masses as well as changes in the kidneys themselves. This test also shows any scarring of the kidney and detects whether there is a blockage of the urine flow anywhere in the kidneys, the ureters (small tubes leading to the bladder), and the bladder. The renal scan may be performed prior to a KIDNEY BIOPSY. It can also show if the kidneys are large, as may occur with AMYLOIDOSIS, diabetes mellitus, the HUMAN IMMUNODEFICIENCY VIRUS ASSOCIATED NEPHROPATHY (HIVAN), or MYELOMA KIDNEY.

### Other Tests

Other tests may be ordered by the physician if he or she suspects particular diseases; for example, a kidney biopsy may be ordered if glomerulonephritis is suspected or in cases when the cause of kidney damage is unknown.

*Kidney biopsy*   A kidney biopsy involves removing a sample of tissue from the kidney that is about $\frac{1}{10}$ of an inch in diameter and is from $\frac{1}{2}$ to $\frac{3}{4}$ inch in length, removed through a special needle. This is an invasive test and is reserved for conditions in which either the correct diagnosis is unknown or treatment regimens are being considered with the potential for significant toxicity. A kidney biopsy is evaluated by a pathologist, who determines how advanced any existing cancer is, a process also known as staging. Imaging tests used prior to the kidney biopsy indicate whether a tumor is likely to be present. A kidney biopsy is also used to diagnose ALPORT SYNDROME, GOODPASTURE SYNDROME, IgA NEPHROPATHY, LUPUS NEPHRITIS, MEMBRANOUS NEPHROPATHY, MINIMAL CHANGE DISEASE, and nephrotic syndrome.

*Intravenous pyelogram (IVP)*   Used less frequently in the United States than in past years, the intravenous pyelogram (IVP) is a test that uses special dye known as contrast dye which is injected into the vein to image the kidneys. It can detect kidney stones and other abnormalities; however, many doctors prefer to use noninvasive tests, such as imaging of the kidneys with ultrasound. The contrast dye used for an IVP can itself cause kidney damage, limiting the conditions in which this imaging procedure is used. The IVP is not performed if there is already at least some kidney failure because the dye could be harmful to patients with kidney failure. Some patients are allergic to the contrast dye used in the IVP.

*Cystoscopy*   A CYSTOSCOPY, or an internal examination of the bladder with a special scope, may indicate damage, cancer, or infection. Of course, it may also indicate a healthy bladder.

If infections of the bladder are untreated, they may rise into the kidneys and infect them as well.

See also KIDNEYS AND KIDNEY DISEASE.

**complications of common kidney diseases**   A variety of complications may occur with kidney diseases, such as with PYELONEPHRITIS (kidney infection), KIDNEY STONES, and other kidney diseases and disorders, particularly when they are undiagnosed and/or untreated. For example, untreated kidney stones are extremely painful and often also lead to a kidney infection. The individual may pass the stone but damage could be caused if medical treatment is not received. With regard to another common complication, the risk for metabolic disorders is increased with CHRONIC KIDNEY DISEASE (CKD), and it is particularly elevated among those with kidney failure, according to Czech physicians R. Cibulka and J. Racek in their article for *Physiological Research* in 2007. Other common complications that may occur with chronic kidney disease are ANEMIA, deficiencies of VITAMIN D, and the development of secondary HYPERPARATHYROIDISM. Bone abnormalities and fractures may also occur as complications of CKD, especially among patients who are in the later stages of CKD or those who are receiving dialysis. NEPHROTIC SYNDROME is another common complication of kidney disease.

### Untreated Pyelonephritis

Pyelonephritis typically causes significant symptoms, such as pain with urination (dysuria), frequent urination, and the inability to delay urinating, that typically lead the patient to seek medical attention. If not treated effectively, pyelonephritis can lead to progressive scarring and damage to the kidneys and to the development of kidney stones, which, if the stones become infected, becomes increasingly difficult to treat. It may also lead to high blood pressure and in some cases, the spread of the infection from the kidneys into the bloodstream and the development of sepsis.

### Complications of Kidney Stones

If kidney stones are untreated, they will continue to grow and enlarge. If they become infected, treatment becomes more difficult. If kidney stones enlarge, they become increasingly difficult for the person to pass through urination. They may completely block the ureter (the tube connecting the kidneys to the bladder), causing urinary tract obstruction and hydronephrosis. This can cause damage to the kidney, and this damage may become irreversible if it is allowed to persist for too long. If there is an infection of the blocked urine, antibiotics frequently will be ineffective, and surgical drainage of the infected urine may be necessary.

According to Neil M. Paige, M.D., and Glenn T. Nagami, M.D., in their article on 10 things nephrologists wish primary care physicians knew, the doctors stated that when patients have recurrent stone disease, then patients need a metabolic evaluation to find and treat modifiable risk factors. They recommend that patients with recurrent kidney stones who also have a family history of stones and frequent urinary tract infections or inflammatory bowel disease should be referred to a nephrologist. Patients who do not have such risk factors should have an evaluation of their diet and a review of their medications to determine if they take any drugs that promote kidney stone development. They should also have a urinalysis and blood test for their levels of calcium, phosphorus, electrolytes, and uric acid.

### Complications of Chronic Kidney Disease

Chronic kidney disease presents with many potential complications, particularly if it is untreated. Because CKD has few or no symptoms in its early stages, often it is not diagnosed or treated until the later stages. Even when CKD *is* identified and treated, serious complications may occur, particularly if the disease worsens to END-STAGE RENAL DISEASE (ESRD) or kidney failure; for example, the risk for CARDIOVASCULAR DISEASE is elevated among patients with CKD, as is the risk for the development of secondary hyperparathyroidism. Vitamin D deficiencies are present in nearly all patients undergoing dialysis, and this deficiency leaves patients at risk for bone disorders.

**Cardiovascular complications with CKD** It is known that there is a bidirectional aspect to CKD: Kidney disease causes cardiovascular disease and cardiovascular disease itself is a risk factor for the development of kidney disease. Stinghen and colleagues noted in their 2010 article that elevated levels of inflammatory mediators as well as an activated immune system are present with early chronic kidney disease. According to the researchers, "This chronic inflammatory state is closely linked to several complications of CKD, such as vascular degeneration, myocardial fibrosis, loss of appetite, insulin resistance, increased muscle catabolism and anemia. Potentially, these consequences of a chronically activated immune system impact on the acceleration of atherosclerosis, vascular calcification and development of heart dysfunction."

Some ANTIHYPERTENSIVE DRUGS with proven anti-inflammatory action have been tested on patients undergoing dialysis, such as angiotensin-converting enzyme inhibitors (ACEIs) and angiotensin II receptor blockers (ARBs), showing a benefit compared to placebo, and that this effect is separate from their effect to improve blood pressure control.

Oxidative stress is another problem among patients with kidney disease, and in one study, providing a high dose of vitamin E reduced the risk for cardiovascular disease and myocardial infarction (heart attack).

*Secondary hyperparathyroidism with CKD*
Secondary hyperparathyroidism, or an excessive level of parathyroid hormone (PTH), is a common complication among patients with CKD, caused by changes in the metabolism of vitamin D, CALCIUM, and PHOSPHORUS which occur in the course of kidney disease. CHRONIC KIDNEY DISEASE–MINERAL BONE DISORDER (CKD-MBD), formerly known as renal osteodystrophy, is a further complication of secondary hyperparathyroidism.

Secondary hyperparathyroidism (SHPT) generally has no symptoms which the patient can notice, and is detected only by measuring the level of PTH in the blood. Occasionally, SHPT can cause muscle aches and pains as well as fractures with minimal (or no) trauma. Some studies indicate that there is a low level of bone density that is demonstrated in the bone mineral

density test as well as by the higher incidence of fractures occurring among patients with CKD. SHPT is prevented or managed with the attempt to reduce excessively high levels of PTH, normalize serum calcium and vitamin D, and manage HYPERPHOSPHATEMIA (high levels of phosphorus in the blood) with dietary changes as well as medications that are phosphate binders. Excessive treatment of SHPT may lead to another type of CKD-related bone disease, adynamic bone disease, in which the normal remodeling of bone does not occur. This leads to increased bone pain and fractures.

*Metabolic abnormalities with CKD and ESRD*
R. Cibulka and J. Racek noted in their 2007 article that patients with ESRD are at risk for metabolic disorders and nutritional abnormalities, such as atherosclerosis, anemia, and malnutrition, as well as hyperparathyroidism. They may also experience elevated triglyceride levels and low levels of high-density lipoprotein (HDL, or the "good" CHOLESTEROL).

Renal anemia, common among individuals with CKD, causes fatigue and decline in cognitive abilities (thinking and reasoning) as well as sexual capacity. In addition, patients with CKD and anemia have an increased risk of death from cardiovascular causes. The anemia can be treated with erythropoiesis-stimulating agents (ESAs), such as erythropoietin. Unfortunately, correcting the anemia with ESA therapy does not seem to substantially alter the increased mortality risk as compared to insuring that the anemia does not become severe (a hemoglobin level less than 9 grm/dl is severe).

Cibulka and Racek also note that most patients with kidney failure have hyperhomocysteinemia, or elevated levels of homocysteine that are three or four times above the normal rate. It is unknown what causes this elevated level in patients with kidney failure. It is known, however, that high levels are problematic; for example, hyperhomocysteinemia is itself a risk factor for the development of cardiovascular disease. Interestingly, patients with malnutrition do not have hyperhomocysteinemia. At present, effective treatments of hyperhomocysteinemia that also decrease cardiovascular risk have not yet been developed.

Metabolic acidosis is another common complication occurring in CKD. This complication develops because the kidneys produce bicarbonate, which treats the acidosis, and this may not occur sufficiently in patients with CKD. Treating the acidosis with oral sodium bicarbonate medication appears to improve nutritional status and may also decrease the risk of progression of the CKD.

*Vitamin and mineral abnormalities with kidney disease* According to Samina Khan, M.D., vitamin D deficiency is common among patients with CKD because changes in the metabolism of vitamin D occur in the early stages of the disease along with declining kidney function. Khan noted that vitamin D deficiency (also known as hypovitaminosis D) was common among nearly half of young adults; however, the deficiency among patients with CKD is greater. Some studies have shown that 97 percent of dialysis patients have vitamin D deficiencies. A deficiency of vitamin D correlates with impaired immune resistance, an increased risk for fractures, and other medical risks. Vitamin D deficiency can be tested for and treated. Patients with ESRD who are treated with vitamin D analogues have a decreased risk of cardiovascular or infection-related mortality and a decreased risk of hospitalization. These patients may need special forms of vitamin D that do not require processing in the kidney to activate the vitamin D, as is necessary for the body's naturally produced vitamin D.

Cibulka, R., and J. Racek. "Metabolic Disorders in Patients with Chronic Kidney Failure." *Physiological Research* 56 (2007): 697–705.

Khan, Samina, M.D. "Vitamin D Deficiency and Secondary Hyperparathyroidism among Patients with Chronic Kidney Disease." *American Journal of the Medical Sciences* 333, no. 4 (2007): 201–207.

Paige, Neil M., M.D. and Glenn T. Nagami, M.D. "The Top 10 Things Nephrologists Wish Every Primary Care Doctor Knew." *Mayo Clinic Proceedings* 84, no. 2 (2009): 180–186.

Stinghen, Andréa E. M., et al. "Immune Mechanisms Involved in Cardiovascular Complications of Chronic Kidney Disease." *Blood Purification* 29 (2010): 114–120.

**crystal nephropathy** A condition caused by the precipitation of crystals in the renal tubules that obstructs the urine flow and that can lead to acute renal failure. The most common causes of crystal nephropathy include acute uric acid nephropathy and high doses of intravenous acyclovir. Less common causes include the use of sulfonamide antibiotics, ethylene glycol (present in antifreeze), the ingestion of very high doses of vitamin C, and the use of methotrexate or indinavir.

### Symptoms and Diagnostic Path

Patients with crystal nephropathy typically present with symptoms and signs that include flank pain, blood in the urine (hematuria), pyuria (pus in the urine), and crystalluria (the presence of crystals in the urine that can be seen with microscopes). Diagnosis is made based on symptoms, signs, and laboratory tests.

### Treatment Options and Outlook

Patients with crystal nephropathy should have regular checks of their kidney function. Patients may also benefit from an increased oral fluid intake. This additional fluid will increase the urine volume, which in turn decreases the concentration of medications causing the condition and thereby limits their likelihood of precipitating out of solution and causing crystal nephropathy. Also, by increasing the urine volume, this speeds up the urine flow through the renal tubules, thereby making any crystals that are present less likely to obstruct the tubules and cause kidney damage.

### Risk Factors and Preventive Measures

Patients with acute acid nephropathy and who take high does of intravenous acyclovir are at the greatest risk for crystal nephropathy. Some medications also lead to the development of crystal nephropathy. This does not mean that everyone who takes one or more of these medications will inevitably develop crystal nephropathy; instead, it simply means that the risk is elevated compared to the risk of not taking the medications. It may be further elevated if individuals frequently use any of these medications. As a result, if chronic use is needed, it is important to have regular checks of the kidney function.

**cystic kidney disease**   See ACQUIRED CYSTIC KIDNEY DISEASE; POLYCYSTIC KIDNEY DISEASE.

**cystic kidney disease, acquired**   See ACQUIRED CYSTIC KIDNEY DISEASE.

**cystitis**   Usually refers to a bacterial infection of the bladder, although cystitis technically means the inflammation of the bladder, with or without infection. Cystitis is also alternatively known as a urinary tract infection (UTI) or a bladder infection. If a bladder infection is not treated with appropriate ANTIBIOTICS, then the bacteria may ascend into the kidneys and cause a kidney infection (PYELONEPHRITIS), a potentially more serious condition. According to the National Kidney and Urologic Diseases Information Clearinghouse (NKUDIC), 429,000 people were ill enough that they had to be hospitalized for UTIs in 2004, the most recent data available as of this writing. However, most people with a UTI can be treated as outpatients with appropriate antibiotics.

Some people develop chronic recurrent bladder and/or kidney infections, and the doctor needs to investigate possible causes, such as undiagnosed Type 2 DIABETES or another illness that may be responsible.

### Symptoms and Diagnostic Path

Common symptoms and signs of cystitis include the following:

- pain or a burning sensation while urinating
- cloudy urine
- urinating small amounts of urine
- a feeling of urgency and the need to urinate when little urine is present

The physician diagnoses cystitis on the basis of the patient's symptoms as well as the results of laboratory tests. A simple urinalysis can detect most cases of cystitis with dipsticks that are used to detect the presence of nitrates and/or white blood cells; however, in some cases, the urine is cultured to determine the specific bacteria that are causing the infection. With a culture, the urine is placed in a special bacteria-friendly environment to see if bacteria grow and if so, to identify the type of bacteria that is present. *Escherichia coli (E. coli)* is a bacterium that is a common cause of cystitis.

### Treatment Options and Outlook

In most cases, treatment with an antibiotic for seven to 10 days will eradicate the bacteria. Symptoms usually disappear within two to three days; however, the individual should continue the treatment until the medication is completely gone. Discontinuing treatment too early could cause a regrowth of the bacteria and a return of the symptoms, and could also complicate treatment and recovery. It also increases the risk of bacteria that are not completely eradicated developing resistance to that antibiotic. In this case, recurrence of the bacteria can develop, and the antibiotic that was previously used would no longer be effective. Because there are only a limited number of antibiotics available for use, this can lead to substantial complications in susceptible patients. Despite these problems that can result from early discontinuation of antibiotics, it is very common for people to stop taking the medication for cystitis when they feel better.

### Risk Factors and Preventive Measures

Cystitis is common among females, especially in women of childbearing or sexual activity age.

Elderly males and females are also at risk for cystitis. In addition, some individuals are prone to recurrent bouts of cystitis for a variety of reasons.

To prevent bladder infections, individuals should drink plenty of fluids: at least 10 glasses per day. This will encourage more frequent urination. Some individuals with recurrent infections find that drinking cranberry juice, which is highly acidic, helps to limit their instances of infections. However, individuals who are taking warfarin (Coumadin), a blood thinner, should avoid cranberry juice. In addition, those who have interstitial cystitis, a painful spastic bladder condition, should also generally avoid cranberry juice or cranberry juice tablets because the high acidity of cranberry juice may cause bladder spasms. In women who find that sexual activity precipitates cystitis, urination shortly after intercourse can help decrease the frequency of infections.

See also INFECTIONS; URINE/URINALYSIS/URINE CULTURE.

Griebling, Tomas L., M.D. "Urinary Tract Infection in Men." In *Urologic Diseases in America,* edited by M. S. Litwin and C. S. Saigal, 623–645. Bethesda, Md.: National Institute of Diabetes and Digestive and Kidney Diseases (NIDDK), 2007.
———. "Urinary Tract Infection in Women." In *Urologic Diseases in America,* edited by M. S. Litwin and C. S. Saigal, 587–620. Bethesda, Md.: National Institute of Diabetes and Digestive and Kidney Diseases (NIDDK), 2007.

**cystoscopy**   A procedure in which a special device, a cystoscope, is inserted directly into the urinary bladder for the purpose of inspecting the urethra, the bladder, and the entry of the ureters into the bladder. This procedure is performed by a urologist, a specialist in diseases and disorders of the urogenital system. A cystoscopy may be performed if the doctor suspects a serious problem within the bladder. Sometimes individuals who have recurrent bouts of CYSTITIS (urinary tract infections) are given a cystoscopy to help the physician determine whether a problem within the bladder itself is somehow causing chronic infections; for example, the bladder should be smooth and not rough or pitted. If it is rough or pitted, this provides more places for bacteria to lodge themselves. Cystoscopy is also performed routinely as a component of the evaluation of hematuria (blood in the urine).

Cystoscopes are fiberoptic devices, and are user-friendly for the patient as well as for the urologist. However, the cystoscopy can be performed under local, general, or spinal anesthesia, if needed.

### Procedure

The procedure is usually performed on an outpatient basis in the urologist's office. The patient empties his or her bladder before the procedure. The physician uses a catheter to remove any remaining urine from the bladder before inserting the cystoscope to inspect the bladder.

The cystoscopy is not only a diagnostic tool but also a tool that can be used to treat patients; for example, the cystoscope can be used to remove bladder stones and bladder polyps, and to sample tissue to be biopsied from bladder tumors. It can also be used to instill chemotherapy medications to treat bladder cancer.

### Risks and Complications

The cystoscopy may be painful in individuals who are having bladder pain or spasms but there should be no serious risks with the procedure itself. The physician may give the patient a one-day course of antibiotic should any bacteria have inadvertently entered the bladder during the procedure. At times, the cystoscopy can lead to urethral or bladder injury. If this happens, a Foley catheter may need to be placed into the bladder to allow the natural healing of the urethral or bladder injury.

### Outlook and Lifestyle Modifications

There are no major outlook or lifestyle modifications that are associated with the cystoscopy procedure.

See also COMMON MEDICAL TESTS AND PROCEDURES; PYELONEPHRITIS.

**daily living with major kidney diseases** Individuals with severe or chronic kidney disease often must make major adaptations to their lives in order to cope with their illness. This is particularly true among those with kidney failure caused by END-STAGE RENAL DISEASE or ACUTE KIDNEY INJURY (AKI) and who must have DIALYSIS or KIDNEY TRANSPLANTATION in order to survive. For example, they must be sure to take the medications on a schedule that is ordered by the physician and they must also take IMMUNOSUPPRESSIVE drugs to prevent the body from rejecting the transplanted organ. One problem with taking immunosuppressants is that the individuals who take them are at an increased risk for developing infections and diseases and even cancer, because the suppression of their immune system that keeps it from rejecting the transplanted kidney has also impeded their resistance.

### Managing Diabetes: Keeping Blood Sugar Levels as Close to Normal as Possible

Many people with chronic kidney disease also have DIABETES MELLITUS, and studies have documented that when the individual's blood glucose levels are as close to normal as possible, then the person's risk for worsening kidney disease and other diseases that are linked to diabetes are decreased. In contrast, if diabetes is not managed sufficiently, then the individual is at risk for numerous diabetic complications, including eye disease up to and including blindness, the amputation of the feet and limbs, kidney failure, digestive complications such as gastroparesis, which causes delayed emptying of the stomach, and many other complications. In the worst case, the failure to manage the hyperglycemia

can lead to coma and death. There may be an increased risk for hypoglycemia (low blood sugar) with very tight glucose control, but regular blood testing should detect any trends toward excessively low levels of blood sugar.

Medications often help individuals manage their diabetes when they are unable to maintain close to normal blood sugar levels by diet alone. There are many different types of medications used to treat diabetes, although most frequently metformin (Glucophage) is used as the first treatment.

In 2010, the Food and Drug Administration issued guidelines in the case of the diabetes medication rosiglitazone maleate (Avandia). This drug can either cause or worsen heart failure. In addition, patients with any heart problems or who take medications for hypertension should inform their doctors of these medical problems before starting rosiglitazone maleate. This drug should not be taken with insulin or nitrate medications. Patients with diabetic eye disease, particularly macular edema, should tell their doctors before they start rosiglitazone maleate. Women who are pregnant or planning to become pregnant should advise their physicians before starting this drug. The drug can also cause anemia and hypoglycemia.

### Managing Hypertension

Another important aspect of living with kidney disease is keeping one's blood pressure as close to normal as possible. Many people with kidney disease, especially those with chronic kidney disease, have high blood pressure. Most people with HYPERTENSION need to take ANTIHYPERTENSIVE DRUGS to decrease their blood pressure.

Lifestyle choices can also help considerably, such as weight loss among the overweight and obese and regular exercise based on the doctor's recommendation for an individual. For most types of kidney diseases, treatment with an ACE inhibitor has beneficial effects of lowering blood pressure and also protecting the kidneys. As with all drugs, there are risks and benefits with antihypertensive medications, and all individuals should advise their doctors of any health problems before starting antihypertensives.

### Managing Hyperlipidemia

High CHOLESTEROL levels (hyperlipidemia) are a frequent problem among many people with kidney disease, and this problem can be managed with medications in the "statin" class of drugs as well as with an improved diet and regular exercise. A physician's monitoring of the cholesterol levels is also crucially important.

### When Emotional Disorders Intrude: Depression and Anxiety

Individuals with chronic kidney disease have a higher rate of depression than others, and the rate is particularly pronounced if they are undergoing dialysis treatments or are waiting for (or have already received) a kidney transplantation. In addition, some research has shown that people with recurrent kidney stones experience both anxiety and depression. It is important to resolve these issues as part of effective daily living.

In an observational study of 854 kidney transplant recipients and 176 dialysis patients in Hungary who were on a waiting list to receive a kidney transplant, researchers Lilla Szeifert, M.D., and colleagues found that the patients who had received a transplant were significantly less depressed than were those on the waiting list for a transplant: In fact, one-third of the waiting list patients were clinically depressed. This high prevalence of depression is not too surprising, since the individuals who are waiting for a transplant may be fearful that the transplant will not occur within a reasonable time, or they may be having complications and adverse symp-

toms related to the dialysis procedure. However, the researchers also found 20 percent of the transplant patients were clinically depressed and receiving the transplanted organ did not obviate all depression.

Of the subjects, only 1.2 percent of the transplant recipients and 1.7 percent of the patients wait-listed for a transplant were taking antidepressant medications, although clearly a higher percentage of them should have been receiving antidepressants, based on the research findings. Higher percentages were receiving antianxiety drugs, or 6.7 percent of the waiting patients and 5.7 percent of the transplant recipients.

The researchers found that the individual's perceived financial system was directly correlated to the risk for depression and that a lower socioeconomic status is linked to an increased risk for depression. In addition, patients with a greater number of comorbidities (other diseases) were more depressed than patients coping with fewer diseases in addition to their kidney disease. The researchers also found that some factors increased the risk for depression, including socioeconomic status, other health problems, and the type of treatment received.

Nonadherence to treatment regimens increases the risk for depression, based on a study by Daniel Cukor and colleagues in *Kidney International* in 2009. The researchers studied 94 kidney transplant recipients and 65 patients receiving hemodialysis, and found that subjects with depression had a significantly lower rate of medication adherence than nondepressed patients. They also found that the dialysis patients were significantly more depressed than the patients who had undergone a transplant.

Some patients with recurrent painful incidents of kidney stones can develop both anxiety and depression, according to a study by D. H. M. P. Diniz and colleagues. In this study, there were 32 subjects with recurrent kidney stones and 32 controls. The patients with kidney stones had experienced at least two episodes of stones over a three-year period, and the control group were eye patients seen in an ophthalmology outpatient clinic. The patients with kidney stones were significantly more anxious and depressed than the subjects in the control group. Of the patients in the kidney stone group, 6.2 percent were severely depressed and 34.4 percent were moderately depressed. In contrast, in the control group, none of the subjects were severely depressed and 9.4 percent were moderately depressed.

### Making Major Lifestyle Changes

Medications alone cannot manage kidney disease sufficiently, and most people must make changes to their daily lives, such as ending bad habits and carefully monitoring diet and nutrition.

*Ending a smoking habit* Experts report that SMOKING is the single most reversible cause of serious disease. Smoking can seriously exacerbate kidney disease and limit the benefits that can be made by many other important actions individuals take, such as managing their blood sugar and blood pressure and cholesterol levels, losing weight, or carefully monitoring their diet.

*Losing weight if overweight or obese* Some people with kidney disease are overweight or obese, which is not surprising, since the majority of Americans are considered either overweight or obese based on their body mass index (BMI). However, weight loss and dietary changes can improve the outcome for many people with kidney disease and decrease the risks accruing from complications from their kidney disease. (See OBESITY.)

*Monitoring the diet for those on dialysis* Individuals on dialysis must very carefully monitor their diets, ensuring that they do not consume too many foods that would cause excess fluid to form in their bodies, as well as limiting fluid consumption itself. Some foods contain a great deal of fluid, such as soup, ice cream, melons, grapes, apples, oranges, tomatoes, lettuce, and celery, as well as gelatin desserts. Patients on dialysis often need to limit their fluid levels.

It is important to limit the consumption of foods that contain POTASSIUM because excess potassium levels can be dangerous to a dialy-

sis patient. Potassium is present in fruits and vegetables, milk, and many other foods. Some foods that contain large amounts of potassium and, consequently, are especially important for those on dialysis to limit carefully are as follows: tomatoes and tomato sauce, avocadoes, bananas, kiwis, and dried fruit. Note that some foods that are high in potassium can be altered so that they are acceptable for the dialysis patient; removing the peel from potatoes also removes most of the potassium. They then need to be soaked for several hours and then drained and rinsed before cooking. HYPERKALEMIA (excessive levels of potassium in the blood) can be harmful to the heart and can even cause a heart attack.

Dietary salt restriction is critical for patients with almost all types of kidney disease. Salt (sodium chloride) ingestion increases blood pressure, which both directly increases the rate of damage to the kidney and can lead to edema formation, both in the ankles and legs and, more importantly, in the lungs where it can interfere with breathing. Increased salt intake also increases urinary protein excretion, which is associated with increased cardiovascular risk and increased rates of progression of kidney disease that are over and above those due to changes in blood pressure.

People on dialysis need to eat sufficient amounts of high-quality protein to maintain adequate nutrition and to help the immune system work more efficiently. Protein builds up muscle and repairs tissue. Protein itself is broken down into urea, but an excessive level of urea in the blood is problematic. Limiting proteins to such foods as meat, fish, poultry, and eggs can help to reduce the overall level of urea in the blood. However, excessive amounts of protein intake can be damaging to the kidney in the patient with chronic kidney disease and can lead to worsening rates of progression of the kidney disease and a need to start dialysis or receive a kidney transplant at an earlier time than would otherwise be necessary. Close consultation with both the nephrologist and the dietitian may be necessary to identify the appropriate amount of protein intake and then to design a diet which provides this amount.

People receiving dialysis need to keep their dry weight within balance. Their dry weight is their weight directly after a dialysis session and when all the extra fluid has been removed from the body. The dry weight may fluctuate somewhat. The individual's physician can tell the dialysis patient what their dry weight should be.

According to the National Institute of Diabetes and Digestive and Kidney Diseases (NIDDK), individuals on dialysis should not take over-the-counter (OTC) vitamin pills because they may contain vitamins or minerals that are harmful to people on dialysis. Instead, the doctor may wish to prescribe vitamins when they are needed.

Changes in thinking are also required with dialysis; for example, most people are used to physicians urging them to drink plenty of fluids and lots of water; however, when one is on dialysis, it is important to limit fluid consumption because extra fluid makes the job of dialysis more difficult.

***Monitoring the diet for individuals who have had kidney stones*** Many kidney stones are made of calcium oxalate, and if an individual learns that his or her stones were comprised of this substance, then restricting the consumption of items high in oxalate can decrease the risk of the formation of new kidney stones. Oxalate is found in many fruits and vegetables, and spinach, rhubarb, nuts, and wheat bran have been demonstrated to particularly increase oxalate in the urine. Some fluids should be avoided by a person who has produced oxalate kidney stones, especially grapefruit juice, cranberry juice, and dark colas. Individuals who form calcium oxalate stones should not avoid calcium, and instead should obtain calcium from their food.

If an analysis of the kidney stone reveals that the stones were comprised of uric acid, then a diet high in purines should be changed, which means restriction of organ meats, fish, and shellfish. In addition, people who form uric acid kidney stones should avoid eating more than six ounces of meat each day.

It is also important for all individuals who have formed kidney stones to drink plenty of water, whatever type of stone is found, because water can help prevent the formation of many types of kidney stones. In addition, water can help flush out smaller stones before they develop into large stones which are difficult to pass. Individuals who have had kidney stones should drink enough fluid to produce at least two quarts of urine a day, and a greater fluid consumption is needed if the individual participates in physical activities that generate excessive perspiration. A simple rule physicians often give patients with recurrent kidney stones is that they should drink enough fluids so that their urine does not turn yellow and is instead clear or almost clear.

If the individual formed cystine stones, diet cannot help but consuming a greater amount of water, or more than a gallon every 24 hours, will help limit the formation of further kidney stones.

### Changes Needed with Kidney Transplantation

Numerous changes are needed with kidney transplantation, largely because immunosuppressive drugs must be taken to prevent the rejection of the kidneys and consequently, the risk for INFECTION or even for the development of cancer is elevated. Frequent physician visits are required in the early stages of the new transplant. The patient must also adapt to the emotional issues that precede the kidney transplantation as well as the concerns that occur subsequent to the transplantation.

See also DEPRESSION.

Corruble, E., et al. "Progressive Increase of Anxiety and Depression in Patients Waiting for a Kidney Transplantation." *Behavioral Medicine* 36, no. 1 (2010): 32–36.

Cukor, Daniel, et al. "Depression Is an Important Contributor to Low Medication Adherence in Hemodialyzed Patients and Transplant Recipients." *Kidney International* 75 (2009): 1,223–1,229.

Diniz, D. H. M. P., S. L. Blay, and N. Schor. "Anxiety and Depression Symptoms in Recurrent Painful Renal Lithiasis Colic." *Brazilian Journal of Medical and Biological Research* 40 (2007): 949–955.

Szeifert, Lilla, M.D., et al. "Symptoms of Depression in Kidney Transplant Recipients: A Cross-Sectional Study." *American Journal of Kidney Diseases* 55, no. 1 (2010): 132–140.

**dehydration-induced acute renal failure**   See MYELOMA KIDNEY.

**Denys-Drash syndrome**   A rare genetic disorder that occurs on the WT1 gene on chromosome 11p13. It is characterized by the triad of progressive renal disease, male pseudohermaphroditism, and Wilms tumor. Only about 60 cases have been reported worldwide. PROTEINURIA (a sign of kidney disease) develops shortly after birth, and the child develops kidney failure within one to four years. Male pseudohermaphroditism refers to ambiguous male genitals and difficulty determining the individual's gender. Denys-Drash syndrome is also known as Drash syndrome. The syndrome was first reported by Drash in 1970. The name of the disorder was subsequently changed to Denys-Drash syndrome in 1985 because the anomalies were first reported by Denys in France in 1967.

### Symptoms and Diagnostic Path

The child with Denys-Drash syndrome has a serious life-threatening kidney disease and may also have abnormal male genitals. Proteinuria can be identified with laboratory testing, as can kidney failure.

### Treatment Options and Outlook

Denys-Drash syndrome does not respond to IMMUNOSUPPRESSIVE DRUGS or to corticosteroids. Treatment is comprised of maintaining proper electrolyte balance and nutrition and also management of infections and of kidney failure. If KIDNEY TRANSPLANTATION is performed, the NEPHROTIC SYNDROME abates, according to Patrick Niaudet.

### Risk Factors and Preventive Measures

This disorder is extremely rare and the only risk factor is a genetic inheritance. There are no known preventive measures.

Niaudet, Patrick. "Denys-Drash Syndrome." *Orphanet.* March 2004. Available online. URL: www.orpha.net/data/patho/GB/uk-Drash.pdf. Accessed February 15, 2010.

Online Mendelian Inheritance in Man (OMIM). "Denys-Drash Syndrome." Available online. URL: http://www.ncbi.nlm.nih.gov/entrez/dispomim.cgi?id=194080. Accessed February 15, 2010.

**depression**   Depression is a psychiatric disorder which is a serious chronic state of low mood that is accompanied by feelings of hopelessness and/or worthlessness and a loss of interest in activities that the individual formerly found enjoyable. Many people with serious chronic diseases are at risk for the development of depression, as are patients who know that they have CHRONIC KIDNEY DISEASE (CKD). This is particularly true in the case of patients with END-STAGE RENAL DISEASE (ESRD) and who must eventually undergo DIALYSIS or KIDNEY TRANSPLANTATION in order to survive. The presence of depression itself often makes the medical burden of coping with kidney disease even more difficult.

### Symptoms and Diagnostic Path

Depression is characterized by a variety of different symptoms, including both psychological and physical symptoms. For example, physical symptoms may include either sleeping too much or too little, as with severe insomnia, as well as extreme fatigue and an overall lack of energy. The depressed person may experience a significant weight loss or gain from eating too little or too much.

The psychological symptoms of depression include feelings of sadness that are experienced most of the time, and the individual may also have thoughts of suicide. The depressed person may also feel worthless or guilty, and he or she often has difficulty making decisions and concentrating. The depressed person may also cry frequently or may seem apathetic and emotionless. It is also important to note that depressed individuals with chronic kidney disease have more frequent and longer hospital stays, and they are also more likely to stop taking their medication, which is very dangerous.

The severely depressed person not only often has thoughts of suicide but he or she may have a plan to carry out the suicide. In the case of the individual who is receiving dialysis, choosing to end dialysis will ultimately have the effect of ending the person's life; however, researchers do not consider this to be a passive form of suicide and only consider other active means to end the person's life as a "suicide."

### Treatment Options and Outlook

Patients with kidney disease who are depressed may receive psychotherapy as well as antidepressant medications to treat their depression. Even for those with poor kidney function, many antidepressants are safe for them to take, such as fluoxetine (Prozac), amitriptyline (Elavil), and many other antidepressants that are available today. These medications are primarily metabolized by the liver rather than by the kidneys, and thus they do not present a risk to the kidneys. Some individuals need more than one antidepressant to resolve their depression. The physician who prescribes the antidepressants should coordinate the medication treatment plan with the patient's nephrologist.

Cognitive-behavioral therapy (CBT) is the most common form of therapy that is used with depressed patients. With CBT, the depressed person is taught to challenge irrational and negative thoughts and learn to replace them with more positive yet realistic thoughts. For example, the person who tells herself or himself, "I am no good to anyone any more" or "I am worthless" can learn to challenge these thoughts and affirm his or her value to the self as well as to family members and friends. There are many other forms of psychotherapy which may be useful. The physician should be consulted for recommendations to therapists or the prescribing psychiatrist can make recommendations.

### Risk Factors and Preventive Measures

According to the American Association of Kidney Patients (AAKP), the depression rate among all Americans is about 10 percent, but for those patients who are receiving dialysis, depression rates increase to 20–30 percent. Depression is the most serious psychiatric problem that occurs among dialysis patients, and its presence and also its treatment can directly affect their survival rate. Fortunately, depression is also a highly treatable disorder.

### Chronic Kidney Disease, Depression, and Anxiety

Research has shown that people with chronic kidney disease are at risk for the development of serious psychiatric disorders; for example, in a study of depression in 272 subjects with chronic kidney disease (none of whom were on dialysis) published in the American Journal of Kidney Diseases in 2009 by S. Susan Hedayati and colleagues, the researchers found that 21 percent of the subjects were experiencing a current major depressive episode. The researchers found that 18.4 percent of the subjects also had an anxiety disorder, including such anxiety disorders as panic disorder, social anxiety disorder, posttraumatic stress disorder, obsessive-compulsive disorder, or generalized anxiety disorder. Anxiety disorders are also treatable with medications.

The researchers found several significant patterns among those who were depressed; for example, the subjects who were depressed were younger and less likely to be employed than the individuals with CKD but without depression. A significant percent of the depressed subjects had a history of alcohol or drug abuse, as well as a history of lifetime depression and other psychiatric illnesses. The researchers also found that the diagnosis of DIABETES MELLITUS was significantly related to an incidence of a major depressive episode.

The researchers said, "The principal new finding in this study is that a major depressive episode is common in patients with earlier stages of CKD, before the onset of ESRD [end-stage renal disease, or kidney failure] and dialysis therapy. We also found that the prevalence of a major depressive episode does not vary with stage of predialysis CKD."

They added

Earlier screening of patients with CKD for depression before dialysis therapy initation becomes particularly important in light of the strong and independent association of depression with poor outcomes reported in multiple studies of patients with ESRD on long-term dialysis therapy. Long-term hemodialysis patients with a clinical diagnosis of depression are twice as likely to die or require hospitalization compared with their nondepressed counterparts. Depression also is associated with peritonitis in long-term peritoneal dialysis patients and with increased numbers of hospitalizations and lengths of stay in hemodialysis patients.

### Social Support, Agreeableness, and Depression in Chronic Kidney Disease

Most people assume that patients with chronic kidney disease need social support and a network of people on whom they can rely; however, the level of support that is needed may vary considerably from individual to individual. Researchers Karin F. Hoth and colleagues performed a longitudinal study of the relationship between social support, agreeableness, and depressive symptoms among those with chronic kidney disease (CKD), reporting on their findings in the *Journal of Behavioral Medicine* in 2007. The researchers studied 59 subjects with CKD, assessing them on the Social Provisions Scale, the Beck Depression Inventory, and other psychological scales, and following the subjects up a year and a half later.

The researchers found that a greater level of social support among the subjects who also ranked high in the trait of agreeableness was predictive for a lower level of depression over time. However, among those subjects who were rated *low* in agreeableness, their level of social support had little effect on their level of depression. The researchers said that these findings revealed the importance of considering personality as well as social support in relation to the patient's illness. Some people need more social

support than others, including those with kidney disease.

They also said

Another important implication of the current study is that while it is generally assumed that interventions aimed at increasing social support are beneficial, our findings suggested that individual differences should be considered. The findings suggest that agreeable individuals are most likely to benefit from interventions aimed at increasing social support. In contrast, it might be helpful to determine additional intervention strategies for individual low in agreeableness (e.g. individual coping or information oriented interventions) to maximize coping. Thus, a variety of strategies to provide support to patients both via social interaction, teaching of individual coping strategies, and availability of information may be beneficial so that patients have access to the approaches that match their preferred style of interaction.

### Depression, Quality of Life, and Stress in Patients with CKD and ESRD

In a 2009 study by Khaled Abdel-Kader and colleagues, published in the *Clinical Journal of American Society of Nephrology*, the researchers compared 90 subjects with ESRD and 87 subjects with advanced CKD, comparing their symptoms of depression. They found that both groups of subjects were alike in terms of their number of depressive symptoms as well as in their symptom severity.

The researchers said, "Past studies demonstrated that patients receiving maintenance dialysis experience a multitude of physical and emotional symptoms, a particularly high prevalence of depression, and significant impairments in QOL [quality of life]. The findings of the present study suggest that patients with advanced CKD who are not dependent on chronic renal replacement therapy experience a comparable overall burden of symptoms and depression and low QOL."

In another analysis of 226 patients with ESRD but who were not yet receiving dialysis, researchers Lori Harwood and colleagues reported their findings in 2009 in *Nephrology Nursing Journal*. The average age of the subjects was 64.5 years. The researchers found that the greatest stressors on the subjects were fatigue, sleep problems, parasthesia (the feelings of pins and needles in the hands and feet), and muscle cramps.

Coping strategies that the researchers identified in the majority of subjects included the attempt to keep life as close to normal as possible, used by 82 percent of the subjects, followed by trying to think positively (80.9 percent). Interestingly, the researchers found that the number of stress factors was inversely proportionate to the individual's age, which means that the older patients reported fewer stressors than younger patients. The researchers speculated that this may have been due to a greater acceptance of the unknown and the uncontrollable among the older patients compared to their younger cohorts, as well as the use of familiar coping strategies that had worked for older subjects in the past.

### Depression and Anxiety among Hemodialysis Patients

Receiving dialysis treatments can lead to the development of depression and/or anxiety. In a study of 70 predominantly black patients who were undergoing hemodialysis, researchers Daniel Cukor and colleagues analyzed the presence of depression and anxiety among the subjects, reporting their findings in 2007. They found that 20 percent of the subjects had major depression and 9 percent had dysthymia (a low level of depression) or another lesser form of depression. In addition, 27 percent of the subjects had an anxiety disorder. Nineteen percent of the subjects had a current substance abuse diagnosis, and 10 percent had a psychotic disorder.

Of those with a psychotic disorder, 80 percent were receiving psychiatric treatment, but only 12 percent of the patients with depression or an anxiety disorder were receiving treatment from a mental health professional. The authors stated, "This highlights how underrecognized depression and anxiety are and perhaps suggests a tolerance of depression and anxiety by physicians

and staff, accepting them as part of the ESRD experience."

The researchers also noted that among those patients who had no psychiatric illness, their scores of assessment placed them within the normal range for depression and their quality of life scores placed them much higher than among those patients with anxiety or depression. The authors stated, "It seems that despite all of the medical and psychologic challenges of living on dialysis, people without a comorbid [co-occurring] psychiatric condition, particularly depression, can enjoy a much greater quality of life. These finding have strong implications for the need for treatment of depression in patients with ESRD, because now there is indication that treatment might not only decrease depression but also improve quality of life."

In another study of depression and the risk of death among chronic HEMODIALYSIS patients, reported by Edgar C. Diefenthaeler and colleagues in 2008, the researchers followed 40 dialysis patients for about two years. They used the Beck Depression Inventory to identify those patients who were depressed. They found that 39 percent of the depressed patients had survived after two years, compared to the much larger percentage of 95 percent of the non-depressed patients who had survived after two years. This finding clearly indicates that depression itself is likely a risk factor that affects survival among hemodialysis patients.

The researchers said, "Depression is a frequent problem in HD [hemodialysis] patients. Despite being underdiagnosed, it appears to exert an important influence on clinical outcomes." They added, "Our study suggests that an increased intensity of depressive symptoms is associated with mortality in HD patients independently of other factors such as age, concurrent systemic disease, clinical variables, and efficacy of dialysis treatment."

### The Decision to End Dialysis: Suicide or a Rational Choice

Patients who are receiving dialysis sometimes choose to end their dialysis treatments, which will result in ending their lives. They may be depressed, or they may have decided that the pain and aggravation of their illness is too difficult to stand. It may be difficult to determine whether the person is depressed or has made what, to him or her, seems like a rational choice. Some patients take other actions to end their lives, committing suicide, and the risk for suicide among patients with ESRD is about 84 percent higher than among individuals in the general population. Researchers Kurella and colleagues found that the risk for suicide among ESRD patients was the highest among male whites and Asians.

In contrast, withdrawal from dialysis (which is not generally considered suicide), occurs in 9–20 percent of patients, primarily among those who are female, older, and white. They are also more likely to be very ill with cancer, malnutrition, physical impairments, and chronic diseases.

Physicians must determine whether the decision to end dialysis is made by a severely depressed person who is untreated for depression or if it is made by a rational person who no longer wishes to undergo the difficulties of dialysis. This is the issue that is discussed by John Michael Bostwick, M.D., and Lewis M. Cohen, M.D., in their 2009 article in *Psychosomatics*. The authors discuss deaths other than kidney failure that are hastened by the decision to terminate treatment but they use chronic kidney disease and dialysis as their model.

Some patterns are seen among those who choose to end their dialysis. According to the authors, those individuals who discontinue their dialysis are usually diabetic, white, and elderly, and they are also extremely ill. From a third to a half of the decisions in these situations are actually made by the family members or other individuals rather than the patient. The authors say

Although death is inevitably sad, a prospective study of the qualitative aspects of dying after dialysis cessation has found that 85% of the deaths are judged to be good. Especially when medical and familial interests concur, many of these deaths are not only good but "very good."

When symptoms are well-managed and where all participants collaborate and achieve agreement, death is often recalled as being merciful, compassionate, and even uplifting. Families and loved ones may find such deaths to be an epiphany and not a trauma. This stands in stark contrast to descriptions by families after true suicides.

However, the authors also noted that "contemporary medical practitioners can benefit from guidelines to help ensure that when they acquiesce to requests to facilitate dying, they are not abetting suicide or committing homicide." It should also be noted that it is important for the physician to avoid substituting his or her own values and how he or she believes they would feel in the same situation, because patients may feel very differently and their wishes should be respected.

In their article on the role of depression in the survival of hemodialysis patients, published in the *Journal of the American Society of Nephrology* in 1993 and which is still valuable today, Paul L. Kimmel and colleagues recommended that doctors and nurses look for evidence of depression in patients, either direct or indirect evidence.

For example, as some examples of indirect evidence of depression, the authors say, "The indirect presentation for depressive symptoms requires the professional staff to take note of changes in nonverbal behavior. Speech that is soft, slow, or faltering in tone may indicate depressed mood. A less-common presentation is agitated speech, sometimes accompanied by disorganized thinking and distractibility. Body posture that is slumped, slowing of movements, and drowsiness are also diagnostic signs of depression. Lack of care with grooming, housekeeping, and social habits, such as greetings and courtesies, and poor attendance at dialysis treatment may indicate apathy. Forgetfulness about otherwise routine activities may suggest problems with concentration. Increased requests for help, indecisiveness, or complaints that treatment is too burdensome or not useful may indicate feelings of helplessness."

In a study of suicide committed among those with ESRD performed by Manjula Kurella and colleagues and reported in 2005 in the *Journal of the American Society of Nephrology,* the authors considered 463,563 subjects ages 15 and older who started dialysis from 1995–2000. They compared those subjects who withdrew from dialysis before their deaths (9.6 percent) to subjects who committed suicide (less than 1 percent). The researchers found that those individuals who committed suicide were more likely to be male, younger, uninsured, and with either an alcohol or a drug dependence. They were also less likely to be black, nonambulatory (unable to move about), or to have diabetes mellitus, congestive heart failure, or stroke. A prior hospitalization with a mental illness increased the risk for suicide by five times.

The researchers found that the risk for suicide was the greatest in the first three months of dialysis initiation and that it decreased over time. The researchers said, "These data establish a high-risk profile for suicide in ESRD patients for whom it may be advisable to seek counseling and other interventions in an effort to reduce risk." The probability of dialysis withdrawal was high for the first year of treatment and decreased greatly thereafter.

See also DAILY LIVING WITH MAJOR KIDNEY DISEASES; SLEEP PROBLEMS.

Abdel-Kader, Khaled, Mark L. Unruh, and Steven D. Weisbord. "Symptom Burden, Depression, and Quality of Life in Chronic and End-Stage Kidney Disease." *Clinical Journal of the American Society of Nephrology* 4 (2009): 1,057–1,064.

Bostwick, John Michael, M.D., and Lewis M. Cohen, M.D. "Differentiating Suicide from Life-Ending Acts and End-of-Life Decisions: A Model Based on Chronic Kidney Disease and Dialysis." *Psychosomatics* 50, no.1 (2009): 1–7.

Cukor, Daniel, et al. "Depression and Anxiety in Urban Hemodialysis Patients." *Clinical Journal of the American Society of Nephrology* 2 (2007): 484–490.

Cukor, Daniel, et al. "Depression Is an Important Contributor to Low Medication Adherence in Hemodialyzed Patients and Transplant Recipients." *Kidney International* 75 (2009): 1,223–1,229.

Diefenthaeler, Edgar C., et al. "Is Depression a Risk Factor for Mortality in Chronic Hemodialysis Patients?" *Revista Brasileira de Psiquiatria* 30, no. 2 (2008): 99–103.

Harwood, Lori. "Stressors and Coping in Individuals with Chronic Kidney Disease." *Nephrology Nursing Journal* 36, no. 3 (2009): 265–277.

Hedayati, S. Susan, M.D. "Prevalence of Major Depressive Episode in CKD." *American Journal of Kidney Diseases* 54, no. 3 (2009): 424–432.

Hoth, Karin F., et al. "A Longitudinal Examination of Social Support, Agreeableness and Depressive Symptoms in Chronic Kidney Disease." *Journal of Behavioral Medicine* 30, no. 1 (2007): 69–76.

Kimmel, Paul L., and Rolf A. Peterson. "Depression in Patients with End-Stage Renal Disease Treated with Dialysis: Has the Time to Treat Arrived?" *Clinical Journal of the American Society of Nephrology* 1 (2006): 349–352.

Kimmel, Paul L., Karen Weihs, and Rolf A. Peterson. "Survival in Hemodialysis Patients: The Role of Depression." *Journal of the American Society of Nephrology* 4, no. 1 (1993): 12–27.

Kurella, Manjula, et al. "Suicide in the United States End-Stage Renal Disease Program." *Journal of the American Society of Nephrology* 16 (2005): 774–781.

**diabetes insipidus (DI)** A disorder that is characterized by an unusually large volume of excreted urine which cannot be reduced by drinking less fluids. This disorder is caused by the inability of the kidneys to concentrate urine. It may lead to extreme thirst despite the fact that the individual may be drinking plenty of water and may also be urinating frequently. Note that diabetes insipidus (DI) is *not* associated in any way with either Type 1 or Type 2 DIABETES MELLITUS, despite its similar-sounding name.

Individuals with DI should wear a medical alert bracelet or carry information in their wallet or purse that can alert others to their condition should they become unconscious or unable to communicate for any reason. One of the complications of DI is the rapid development of very high levels of blood sodium concentration, which can lead to confusion, coma, and in some cases, irreversible neurologic damage. In the event that a person with DI is injured, it is essential that medical personnel caring for the individual are aware of this condition.

There are several forms of diabetes insipidus, according to Daniel G. Bichet in his chapter on polyuria (frequent urination) and diabetes insipidus in *Seldin and Giebisch's The Kidney: Physiology and Pathophysiology* (2008). The most common form of DI is caused by the insufficient secretion of the antidiuretic hormone, arginine vasopressin (AVP). This form of DI is also called central DI, neurogenic DI, or hypothalamic DI. This defect is caused by the central nervous system's failure to make AVP. Another common form of DI is nephrogenic diabetes insipidus (NDI), which is caused by the kidney's insensitivity to the AVP. Some forms of nephrogenic DI are inherited.

Much less common is dipsogenic DI, which leads to extremely heavy consumption of fluid, thus causing excessive urination. (Note that it is possible to drink too much water; in rare cases, this can lead to water intoxication and even death.) After the consumption of large amounts of fluids for prolonged periods of time, the kidneys have a gradual decrease in their ability to concentrate the urine and may be unable to decrease urine volume in the event that the person rapidly decreases fluid intake.

Psychogenic DI is another form of DI, and it is related to a severe emotional disorder. Last is gestational diabetes insipidus, or an increased metabolizing of vasopressin during the pregnancy. (This does not refer to the frequent urination that many pregnant women experience during pregnancy.)

According to Bichet, some medications and drugs can cause an acquired form of NDI, such as lithium, nonpeptide vasopressin receptor antagonist medications, demeclocycline (Declomycin), Amphotericin B, methoxyflurane, diphenylhydantoin (Phenytoin), nicotine from SMOKING, and alcohol. Bichet says lithium use is the most common cause of acquired NDI, and some studies have shown that more than half of patients on lithium therapy have developed NDI.

If patients must continue to take lithium rather than be prescribed another medication, then they may be able to take amiloride (Midamor) to reverse or minimize their acquired NDI. Patients with lithium-induced nephrogenic DI have a slow onset of their disease, and often do not tell their health care personnel about their large urine volumes unless they are specifically asked.

### Symptoms and Diagnostic Path

The person with untreated diabetes insipidus (DI) has a frequent urge to consume fluids and typically awakens at night to urinate. He or she may have also an intense craving for ice water. (This is not the same situation as when a person who is normally thirsty chooses to drink ice water.) The individual also produces a very high volume of urine: from three to 15 liters of urine per day. The healthy adult produces less than two liters of urine daily.

Mild dehydration is a common symptom of DI, and it is related to the excessive urination that is associated with this disorder. Children with DI are at particular risk of recurrent, severe dehydration that may lead to irreversible neurologic damage. Identification of DI in these children and appropriate treatments can prevent neurologic disease that was previously thought to be an inevitable component of pediatric DI.

Other symptoms of DI in an adult may include

- weight loss
- rapid heart rate
- low body temperature
- muscle pain
- fatigue
- irritability
- dry skin

An electrolyte imbalance may occur in individuals with DI because of their excessive levels of urination. The symptoms of DI are essentially the same in all forms of DI, despite the cause of the disorder.

The symptoms of DI in an infant include vomiting, fever, and seizures, and the child's blood shows high levels of sodium (HYPERNATREMIA). Note that hypernatremia is often avoided in most individuals with DI because they are able to consume very large quantities of fluids in response to their thirst, but this is not an option that is available to the infant.

In order to distinguish DI from other causes of excess urination, laboratory tests are ordered and the individual's blood glucose levels, bicarbonate levels, and calcium levels are tested.

A fluid deprivation test is the best laboratory test for DI, and it should be administered in a closely monitored clinical setting. In this test, patients are monitored closely while not being allowed to ingest any fluids. The urine volume and concentration and the blood sodium and other electrolytes are measured every one to two hours. If the individual continues to excrete large volumes of dilute urine despite not taking in any fluids for several hours, then he or she will be given exogenous antidiuretic hormone (ADH).

If the person has central DI, then administering the ADH rapidly corrects the problem; the urine volumes will quickly decrease, and the urine concentration will also increase. However, if the person has nephrogenic DI, the exogenous ADH will have no effect. Because there is the possibility of substantial fluid losses and development of volume depletion, hypotension (low blood pressure), and hypernatremia during this test, it is important that it be performed only in a closely monitored setting where there is an ability to make a rapid determination of the urine volume and concentration and the serum sodium and the opportunity to provide emergency medical care, if needed.

### Treatment Options and Outlook

If the disorder is mild, advising the individual to drink much more water may be all that is required to treat the cause, and the consumption of 2–2.5 liters of water per day may be sufficient. However, in many cases of central DI,

desmopressin is the recommended treatment. This drug is given with a transdermal injection or nasal spray or an oral pill. Note that when the individual with DI takes desmopressin, he or she is advised to drink fluids *only* when thirsty in order to avoid an excess of fluids.

Desmopressin is *not* prescribed for the individual with nephrogenic DI. Instead, with nephrogenic DI, the individual is prescribed hydrochlorothiazide (HCTZ) and/or indomethacin. HCTZ is a diuretic medication, but paradoxically, it is also the drug of choice for nephrogenic DI, and it can result in *decreased* urination in the case of a person with nephrogenic DI. As with central DI, the person with nephrogenic DI who is taking medication for this disorder should *not* drink fluids unless he or she is thirsty.

### Risk Factors and Preventive Measures

Sometimes DI is inherited, but there are no known means to prevent inherited diabetes insipidus or other forms of DI. Once the cause of the diabetes insipidus is identified, it is treated to prevent the development of any further symptoms.

See also ELECTROLYTES AND ELECTROLYTE IMBALANCES; MEDICATIONS THAT CAN HARM THE KIDNEYS.

Bichet, Daniel G. "Polyuria and Diabetes Insipidus." In *Seldin and Giebisch's The Kidney: Physiology and Pathophysiology*. Vol. 1, edited by Robert J. Alpern and Steven C. Hebert, 1,225–1,247. Burlington, Mass.: Academic Press, 2008.

Palevesky, Paul. "Hypernatremia." In *Primer on Kidney Diseases*, 4th ed., edited by Arthur Greenberg, M.D., 66–73. Philadelphia, Pa.: Saunders, 2005.

Petit, William A., Jr., M.D., and Christine Adamec. *The Encyclopedia of Endocrine Diseases and Disorders*. New York: Facts On File, 2005.

Rivard, Christopher J., and Laurence Chan, "Hypernatremic States." *Seldin and Giebisch's The Kidney: Physiology and Pathophysiology*. Vol. 1, edited by Robert J. Alpern and Stephen C. Hebert, 1,203–1,224. Burlington, Mass.: Academic Press, 2008.

**diabetes mellitus** A serious disease that is related to either an insufficiency of the insulin that is made by the body (Type 1 diabetes) or to a decreased ability of the body to use the insulin that is present (Type 2 diabetes). Individuals with either type of diabetes have an increased risk for CHRONIC KIDNEY DISEASE as well as for kidney failure (END-STAGE RENAL DISEASE); in fact, diabetes is the number one cause for kidney failure in the United States, followed by hypertension. Many individuals with diabetes also have hypertension, further exacerbating their risk for chronic kidney disease and kidney failure. However, according to the National Institutes of Health (NIH), with good care, less than 10 percent of diabetics will ultimately develop kidney failure.

Type 1 diabetes is usually first identified in children and adolescents, and it is treated with the administration of insulin. Regular testing of blood glucose levels and the adjusting of insulin doses and dietary food intake is the cornerstone of therapy. In general, the closer that the blood glucose is maintained to normal, the fewer long-term complications that will ensue. The patient with diabetes must also be monitored for common complications, such as kidney disease and eye disease. Type 1 diabetes represents about 5 percent of all the cases of diabetes in the United States.

In contrast, Type 2 diabetes is often associated with OBESITY and/or elderly age, and often does not develop until adulthood, although obese adolescents can develop Type 2 diabetes. Type 2 diabetes is increasing in prevalence in the United States as more people are overweight or obese; for example, according to the Centers for Disease Control and Prevention (CDC), about two-thirds of all Americans are overweight and about 25 percent are obese. Type 2 diabetes represents about 95 percent of all cases of diabetes mellitus.

During pregnancy, some women will develop gestational diabetes mellitus (GDM), a form of diabetes that presents only during pregnancy. Women with GDM must be very careful about their diet and may need to use insulin during the pregnancy. They are likely to develop GDM with each pregnancy, and they are also at an increased risk for developing Type 2 diabetes at some point subsequent to their pregnancy. The high blood glucose levels during pregnancy can lead to the increased risk of complications during delivery and can cause growth abnormalities in the fetus.

### Symptoms and Diagnostic Path

Common symptoms of diabetes mellitus include the following indicators:

- frequent urination
- extreme thirst
- chronic fatigue
- itching skin

If the physician suspects that a patient has diabetes, he or she will order laboratory tests to determine its presence, such as the oral glucose tolerance test (OGTT) or the fasting plasma glucose test (FPGT). Another test is the Hemoglobin A1c test, which shows an approximation of the average blood glucose levels over a period of about three months. This test is particularly useful in assessing the individual's long-term response to therapy.

It is also important for the person with diabetes to keep his or her blood pressure under good control, and the goal for most people with diabetes is a blood pressure reading of approximately 120/80. Hypertension in combination with diabetes can lead to an increased chance of developing severe kidney disease (including kidney failure) as well as a stroke or heart attack.

### Treatment Options and Outlook

Diabetes is treated based on the form of the disease as well as its severity. Individuals with Type 1 diabetes must receive insulin. In most cases, individuals with Type 2 diabetes may be treated with oral medications; however, some individuals will need insulin as well. It is also extremely important that all patients with diabetes monitor their blood sugar levels by testing their blood at least once per day. (The individual's doctor will tell him or her how frequently the blood should be tested.)

According to the National Diabetes Education Program (NDEP), whole blood values before meals should be in the range of 80–120, and the levels one to two hours just after meals should be below 170.

Some actions that may cause blood glucose levels to increase include

- eating foods that are high in sugar or easily processed carbohydrates
- exercising less than usual
- infections
- stress
- eating more than usual
- some medications
- not taking diabetes medications

Blood sugar levels can also drop too low (hypoglycemia), and some things that can make the blood glucose levels fall are

- exercising more than usual
- eating less than usual or skipping a meal
- taking more insulin than needed
- taking too much diabetes medication

### Risk Factors and Preventive Measures

Type 1 diabetes cannot be prevented yet, but ongoing research is investigating new treatment options in those at risk. However, Type 2 diabetes can be avoided by many people at risk by losing weight, increasing physical activity, and decreasing carbohydrate intake. Other risk factors for individuals developing Type 2 diabetes include the following:

- age greater than 45 years
- having a baby that weighs more than 9 pounds at birth
- hypertension

- high-density cholesterol levels of under 35
- high blood levels of triglycerides
- a low activity level
- a poor diet
- a past history of gestational diabetes, or diabetes that occurred only during pregnancy
- the race or ethnicity of African American, Hispanic American, or Native American

SMOKING cigarettes also appears to be related to an increased risk for the development of Type 2 diabetes.

Specialists can help improve the outcome of patients with diabetes who develop complications. For example, research has shown that patients with both diabetes and moderately severe to severe chronic kidney disease who are treated by a NEPHROLOGIST for their kidney disease have a lower risk of death than other patients.

Diabetes of either Type 1 or Type 2 is a risk factor for the subsequent development of kidney disease and also for kidney failure. If diabetes is primarily implicated in kidney disease, this condition is known as DIABETIC NEPHROPATHY. With diabetic nephropathy, both kidneys are affected. The highest risk for kidney failure occurs when individuals with diabetes have HYPERTENSION as well. This condition may lead to protein in the urine (PROTEINURIA). At least an annual test for microalbuminuria is indicated for patients diagnosed with diabetes mellitus.

It is very important for patients with diabetes to keep their hypertension under the best control that is possible with both diet and medications. In addition, if a patient with diabetes has or may have a bladder infection (CYSTITIS), then he or she should immediately inform the physician. An untreated bladder infection can ultimately lead to a kidney infection (PYELONEPHRITIS).

In contrast to what is believed by most people, individuals with diabetes can safely eat some foods that contain sugar as long as their glucose levels are not very high. In addition, some people with diabetes experience a rapid dropping of their glucose levels to hypoglycemia, in which case they need emergency doses of sugar or other carbohydrates.

Although kidney disease cannot always be prevented by individuals with diabetes, there are some steps that individuals can take to reduce the likelihood of kidney disease. These include the following:

- Keep the blood glucose as close to normal as possible. Use daily testing to determine the glucose level and make dietary adjustments as needed.
- Keep the blood pressure approximately 120/80 in order to help prevent kidney damage. Individuals who take medication for their blood pressure should be sure to take the medicine as directed.
- Follow the dietary program recommended by the doctor. If an individual with diabetes already has kidney problems, the dietitian may recommend that the person should cut back on foods high in protein, such as meat.
- Have urine checked at least annually for microalbuminuria (small amounts of protein in the urine), which could indicate a kidney problem.
- Have the blood tested at least annually for creatinine levels. This laboratory test is used to estimate the GLOMERULAR FILTRATION RATE (GFR), which measures kidney function and can detect problems.
- When possible, avoid taking painkillers on a regular basis, such as aspirin or acetaminophen (Tylenol). Frequent use of these over-the-counter drugs can be harmful to the kidneys. Note that some doctors may recommend a low dose of daily aspirin to protect the heart.
- If there are symptoms of a bladder infection (cystitis) or a kidney infection, the individual should see the doctor immediately for testing. If an infection is present, it should be treated right away.
- If early signs of kidney disease develop, certain medications, specifically ACEIs and ARBs

have been shown to decrease the risk of worsening kidney disease. In general, patients with diabetes and proteinuria or an impaired glomerular filtration rate should use either an ACEI or ARB unless there is a significant countervening reason.

See also DIALYSIS; KIDNEY TRANSPLANTATION; MEDICATIONS THAT CAN HARM THE KIDNEYS; PREDIABETES.

Beaser, Richard S., M.D., and the Staff of Joslin Diabetes Center. *Joslin's Diabetes Deskbook: A Guide for Primary Care Providers*. 2nd ed. Boston, Ma.: Joslin Diabetes Center, 2007.
*Diabetes Mellitus: A Guide to Patient Care*. Ambler, Pa.: Lippincott Williams & Wilkins, 2007.
Petit, William A., Jr. M.D., and Christine Adamec. *The Encyclopedia of Diabetes*. 2nd ed. New York: Facts On File, 2011.
Tseng, Chin-Lin, et al. "Survival Benefit of Nephrologic Care in Patients with Diabetes Mellitus and Chronic Kidney Disease." *Archives of Internal Medicine* 168, no. 1 (January 14, 2008): 55–62.

**diabetic nephropathy**  Kidney damage that is related to or or caused by DIABETES MELLITUS, whether it is caused by Type 1 diabetes or Type 2 diabetes. Diabetic nephropathy is the leading cause of kidney failure (END-STAGE RENAL DISEASE) in the United States and it is also a leading cause of morbidity (illness) and mortality (death) in both Type 1 and Type 2 diabetic patients. The likelihood of developing kidney failure is similar in patients with Type 1 and Type 2 diabetes. Because 90–95 percent of all diabetics have Type 2 diabetes, the prevalence of diabetic nephropathy is much greater with Type 2 diabetes. It should also be noted that patients who develop diabetic nephropathy often have diabetic retinopathy, a severe eye disease which leads to blindness if not identified and treated in time. Thus, the problem of blindness may be added to that of kidney failure.

According to the United States Renal Data System (USRDS) Annual Report published in

**TABLE 1: INCIDENCE OF REPORTED DIABETIC ESRD PATIENTS, BY STATE AND TERRITORY, 2007**

| State or Territory | Number |
|---|---|
| **States** | |
| Alabama | 899 |
| Alaska | 59 |
| Arizona | 1,052 |
| Arkansas | 427 |
| California | 6,061 |
| Colorado | 441 |
| Connecticut | 409 |
| Delaware | 146 |
| District of Columbia | 132 |
| Florida | 2,873 |
| Georgia | 1,595 |
| Hawaii | 368 |
| Idaho | 157 |
| Illinois | 1,975 |
| Indiana | 959 |
| Iowa | 313 |
| Kansas | 308 |
| Kentucky | 690 |
| Louisiana | 960 |
| Maine | 119 |
| Maryland | 892 |
| Massachusetts | 686 |
| Michigan | 1,629 |
| Minnesota | 498 |
| Mississippi | 563 |
| Missouri | 917 |
| Montana | 79 |
| Nebraska | 233 |
| Nevada | 361 |
| New Hampshire | 103 |
| New Jersey | 1,585 |
| New Mexico | 373 |
| New York | 3,095 |
| North Carolina | 1,548 |
| North Dakota | 90 |
| Ohio | 2,134 |
| Oklahoma | 638 |
| Oregon | 366 |
| Pennsylvania | 2,149 |
| Rhode Island | 112 |
| South Carolina | 836 |
| South Dakota | 100 |
| Tennessee | 1,035 |
| Texas | 4,668 |
| Utah | 218 |
| Vermont | 46 |
| Virginia | 1,233 |
| Washington | 660 |
| West Virginia | 385 |
| Wisconsin | 642 |
| Wyoming | 37 |
| **Territories** | |
| American Samoa | 12 |
| Guam | 76 |
| Puerto Rico | 868 |
| Saipan | 21 |
| Virgin Islands | 30 |
| **All** | **48,871** |

Source: Adapted from United States Renal Data System. *USRDS 2009 Annual Data Report.* Vol. 3: *Reference Tables on ESRD in the United States.* Bethesda, Md.: National Institutes of Health, National Institute of Diabetes and Digestive and Kidney Diseases, 2009, p. 445.

The data reported here have been supplied by the United States Renal Data System (USRDS). The interpretation and reporting of these data are the responsibility of the authors and in no way should be seen as an official policy or interpretation of the U.S. government.

2009, in the year 2007, 48.5 percent of Medicare patients with end-stage renal disease had diabetes as the cause of their kidney disease.

There was an incidence (new cases) of 48,871 individuals in the United States with diabetes and end-stage renal disease (ESRD) in 2007, according to the USRDS. The largest numbers of individuals with diabetic nephropathy were located in California (6,061), Texas (4,668), and New York (3,095). (See Table 1 for more information.)

In terms of the prevalence (all cases) of diabetic ESRD, there were 634.8 patients per million population with this disorder who were alive on December 31, 2007, according to the USRDS. The highest prevalence of diabetic nephropathy was found among individuals ages 65–74 years or 2,562.7 per million. There were also gender and racial and ethnic differences: Males were more likely to have diabetic ESRD than females in 2007, and African Americans had the highest rate of diabetic ESRD (1,492.3 per million), followed by Native Americans (1,363.5 per million). See Table 2 for more information.

**TABLE 2: POINT PREVALENT RATES OF REPORTED DIABETIC ESRD IN 2007**

(Patients Alive on December 31, 2007) per Million Population, by Age, Gender, Race, and Ethnicity

| Factor | Rate |
|---|---|
| **Age** | |
| 0–4 | 0.5 |
| 5–9 | - |
| 10–14 | - |
| 15–19 | 0.8 |
| 20–29 | 26.7 |
| 30–39 | 211.0 |
| 40–49 | 542.0 |
| 50–59 | 1,232.9 |
| 60–64 | 1,976.9 |
| 65–69 | 2,516.9 |
| 70–79 | 2,435.4 |
| 80–84 | 1,652.4 |
| 85+ | 743.8 |
| **Gender** | |
| Male | 691.0 |
| Female | 580.2 |
| **Race and ethnicity** | |
| White | 486.1 |
| African American | 1,492.3 |
| Native American | 1,363.5 |
| Asian | 599.2 |
| Hispanic | 740.8 |
| Non-Hispanic | 615.8 |
| **All** | **634.8** |

Source: Adapted from United States Renal Data System. *USRDS 2009 Annual Data Report.* Vol. 3: *Reference Tables on ESRD in the United States.* Bethesda, Md.: National Institutes of Health, National Institute of Diabetes and Digestive and Kidney Diseases, 2009, p. 459.

The data reported here have been supplied by the United States Renal Data System (USRDS). The interpretation and reporting of these data are the responsibility of the authors and in no way should be seen as an official policy or interpretation of the U.S. government.

## Symptoms and Diagnostic Path

Diabetic nephropathy is characterized by the development of urinary protein losses (PROTEIN-URIA) that are due to the effects of the associated hyperglycemia on the kidneys. In the very earliest stages of diabetic nephropathy, abnormal amounts of albumin, a protein normally found in the blood and not in the urine, can be detected in the urine. Low concentrations of albumin (30–300 mg/gm creatinine) are termed microalbuminuria and higher concentrations (greater than 300 mg/gm creatinine) are termed macroalbuminuria. This sign is readily there to be identified, but the test must be ordered.

In the early stages of diabetic nephropathy, the glomerular filtration rate (GFR) may be normal or even increased. As the condition progresses, both albuminuria and proteinuria increase and the GFR decreases. Patients with early stages of diabetic nephropathy may have normal blood pressure, but as the condition advances, almost all will develop HYPERTENSION. Otherwise, there are no specific symptoms of diabetic nephropathy.

A KIDNEY BIOPSY is generally not needed in this condition. If performed, nodular glomerulosclerosis, also known as Kimmelstiel-Wilson lesion, is characteristic of diabetic nephropathy. Patients with diabetes may also have kidney disease from any of the many other causes of kidney disease. Nevertheless, the most common cause of kidney disease in patients with diabetes mellitus is diabetic nephropathy.

The American Diabetes Association recommends that patients with Type 1 disease be tested for microalbuminuria (low levels of urinary albumin) beginning five years after their initial diagnosis of diabetes and then yearly thereafter. It also recommends that patients diagnosed with Type 2 diabetes mellitus should be screened for diabetic kidney disease when they are first diagnosed with diabetes, and then yearly thereafter.

## Treatment Options and Outlook

Research has established that it is possible to either prevent or delay the progression of diabetic nephropathy in at-risk diabetic patients with the use of intensive control of blood glucose (blood sugar) levels to as close to normal as possible and with intensive blood pressure control as well. In addition, medications that are inhibitors of the renin-angiotensin system, specifically ANGIOTENSIN-CONVERTING ENZYME INHIBITORS (ACEIs) and ANGIOTENSIN II RECEPTOR BLOCKERS (ARBs), have been shown to be protective against kidney disease. Patients need to work closely with their doctors to maintain tight control of their diabetes and of their high blood pressure, if hypertension is present, and also to insure that they are using appropriate medications.

Because microalbuminuria often progresses to the worse stage of macroalbuminuria (a high volume of albumin in the urine), it is important to diagnose microalbuminuria as early in the disease as possible and before macroalbuminuria develops. ACEIs and ARBs can decrease the microalbuminuria and slow the development of macroalbuminuria, and also slow the decrease in GFR. According to the USRDS, about 77 percent of diabetic individuals with chronic kidney disease use ACE inhibitors, ARBs or renin inhibitors.

In rare cases, neither ACE inhibitors nor ARBs can be used by patients. In such cases, other ANTIHYPERTENSIVE DRUGS, often in the classes of CALCIUM CHANNEL BLOCKERS, BETA BLOCKERS, or DIURETICS, are used for hypertension control. They may also be necessary as additional medications for blood pressure control or for treatment of other medical conditions. To the extent that lowering the blood pressure slows the progression of diabetic nephropathy, these medications are also effective in treating diabetic nephropathy. Whether they are effective in slowing the progression of diabetic nephropathy beyond their effect on blood pressure is not known.

### Risk Factors and Preventive Measures

Diabetic kidney disease is a problem occurring more commonly in African-American, Native American, Polynesian, and Maori populations. More than 50 percent of Pima Indian diabetics develop diabetic nephropathy as young as age 20. In addition, more than one-third of diabetic Pima Indians will develop ESRD requiring dialysis therapy. Patients with Type 1 diabetes typically develop diabetic nephropathy beginning 10 to 15 years after the onset of their diabetes. Approximately one in four patients with Type 2 diabetes will have microalbuminuria 15 years after the onset of their diabetes. With Type 2 diabetes, the timing of the onset of renal involvement is more difficult, in part because the onset of their diabetes is more gradual and the time of the onset often cannot be definitively determined. As techniques to control blood glucose have improved,

and angiotensin-converting enzyme inhibitors and angiotensin receptor blockers are used early in patients with diabetic nephropathy, the overall rates of developing renal failure from diabetic nephropathy have decreased.

Ideally, diabetic nephropathy is avoided altogether. Several strategies to try to achieve this goal of avoiding renal failure from diabetic nephropathy include

- tight control of blood sugar
- early detection of microalbuminuria, when effective therapies can still be instituted, by with an annual measurement of the urinary albumin-creatinine ratio
- strict control of hypertension and the early use of medications such as angiotensin-converting enzyme inhibitors or angiotensin receptor blockers
- detection and treatment of abnormal lipid patterns
- whenever possible, avoidance of medications that could cause kidney damage

See also CHRONIC KIDNEY DISEASE; DIALYSIS; KIDNEY TRANSPLANTATION; MEDICATIONS THAT CAN HARM THE KIDNEYS; PREDIABETES.

Beaser, Richard S., M.D. and the Staff of Joslin Diabetes Center. *Joslin's Diabetes Deskbook: A Guide for Primary Care Providers.* 2nd ed. Boston, Ma.: Joslin Diabetes Center, 2007.

Johnson, Susan L., M.D., et al. "Who Is Tested for Diabetic Kidney Disease and Who Initiates Treatment." *Diabetes Care* 29, no. 8 (August 2006): 1,733–1,738.

Maeda, Shiro. "Review: Genetics of Diabetic Nephropathy." *Therapeutic Advances in Cardiovascular Disease* 2 (2008): 363–371.

Radbill, B., B. Murphy, and D. LeRoith. "Rationale and Strategies for Early Detection and Management of Diabetic Kidney Disease." *Mayo Clinic Proceedings* 83, no. 12 (2008): 1,373–1,381.

United States Renal Data System. *USRDS 2009 Annual Data Report: Atlas of Chronic Kidney Disease and End-Stage Renal Disease in the United States.* Bethesda, Md.: National Institutes of Health, National Institute of Diabetes and Digestive and Kidney Diseases, 2009.

**dialysis** The process by which the individual's bloodstream is cleansed of toxins and of extra fluids when his or her kidneys are no longer sufficiently functional to maintain health. Dialysis may be necessary because of END-STAGE RENAL DISEASE (ESRD), the last stage of CHRONIC KIDNEY DISEASE; an ACUTE KIDNEY INJURY; or it may be necessary for treatment of a potentially lethal overdose of a medicine or other chemical. Most people with dialysis must continue receiving dialysis to live unless they receive a KIDNEY TRANSPLANTATION; however, some individuals recover from their kidney failure, and thus, dialysis can be discontinued. Such a situation may occur when medication or disease caused a temporary dysfunction of the kidneys and the cause has been identified, treated, and resolved.

There are two major forms of dialysis that are used to treat individuals with kidney failure in the United States: HEMODIALYSIS and PERITONEAL DIALYSIS. Hemodialysis is a process in which blood is removed from the body and travels through a dialysis machine that both removes the wastes from the blood and adds back compounds which are needed, and then returns the blood back into the body in a continuous process. In contrast, with peritoneal dialysis, a special catheter in the abdominal cavity (the peritoneum) is used to alternately fill and then empty the abdomen with dialysis solution. Compounds and chemicals that are in the body and that are present in excess can diffuse into this fluid, and they are then removed from the body when the fluid is drained. Hemodialysis is the most common therapy for patients diagnosed with ESRD in the United States who receive dialysis, and it is used with more than 90 percent of all dialysis patients.

### Considering the Numbers on Dialysis

According to the National Kidney and Urologic Diseases Information Clearinghouse (NKUDIC), 341,319 individuals in the United States received dialysis treatment in 2005. Statistics from 2005 show that if one looks at those patients who are still alive for 91 days after starting dialysis, 78.3 percent will be alive one year after starting dialysis and 63.6 percent will be alive after two years. However, only 10.3 percent will be alive after 10 years. There are about 3,500 dialysis centers in the United States as of this writing in 2010.

In more recent data, according to the United States Renal Data System (USRDS), 99,886 individuals in the United States with ESRD began receiving hemodialysis in 2007, and 6,376 people began peritoneal dialysis in 2007. (See Table 1.)

**TABLE 1: COUNTS OF DIALYSIS AT INITIATION BY AGE, GENDER, RACE, ETHNICITY, AND PRIMARY DIAGNOSIS IN THE UNITED STATES, 2007, AMONG PATIENTS WITH ESRD**

| Characteristic | Hemodialysis | Peritoneal Dialysis |
|---|---|---|
| **Age** | | |
| 0–19 | 636 | 419 |
| 20–44 | 11,656 | 1,153 |
| 45–64 | 37,141 | 2,717 |
| 65–74 | 23,492 | 1,183 |
| 75 and older | 26,961 | 904 |
| **Gender** | | |
| Male | 56,049 | 3,385 |
| Female | 43,837 | 2,991 |
| **Race and ethnicity** | | |
| White | 64,995 | 4,612 |
| African American | 29,759 | 1,365 |
| Native American | 1,113 | 61 |
| Asian | 4,019 | 338 |
| **Hispanic Status** | | |
| Hispanic | 12,711 | 771 |
| Non-Hispanic | 87,175 | 5,605 |
| **Primary diagnosis** | | |
| Diabetes | 44,664 | 2,565 |
| Hypertension | 28,637 | 1,511 |
| Glomerulonephritis | 6,145 | 809 |
| Cystic kidney | 1,766 | 374 |
| Other urologic | 1,367 | 74 |
| Other cause | 12,693 | 766 |
| Unknown/missing data | 4,614 | 277 |
| **All** | **99,886** | **6,376** |

Adapted from United States Renal Data System. *USRDS 2009 Annual Data Report: Atlas of Chronic Kidney Disease and End-Stage Renal Disease in the United States.* Bethesda, Md.: National Institutes of Health, National Institute of Diabetes and Digestive and Kidney Diseases, 2009, p. 252.

Note: The data reported here have been supplied by the United States Renal Data System (USRDS). The interpretation and reporting of these data are the responsibility of the authors and in no way should be seen as an official policy or interpretation of the U.S. government.

**TABLE 2: PREVALENCE COUNTS AND ADJUSTED RATES PER MILLION POPULATION IN THE UNITED STATES BY AGE, GENDER, RACE, ETHNICITY, AND PRIMARY DIAGNOSIS, AMONG PATIENTS WITH ESRD, 2007**

| Characteristic | Numbers of Patients | | Rate per Million Population | |
|---|---|---|---|---|
| | Hemodialysis | Peritoneal Dialysis | Hemodialysis | Peritoneal Dialysis |
| **Age** | | | | |
| 0–19 | 1,228 | 838 | 14 | 9.8 |
| 20–44 | 46,089 | 5,560 | 432 | 52.3 |
| 45–64 | 136,608 | 11,470 | 2,032 | 161.3 |
| 65–74 | 76,155 | 4,752 | 4,450 | 256.6 |
| 75 and older | 73,535 | 3,132 | 4,686 | 179.1 |
| **Gender** | | | | |
| Male | 183,436 | 13,328 | 1,323 | 93.0 |
| Female | 150,179 | 12,424 | 881 | 76.5 |
| **Race and Ethnicity** | | | | |
| White | 184,527 | 16,967 | 702 | 65.8 |
| African American | 129,084 | 6,848 | 4,050 | 194.9 |
| Native American | 5,022 | 326 | 2,003 | 120.9 |
| Asian | 14,982 | 1,611 | 1,212 | 118.2 |
| **Hispanic status** | | | | |
| Hispanic | 48,268 | 3,124 | 1,774 | 96.8 |
| Non-Hispanic | 285,347 | 22,628 | 1,023 | 82.6 |
| **Primary diagnosis** | | | | |
| Diabetes | 147,272 | 8,758 | 473 | 28.2 |
| Hypertension | 95,420 | 6,388 | 308 | 20.7 |
| Glomerulonephritis | 33,492 | 4,519 | 109 | 14.8 |
| Cystic kidney | 8,276 | 1,353 | 27 | 4.4 |
| Other urologic | 6,641 | 590 | 22 | 1.9 |
| Other cause | 29,753 | 3,078 | 97 | 10.1 |
| Unknown/missing data | 12,761 | 1,066 | 41 | 3.5 |
| All | 333,615 | 25,752 | 1,076 | 83.5 |

Adapted from United States Renal Data System. *USRDS 2009 Annual Data Report: Atlas of Chronic Kidney Disease and End-Stage Renal Disease in the United States.* Bethesda, Md.: National Institutes of Health, National Institute of Diabetes and Digestive and Kidney Diseases, 2009, p. 254.
Note: The data reported here have been supplied by the United States Renal Data System (USRDS). The interpretation and reporting of these data are the responsibility of the authors and in no way should be seen as an official policy or interpretation of the U.S. government.

The prevalence of those receiving dialysis is important. The *prevalence* refers to everyone who receives dialysis in a year; the term *incidence* refers to only those who newly started receiving dialysis in that year. According to the USRDS, the prevalence for hemodialysis in the United States in 2007 was 333,615 people, while 25,752 individuals received peritoneal dialysis. (See Table 2.)

When considering ethnicity, the highest rates of individuals needing dialysis in 2007 occurred among African Americans, according to data from the USRDS, with a rate of 4,050 per million African Americans requiring renal replacement hemodialysis. The next highest rates were seen among American Indians/Native Americans. This is significant data, because if considering only the sheer numbers of the members of a racial group, the majority of individuals in the United States who have ESRD are white, but the proportion of African Americans who have ESRD is greater.

The presence of some diseases increases the risk for kidney failure and the need for dialysis. Among all individuals receiving dialysis in 2007, 37 percent had DIABETES MELLITUS and 24 percent had HYPERTENSION. (See DIABETIC NEPHROPATHY.)

### Elderly Individuals Receiving Dialysis

Some individuals who receive dialysis are elderly; according to the USRDS, 26,961 individuals ages 75 years and older in the United States began receiving hemodialysis and 904 began receiving peritoneal dialysis in 2007. (See Table 1.) Some individuals who are receiving dialysis are *very* elderly, in their late eighties or nineties, although experts report that the patient survival in this group is only modest. The number of octogenarians and nonogenerians receiving dialysis increased from 7,054 people in 1996 to 13,577 in 2003, according to Manjula Kurella, M.D., and colleagues in their article for *Annals of Internal Medicine*.

### Children and Dialysis

When their kidneys fail, children must receive either dialysis or a kidney transplantation to survive, as with adults. Sometimes a preemptive transplantation is used, when experts believe that dialysis will be an imminent issue, and this enables the child to receive a donated kidney before dialysis begins.

If a child does need dialysis, he or she will receive either hemodialysis or peritoneal dialysis, as will adult patients needing dialysis. With hemodialysis, the child usually will receive three treatments per week, but more frequent treatments may be required in small children. Children need at least a few weeks to adjust to dialysis treatments. They will also need considerable emotional support from their parents or other caregivers; in some cases, parents must quit their jobs to provide the care that their child needs. The strain on the family of a child with kidney failure as a whole can be considerable, and it can cause tension within a marriage as well as emotional strains with other children in the family who may receive much less atten-

tion than they have received in the past because of a parental preoccupation with the sick child receiving dialysis.

Dietary changes are often needed with kidney failure as well as dialysis; for example, the child may need to be limited on the consumption of some foods, especially those that contain large amounts of PHOSPHORUS, such as cola drinks, milk, cheese, nuts, dried beans, and peas. The help of a dietitian is often necessary to aid the parent in making the necessary dietary changes. The child will also need to take medications known as phosphate binders, which are needed to lower the phosphate levels in the bloodstream.

Children whose kidneys fail are often eligible for Medicare, despite their youth, because of a Medicare program passed in 1972. (The child may also be eligible for Medicaid, if the parents' income and assets are limited.) However, Medicare alone may be insufficient to cover the medical bills, and a social worker may be able to help the parents identify other sources of financial aid. Even parents who are wealthy could find their funds quickly dissipated with the extensive expenses of dialysis.

### Patients Want Information on Dialysis

According to Adrian Fine and colleagues, based on their research, many physicians fail to provide survival information on dialysis unless it is specifically requested from them by their patients. These researchers studied 100 patients with chronic kidney disease, and the overwhelming majority of patients said that if they needed dialysis, they would want to know what their life expectancy with dialysis would be, as well as know the possible side effects of dialysis and the limitations on their quality of life that dialysis would present. Only 2 percent said that they did *not* want to know the possible side effects of dialysis, while 36 percent said that they would have an "absolute need to know the possible side effects of dialysis." In addition, only 2 percent said they would not want to know the limitations on their quality of life that

TABLE 3: PATIENT PREFERENCE FOR TYPE OF INFORMATION REQUESTED FROM PHYSICIAN

|  | Did Not Want to Know (%) | Would Like to Know (%) | Absolute Need to Know (%) |
|---|---|---|---|
| Possible side effects of dialysis | 2 | 62 | 36 |
| Limitations on quality of life | 2 | 59 | 39 |
| Actual life expectancy on dialysis | 8 | 54 | 38 |
| What dialysis does to the body | 4 | 59 | 37 |
| How effective is dialysis in other patients with similar health problems | 7 | 57 | 36 |
| What will be accomplished by dialysis | 6 | 53 | 41 |

Source: Fine, Adrian, et al. "Patients with Chronic Kidney Disease Stages 3 and 4 Demand Survival Information on Dialysis." *Peritoneal Dialysis International* 27, no. 5 (2007): 590. Permission to reprint granted from Multimed, Inc. in Ontario, Canada.

dialysis would present, while 39 percent said that they would have an absolute need to know this information.

As for their life expectancy on dialysis, only 8 percent of the subjects said that they did *not* want this information while 54 percent said that they would want this information, and 38 percent said that they would have an absolute need to receive this information and would like to receive the information without having to ask for it. (See Table 3 for more information.)

These researchers also found that the most frequently reported reason (89 percent) for individuals wanting information on life expectancy with dialysis was so that they could be more prepared to accept what happens with dialysis. In addition, 82 percent of the subjects said that they would like this information without having to prompt or ask their physicians to provide it to them. The researchers also noted that they found no difference in a desire for information between the subjects who had attended renal education classes and those who did not; the majority said that they would want information on their own specific cases should dialysis later become a necessity for them.

### International Comparisons of Hemodialysis and Peritoneal Dialysis

The percentage of patients who receive hemodialysis versus peritoneal dialysis varies from country to country, but in nearly all countries, the majority of patients receive hemodialysis rather than peritoneal dialysis. According to the USRDS, 92.0 percent of all dialysis patients in the United States receive hemodialysis. Based on data provided by the USRDS for dialysis received in 2007, 100 percent of dialysis patients in Bangladesh receive hemodialysis, followed by Argentina, with 96.1 percent. In contrast, in Jalisco, Mexico, 34.2 percent of dialysis patients received hemodialysis, followed by Hong Kong with 19.4 percent. The balance of the patients received peritoneal dialysis; for example, 7.2 percent of the patients in the United States received peritoneal dialysis and 65.8 percent of the dialysis patients in Mexico received peritoneal dialysis in 2007. (See Table 4 for more details.)

### Deaths of patients on dialysis

The need for dialysis, whether hemodialysis or peritoneal dialysis, is associated with an increased annual risk of dying. For example, according to the USRDS, the annual death rate among all individuals on hemodialysis in the United States in 2007 was 216.6 per 1,000 patient years, this has improved from 236.0 in 2003. The highest rates occurred among people with diabetes or hypertension, largely because most dialysis patients have either diabetes or hypertension. (See Table 5 for more details.) The patient year is a statistical term that considers the number of patients and the number of years

**TABLE 4: PERCENT DISTRIBUTION OF PREVALENT
DIALYSIS PATIENTS, BY MODALITY AND YEAR, 2007\***

| Country | Hemodialysis | Peritoneal Dialysis |
|---|---|---|
| Argentina | 96.1 | 3.9 |
| Australia | 68.4 | 21.8 |
| Austria | 91.2 | 8.7 |
| Bangladesh | 100.0 | 0.0 |
| Belgium, Dutch speaking | 89.2 | 10.6 |
| Belgium, French speaking | 90.5 | 8.3 |
| Bosnia/Herz. | 95.2 | 4.7 |
| Chile | 95.2 | 4.8 |
| Czech Republic | 92.3 | 7.7 |
| Denmark | 71.6 | 24.1 |
| Finland | 76.1 | 20.3 |
| France | 91.2 | 7.7 |
| Greece | 91.7 | 8.3 |
| Hong Kong | 19.4 | 80.4 |
| Hungary | 91.3 | 8.7 |
| Iceland | 72.1 | 26.2 |
| Israel | 92.9 | 7.1 |
| Jalisco (Mexico) | 34.2 | 65.8 |
| Japan | 96.4 | 73.5 |
| Korea | 80.2 | 19.8 |
| Malaysia | 89.9 | 9.1 |
| Netherlands | 76.1 | 21.7 |
| New Zealand | 48.6 | 35.9 |
| Norway | 80.7 | 19.0 |
| Philippines | 87.3 | 12.7 |
| Poland | 92.8 | 7.2 |
| Romania | 81.8 | 18.2 |
| Scotland | 80.4 | 17.7 |
| Spain | 89.4 | 10.5 |
| Sweden | 73.0 | 24.1 |
| Taiwan | 91.5 | 8.5 |
| Thailand | 94.5 | 5.5 |
| Turkey | 88.1 | 11.9 |
| United Kingdom | 78.7 | 19.3 |
| United States | 92.0 | 7.2 |
| Uruguay | 90.6 | 9.4 |

Adapted from United States Renal Data System. *USRDS 2009 Annual
Data Report: Atlas of Chronic Kidney Disease and End-Stage Renal
Disease in the United States.* Bethesda, Md.: National Institutes of
Health, National Institute of Diabetes and Digestive and Kidney
Diseases, 2009, p. 351.

\*According to this source, data for some countries does not represent
100 percent of the ESRD population.
Note: The data reported here have been supplied by the United States
  Renal Data System (USRDS). The interpretation and reporting of
  these data are the responsibility of the authors and in no way should
  be seen as an official policy or interpretation of the U.S. government.

that they are studied. Thus if 100 patients are
studied for 10 years, this is equivalent to 1,000
patient years. This term is used to help show
trends over time.

As can be seen from Table 5, in considering the
annual mortality (death) rates of all individuals
on hemodialysis in 2007, the rate was 216.6 per
1,000 patient years on hemodialysis. The highest
death rate in 2007 was found among those individuals who were ages 85 years and older (524.1
per 1,000). In addition, death rates were higher
among whites (246.6 per 1,000) than among
African Americans and also higher among those
with diabetes or hypertension. Interestingly,
weight is also associated with mortality. Heavier
patients on dialysis actually have a *lower* mortality rate than appropriate weight patients, in
an apparent protective effect, and patients who
are below their desired body weight have even
higher mortality rates.

### The Medicare End-Stage Renal Disease Program and Costs

The Medicare End Stage Renal Disease (ESRD)
Program in the United States helps to cover
the costs of the great majority of individuals
receiving treatment for end-stage renal disease
with either dialysis or a kidney transplant. To
be eligible for coverage, the person must have
ESRD and meet at least one of the following
criteria:

1. The individual must meet the required work
   credits under Social Security, Railroad Retirement, or as a government employee.
2. The individual is receiving Social Security or
   Railroad Retirement benefits.
3. The individual is the spouse or dependent
   child of a person who has met the required
   work credits or is receiving Social Security or
   Railroad Retirement benefits.

In 2006, more than 500,000 patients received
some form of end-stage renal disease therapy
in the United States, and Medicare spent nearly

TABLE 5: ANNUAL MORTALITY RATES AMONG HEMODIALYSIS PATIENTS, PER 1,000 PATIENT YEARS,
2003–2007, UNITED STATES

| Characteristic | 2003 | 2004 | 2005 | 2006 | 2007 |
|---|---|---|---|---|---|
| **Age** | | | | | |
| 0–4 | 262.2 | Unknown | 72.5 | 147.2 | 147.4 |
| 5–9 | 93.5 | 56.7 | 37.1 | 48.4 | 48.9 |
| 10–14 | 66.1 | 37.2 | 43.7 | Unknown | 51.3 |
| 15–19 | 51.5 | 43.4 | 35.1 | 48.8 | 31.1 |
| 20–29 | 60.8 | 58.5 | 58.9 | 57.1 | 53.6 |
| 30–39 | 87.0 | 83.1 | 80.8 | 80.4 | 80.0 |
| 40–49 | 125.1 | 122.1 | 122.1 | 117.2 | 109.7 |
| 50–59 | 167.8 | 165.0 | 158.0 | 159.9 | 151.7 |
| 60–64 | 219.6 | 212.1 | 202.5 | 201.0 | 191.4 |
| 65–69 | 255.5 | 250.3 | 245.3 | 236.7 | 229.9 |
| 70–79 | 331.7 | 328.6 | 324.7 | 314.8 | 303.9 |
| 80–84 | 433.7 | 421.3 | 426.9 | 419.2 | 408.1 |
| 85 and older | 550.9 | 534.7 | 539.3 | 528.2 | 524.1 |
| **Gender** | | | | | |
| Male | 229.5 | 226.6 | 223.6 | 219.9 | 212.2 |
| Female | 243.6 | 237.7 | 234.5 | 229.9 | 221.9 |
| **Race and ethnicity** | | | | | |
| White | 279.8 | 273.4 | 270.5 | 266.2 | 256.6 |
| African American | 186.4 | 185.4 | 181.5 | 177.4 | 170.6 |
| Other race | 180.4 | 174.6 | 172.5 | 166.1 | 161.0 |
| Hispanic | 187.8 | 181.5 | 177.8 | 169.7 | 159.4 |
| Non-Hispanic | 243.9 | 240.3 | 237.5 | 214.4 | 227.2 |
| **Primary diagnosis** | | | | | |
| Diabetes | 263.6 | 256.6 | 251.5 | 245.7 | 234.8 |
| Hypertension | 235.2 | 232.9 | 231.8 | 229.4 | 222.0 |
| Glomerulonephritis | 147.9 | 142.4 | 140.0 | 135.6 | 133.4 |
| Other cause | 229.6 | 227.2 | 222.6 | 218.0 | 211.2 |
| All | 236.0 | 231.7 | 228.6 | 224.5 | 216.6 |

Adapted from United States Renal Data System. *USRDS 2009 Annual Data Report: Atlas of Chronic Kidney Disease and End-Stage Renal Disease in the United States.* Bethesda, Md.: National Institutes of Health, National Institute of Diabetes and Digestive and Kidney Diseases, 2009, p. 633.
Note: The data reported here have been supplied by the United States Renal Data System (USRDS). The interpretation and reporting of these data are the responsibility of the authors and in no way should be seen as an official policy or interpretation of the U.S. government.

$23 billion to care for them, according to the United States Renal Data System's 2008 Annual Data Report. According to the USRDS report, in 2006, Medicare spent about $71,889 per year on a hemodialysis patient. They also spent about $53,327 per year on a peritoneal dialysis patient, and $24,952 per year on a transplant patient (who had already received the transplanted kidney).

Patients who are new to Medicare generally join the original Medicare Plan. If possible, they may join a Medicare Special Needs Plan, which is specific to people with kidney failure and other severe chronic health problems.

Table 6 shows the services and products that were covered by Medicare Part A and Part B in 2007, the most recent data as of this writing. Part A refers to hospital services and Part B refers to

## TABLE 6: DIALYSIS SERVICES AND SUPPLIES COVERED BY MEDICARE

| Service or Supply | Medicare Part A | Medicare Part B |
|---|---|---|
| Inpatient dialysis treatments (if you are admitted to a hospital for special care) | √ | |
| Outpatient dialysis treatments (when you get treatments in any Medicare-approved dialysis facility) | | √ |
| Self-dialysis training (includes instruction for you and for the person helping you with your home dialysis treatments) | | √ |
| Home dialysis equipment and supplies (like alcohol, wipes, sterile drapes, rubber gloves, and scissors) | | √ |
| Certain home support services (may include visits by trained hospital or dialysis facility workers to check on your home dialysis, to help in emergencies when needed, and to check your dialysis equipment and water supply) | | √ |
| Certain drugs for home dialysis (such as heparin to prevent blood clots, topical anesthetics to relieve pain and itching, and Epogea or Epoetin alfa to treat anemia) | | √ |
| Outpatient doctors' services | | √ |
| Most other services and supplies that are a part of dialysis like laboratory tests | | √ |

Source: Centers for Medicare & Medicaid Services. *Medicare Coverage of Kidney Dialysis and Kidney Transplant Services.* Baltimore, Md., 2007, pp. 18–19.

outpatient services. Readers should check with Medicare for the most current information.

### The Decision to Use Dialysis

In the case of patients with advancing kidney failure, prior to the initiation of dialysis, education and counseling on the need for renal replacement therapy is strongly recommended. Patients generally can avoid dialysis until their renal function is below about 15 percent of normal levels. Below this level, the time to initiate dialysis depends upon the evaluation of the patient's health and well-being as well as the results of blood work regarding various metabolic abnormalities associated with progressive kidney failure. The ultimate decision for the onset of dialysis depends on the mutual decisionmaking between the patient and the kidney specialist (NEPHROLOGIST).

Important indications that initiation of dialysis therapy may be needed include the following:

- progressive nausea, possibly vomiting, and anorexia (loss of appetite)
- progressive fatigue and weakness
- progressive weight loss and laboratory studies showing progress malnutrition, such as progressive lowering of the serum albumin level and the serum cholesterol

- an otherwise untreatable development of severely high potassium blood levels (HYPERKALEMIA)
- a lack of bicarbonate or the acidosis of kidney failure.
- progressive fluid accumulation in the lungs or lower extremities that cannot be effectively treated with DIURETICS or other oral medications

Other biochemical complications that may develop as a consequence of advanced renal failure include such medical problems as the development of hypertension, ANEMIA, overactivity of the parathyroid glands (referred to as secondary HYPERPARATHYROIDISM), and vitamin D deficiency. Each of these can be treated with specific medications. However, some patients with severe secondary hyperparathyroidism require surgical removal of most, but not all, of their parathyroid glands (glands that are embedded in the thyroid gland in the neck) in order to return parathyroid gland activity back toward baseline levels.

### Considering Hemodialysis

During hemodialysis therapy, the blood is pumped out of the body and processed through an artifical kidney known as the dialyzer. The dialyzer filters the blood and removes impurities. (Some impurities cannot be removed.) It also enables compounds present in insufficient amounts in the blood to be filtered *into* the blood. Blood is pumped from the body and to the artificial kidney (the dialyzer) and returned to the patient continuously through the dialysis procedure. Although most hemodialysis is provided at outpatient dialysis centers, sometimes hemodialysis is provided to patients in the home.

According to the National Institute on Diabetes and Digestive and Kidney Diseases (NIDDK), individuals who are considering beginning hemodialysis should be sure to ask their health care team the following questions:

- Is hemodialysis the best treatment choice for me? Why?
- If I am treated at a center, can I go to the center of my choice?
- What should I look for in a dialysis center?
- Will my kidney doctor see me at dialysis?
- What does hemodialysis feel like?
- What is self-care dialysis?
- Is home hemodialysis available in my area? How long does it take to learn? Who would train my partner and me?
- What kind of blood access is best for me?
- As a hemodialysis patient, will I be able to keep working? Can I have treatments at night?
- How much should I exercise?
- Who will be on my health care team? How can these people help me?
- With whom can I talk about finances, sexuality, or family concerns?
- How/where can I talk with other people who have faced this decision?

### Peritoneal Dialysis (PD)

Peritoneal dialysis (PD) is a specialized procedure that uses the internal (peritoneal) membrane of the individual's body to help to remove the impurities that the failed kidneys can no longer remove. PD can be either performed during the day, a procedure that is sometimes referred to as continuous ambulatory peritoneal dialysis (CAPD), or it can be managed by an automatic cycler either during either the day or night, a procedure that is called continuous cycle-assisted peritoneal dialysis (CCPD).

Instead of pumping blood out of the body as with hemodialysis therapy, in peritoneal dialysis, the peritoneal membrane in the abdominal cavity functions as the dialysis filter. With PD, a flexible tube (called a PD catheter) is placed in the abdominal cavity. The PD catheter is used to place the PD dialysate fluid within the peritoneal cavity.

The toxic products that have accumulated will diffuse from the blood into the peritoneal dialysate along with excessive water that is present in the blood circulation. When the procedure is complete, this dialysate fluid from the peritoneal cavity is drained through the PD catheter and it is then replaced with the new PD fluid.

The major drawbacks of PD therapy are related to potential infections that may develop within the peritoneal cavity, which are referred to as PD-related peritonitis. In addition, an inability to achieve the correct fluid balance can sometimes be a problem. Most PD fluids are glucose-based, and patients with diabetes mellitus may need more intensive treatment of their blood sugar control as a result. However, non-glucose based PD solutions are also available. Another major issue is that the PD procedure requires the active involvement of the patient and/or an assistant, and it must be performed every day. If the patient and/or their assistant are not very careful with performing the procedure, the risk of infection increases.

With PD, patients must limit their salt and liquid intakes carefully, as is also true with hemodialysis; however, they need not be quite as strict with PD as is required with hemodialysis. However, patients on PD must eat more protein than is required by patients who are on hemodialysis.

According to the National Institute on Diabetes and Digestive and Kidney Diseases (NIDDK), patients who are considering peritoneal dialysis should ask their health care providers the following questions:

- Is peritoneal dialysis the best treatment choice for me? Why? If yes, which type is best?
- How long will it take me to learn how to do peritoneal dialysis?
- What does peritoneal dialysis feel like?
- How will peritoneal dialysis affect my blood pressure?
- How will I know if I have peritonitis (an infection of the peritoneum)? How is it treated?
- As a peritoneal dialysis patient, will I be able to continue working?
- How much should I exercise?
- Where do I store supplies?
- How often do I see my doctor?
- Who will be on my health care team? How can these people help me?
- Who do I contact with problems?
- With whom can I talk about finances, sexuality, or family concerns?
- How/where can I talk with other people who have faced this decision?

### Possible Side Effects of Dialysis

Patients receiving either form of dialysis may suffer from extreme itching (pruritus), which is triggered by the profusion of toxins in the blood. Sometimes, the dialyzer cannot remove all these itch-inducing toxins. Patients may try exposure to ultraviolet light to obtain relief from their extreme itching, or antihistamines may be helpful.

Patients on dialysis often have difficulty with insomnia, and they may also suffer from sleep apnea, which is a sleep disorder that is characterized by temporary cessations of breathing as well as severe snoring. These sleep problems may lead to a day-night reversal in which the person has insomnia at night and is sleepy in the daytime.

Another common problem among patients receiving dialysis is the development of DEPRESSION. It can be extremely difficult for patients to deal with the reality that one's very survival depends on the actions of a machine, and it is also hard to cope with the lack of freedom and the constraints involved with dialysis. Patients on dialysis may also experience anger and confusion.

Muscle cramps are common problems during hemodialysis treatments. The more fluid that is removed during the procedure, the more likely they are to occur, but they can occur even when minimal amounts of fluid are being removed. Typically, muscle cramps respond to temporary changes in the dialysis treatment, such as decreasing the rate of fluid removal. Patients can help to minimize these by limiting the amount of fluid gain between treatments.

Finally, the hemodialysis procedure often leaves a patient feeling tired and fatigued after the procedure. The extent to which this occurs is variable, but seems to parallel the extent of overall health problems that the patient has.

### Diet Is Important in Dialysis

The person receiving dialysis must carefully watch his or her diet, in order to avoid generating any extra fluid. In addition, those foods that are high in phosphorus (such as milk, cheese, dried beans, nuts, and peanut butter) should be limited. Excess phosphorus intake can lead to high serum phosphorus levels, which increase the risk for cardiovascular disease, worsen secondary hyperparathyroidism and lead to increased mortality rates. The consumption of salt should also be limited because salt leads to both higher blood pressure and increased thirst, which then leads to increased fluid intake. With increased fluid intake, more fluid must then be removed during the dialysis procedure, which leads to greater rates of cramping, hypotension (low blood pressure), and, for many patients, fatigue after the procedure. Patients also need to realize that many canned foods are very high in salt. As a result, fresh foods and vegetables are significantly better for the person receiving dialysis.

People on dialysis are generally encouraged to eat a high-quality protein diet, including such foods as fish, meat, poultry, and eggs. Renal failure often causes changes in appetite, which can lead a person to eat less protein, which then leads to worsening nutrition. Maintaining optimal nutrition is essential for maintaining health in the person with renal failure requiring dialysis.

Individuals on dialysis should take only those particular vitamins and minerals that are specifically prescribed or recommended by their physicians, and they should completely avoid all other vitamins or minerals that can be purchased in a store or elsewhere or that could be prescribed by other physicians unless the nephrologist specifically recommends taking these substances. The reason for this constraint is that sometimes over-the-counter (OTC) supplements and items which are regarded as alternative remedies may contain materials that can be very harmful to the person receiving dialysis.

See also GLOMERULONEPHRITIS.

Fine, Adrian, et al. "Patients with Chronic Kidney Disease Stages 3 and 4 Demand Survival Information on Dialysis." *Peritoneal Dialysis International* 27, no. 5 (2007): 589–591.

Kimmel, Paul L., Karen Weihs, and Rolf A. Peterson. "Survival in Hemodialysis Patients: The Role of Depression." *Journal of the American Society of Nephrology* 4, no. 1 (1993): 12–27.

Kurella, Manjula, M.D., et al. "Octogenarians and Nonogenarians Starting Dialysis in the United States." *Annals of Internal Medicine* 146 (2007): 177–183.

National Institute of Diabetes and Digestive and Kidney Diseases. *Kidney Failure: Choosing a Treatment That's Right for You.* Bethesda, Md.: NIDDK, 2007.

United States Renal Data System. *USRDS 2009 Annual Data Report: Atlas of Chronic Kidney Disease and End-Stage Renal Disease in the United States.* Bethesda, Md.: National Institutes of Health, National Institute of Diabetes and Digestive and Kidney Diseases, 2009.

**dialysis, hemodialysis**  See HEMODIALYSIS.

**dialysis, peritoneal**  See PERITONEAL DIALYSIS.

**diet**  See DIETARY CHANGES.

**dietary changes**  With some kidney diseases, it is important for individuials to make changes to their diet to decrease the risk of a recurrence of the disease or to improve their current health and avoid deterioration; for example, individuals who are prone to KIDNEY STONES that are caused by a substance known as oxalate will need to cut back on their consumption of oxalate-rich foods, such as nuts, spinach, rhubarb, wheat bran, chocolate, and sweet potatoes. Doing so should effectively decrease a recurrence of painful kidney stones in the future.

In another case, individuals who are suffering from GOUT should avoid a diet that is heavy in choices of seafood and meat, which are likely to increase their level of uric acid and the risk for a recurrence of the severe pain of gout. (Antigout medications are also usually necessary, such as allopurinol.)

Individuals whose kidneys have failed and who are undergoing DIALYSIS need to avoid foods that are high in PHOSPHORUS, such as milk, cheese, nuts, and cola drinks. Those who must receive dialysis may need to consult with a dietitian to plan their own individual diets effectively. Individuals with CHRONIC KIDNEY DISEASE–MINERAL BONE DISORDER (CKD-MBD) must also be careful to restrict their consumption of foods that are high in phosphorus content to avoid further bone problems.

For those on dialysis, the level of salt consumption should be low to avoid increasing the individual's blood pressure and also triggering thirst, which then increases the overall fluid consumption, a problem with dialysis. In addition, individuals on dialysis are generally advised to eat high levels of protein, as with fish, meat, poultry, and eggs.

Individuals who have HYPERKALEMIA (high potassium levels) will need to decrease their consumption of POTASSIUM-rich foods, in order to avoid making their condition worse. Individuals who have been diagnosed with AMYLOIDOSIS need to restrict their consumption of foods that are high in potassium or SODIUM. In sharp contrast, individuals with either BARTTER'S SYNDROME or GITELMAN SYNDROME need a diet of foods that are *high* in potassium content.

When the kidney disease is diagnosed, physicians will provide patients with advice on any types of foods they should avoid and will often provide a list of such foods. If the needed diet is very restrictive, it may be advisable for individuals to consult with a registered dietitian, who can help them understand what is needed and also help them plan menus.

See also CALCIUM; DAILY LIVING WITH MAJOR KIDNEY DISEASES; MAGNESIUM.

**diuretics** Medications prescribed to treat HYPERTENSION, often in conjunction with other ANTIHYPERTENSIVE DRUGS, and often the first line of therapy for hypertensive patients needing long-term treatment. They are also frequently effective in treating fluid retention that is associated with congestive heart failure, liver disease, CHRONIC KIDNEY DISEASE and NEPHROTIC SYNDROME. Thiazide diuretics have been used since the late 1950s and they continue to be effective at treating high blood pressure. There are also other forms of diuretics, including loop diuretics and potassium-sparing diuretics. Most thiazide diuretics can be prescribed once daily, which increases the likelihood of medication adherence. Thiazide diuretics decrease renal calcium excretion, which suggests the possibility of improved maintenance of bone density as compared with loop diuretics, which can increase urinary calcium loss. Thiazide diuretics interact with NONSTEROIDAL ANTI-INFLAMMATORY DRUGS (NSAIDs) and lead to the retention of SODIUM.

If thiazide diuretics are discontinued, the patient may gain weight, but according to Michael E. Ernst and Marvin Moser, M.D., in their 2009 article on diuretics for the *New England Journal of Medicine,* after discontinuing them, the blood pressure rises slowly and does not quickly reach pretreatment levels. The authors say, "With adherence to lifestyle modifications (e.g., weight loss, reduction in sodium and alcohol intake), nearly 70% of patients may not require antihypertensive medications for up to 1 year after long-term thiazide-based therapy is withdrawn."

Diuretics can lead to the development of some diseases; for example, they cause an elevated risk for GOUT. Because diuretics can cause HYPOKALEMIA, and hypokalemia can worsen blood glucose control, it is possible that these medications can worsen diabetes control. This can usually be minimized by ensuring that hypokalemia does not occur, or if does occur, that it is treated either with dietary maneuvers or with the addition of potassium-chloride containing medications. In addition, if the GLOMERULAR FILTRATION RATE falls significantly, thiazides become less effective. If patients have severe kidney disease or kidney failure, diuretics cannot be used.

| TABLE 1: DIURETICS | |
|---|---|
| **Brand Name** | **Generic Name** |
| Aldactazide | Spironolactone with hydrochlorthiazide |
| Aldactone | Spironalactone |
| Demadex | Torsemide |
| Diuril | Chlorothiazide |
| Enduron | Methylclothiazide |
| Microzide | Hydrochlorothiazide |
| Oretic | Hydrochlorothiazide |
| Lasix | Furosemide |
| | Indapamide |
| Saluron | Hydroflumethizide |
| Thalitone | Chlorthalidone |
| Zaroxolyn | Metolazone |

Another category of diuretics, the loop diuretics, act for only about six hours and often need to be taken twice per day, although some loop diuretics such as torsemide are longer acting and can be taken once per day.

Potassium-sparing agents are not considered effective diuretics for the treatment of hypertension but they are able to reduce potassium loss when used in conjunction with thiazide diuretics. In addition, they avoid urinary loss of magnesium.

Ernst and Moser concluded about diuretics, "With proper attention to appropriate selection, dosing, and monitoring, diuretic-based regimens can greatly improve the ability to achieve blood-pressure goals. Few pharmacologic discoveries have advanced the treatment of any disease in such a profound and enduring manner."

See also DIABETES INSIPIDUS; ELECTROLYTES AND ELECTROLYTE IMBALANCES; LITHIUM AND BIPOLAR DISORDER; MEDICATIONS THAT CAN HARM THE KIDNEYS.

Ernst, Michael E., and Marvin Moser, M.D. "Use of Diuretics in Patients with Hypertension." *New England Journal of Medicine* 361 (2009): 2,153–2,164.

**dyslipidemia**  See CHOLESTEROL; RENAL ARTERY STENOSIS.

**dysplasia, renal**  See RENAL DYSPLASIA.

**ectopic kidney**   A birth defect that causes a kidney to lie in an unusual place in the body. It may cause no problems, and the patient may not even realize that he or she has an ectopic kidney unless it is discovered by accident during an imaging procedure for another problem, or it may cause medical problems such as urinary stones, a urine blockage, or an infection. It is believed that an ectopic kidney develops once in about every 1,000 births. An ectopic kidney can also increase the risk for the development of KIDNEY STONES, kidney infections (PYELONEPHRITIS), and even kidney failure and trauma to the kidney. In most cases, only one kidney is ectopic. Individuals who have ectopic kidneys and who participate in sports may need to wear protective gear around the mid–rib cage area which houses the kidneys.

### Symptoms and Diagnostic Path

Many patients with an ectopic kidney have no symptoms, but some individuals experience infections and/or urinary stones. Some individuals have abdominal pain with an ectopic kidney. The ectopic kidney often has decreased function; since there are two kidneys, a single ectopic kidney with decreased function often does not cause symptoms related to the decreased renal function.

In the most severe cases of ectopic kidney, especially if both kidneys are ectopic, the kidneys may fail altogether, necessitating either DIALYSIS or a KIDNEY TRANSPLANTATION in order to sustain the patient's life. Sometimes the physician may identify a lump within the abdomen during a physical examination and this discovery may lead to the diagnosis of ectopic kidney.

Complications may also occur such as a reflux of the urine from the bladder and back into the kidney. This is termed vesicoureteral reflux and can lead to increased risk of repeated kidney infections (pyelonephritis).

Often the ectopic kidney is unknown until it is discovered during tests that are ordered for other purposes, such as an ultrasound, X-rays, a nuclear scan, a computerized tomography (CT) scan, or a magnetic resonance imaging (MRI) scan.

Ectopic kidneys can occur in association with other developmental abnormalities. Abnormal development of the uterus and vagina can occur in girls and abnormalities in testicular and penis development can occur in boys. Ectopic kidney can also occur in association with adrenal, cardiac, or skeletal abnormalities or as a clinical feature in complex developmental disorders.

### Treatment Options and Outlook

If the ectopic kidney is causing no symptoms or problems, then usually nothing is done; however, if there is hydronephrosis (swelling of the kidney), then surgery may be indicated to remove the ectopic kidney. This should cause no problems as long as the individual's other kidney is functioning normally. In contrast, if the ectopic kidney is damaged extensively, it may need to be surgically removed. If an obstruction is present, surgery may be needed to improve the drainage of the urine. When vesicoureteral reflux leads to repeated infections, prophalyactic (preventive) antibiotics may be helpful.

### Risk Factors and Preventive Measures

There are no known risk factors or preventive measures to an ectopic kidney.

National Kidney and Urologic Diseases Information Clearinghouse. "Ectopic Kidney." April 2007. Available online. URL: http://kidney.niddk.nih.gov/Kudiseases/pubs/pdf/EctopicKidney.pdf. Accessed November 5, 2010.

**elderly and chronic kidney disease**  The elderly are the fastest growing subset of the population in developed countries, and CHRONIC KIDNEY DISEASE (CKD) has been recognized as one of several chronic diseases that primarily affect adults over the age of 65 years. About two-thirds of all patients receiving kidney DIALYSIS are ages 60 years and older, and an estimated 14 percent of these patients are ages 80 years and older.

Elderly people are particularly prone to the development of CKD due to age-related physiological changes. Similarly, age-related changes in the kidneys and the blood supply to the kidneys increase the likelihood of developing CKD; for example, as individuals age, the blood flow to the kidneys decreases. This decreased blood flow in turn decreases the filtration rate from the kidneys, which manifests itself as a decrease in the GLOMERULAR FILTRATION RATE (GFR). In addition, age-related changes in individual functioning units of the kidneys (the nephrons) occur as renal blood flow and GFR diminish over time in elderly persons. Different studies have demonstrated that there is a substantial decrease in kidney function that may start as early as age 30. However, what is not well understood is how much of this decrease in kidney function results from other medical conditions that often develop along with aging, such as HYPERTENSION, DIABETES MELLITUS and CARDIOVASCULAR DISEASE. It would appear that combinations of these factors are important to explain the decrease in kidney function with aging.

In some cases, elderly patients may have CKD despite a normal serum creatinine level. Serum creatinine levels decrease when an individual loses muscle mass. Thus, parallel decreases in both muscle mass, which happens commonly as a result of aging, and in kidney function may result in either no detectable or only minimal change in the serum creatinine level. Using the estimated glomerular filtration rate (eGFR) formula, which takes into account many of the factors that alter the association of the serum creatinine with level of kidney function, is important in order for physicians to accurately assess renal function in the elderly.

### Medications and the Elderly

Prescribed medications should be calibrated to the needs of the individual patient as well as to his or her age. For example, some categories of antidepressants are not indicated for elderly individuals or they are indicated only at lower dosages, including antidepressants in such categories as tricyclics (older antidepressants such as imipramine or desipramine); newer antidepressants (such as serotonin-norepinephrine reuptake inhibitors (SNRIs), including such drugs as venlafaxine/Effexor or duloxetine/Cymbalta); or atypical antidepressants, such as bupropion (Wellbutrin, Wellbutrin XL).

### Aging and the Kidneys

In addition to decreased GFR, aging also decreases and slows the kidneys' ability to respond to normal daily variations. For example, in the younger individual, the absence of fluid intake results in maximal decreases in urine volume within one day, whereas in the elderly individual, the kidney may require three or four days to adapt to new conditions. Since fever and infections can alter fluid intake and losses (in the form of sweat), the elderly individual may be more susceptible to dehydration as a result of the kidney's slowed ability to respond.

### Symptoms and Diagnosis of Kidney Disease in the Elderly

Many people, if not the majority of those with kidney disease, including those who are ages 65 years and older, have no symptoms of kidney disease. However, KIDNEY STONES, if present, can cause severe pain, causing most people to call their doctors or go to a hospital emergency department as soon as possible. Advanced kidney disease typically causes only high blood pressure, fatigue, and decreased appetite, symptoms which may have many other causes, particularly in the elderly.

Kidney disease is diagnosed based on the physician's examination and the laboratory findings. Kidney function is typically measured with simple blood tests. The most commonly used assessment of renal function is the estimated GFR (eGFR), which is based on the serum creatinine and takes into account the individual's age, gender, race, and serum creatinine level to provide an assessment of renal function. A 24-hour urine collection test, a test that was frequently performed in the past, is not routinely necessary at present. A simple urinalysis can detect the presence of bacteria in the urine, and the urine can also be cultured to determine the specific type of bacteria that is present. A renal ultrasound test is frequently performed to assess the size and shape of the kidneys and to identify easily treatable causes of kidney disease.

### Treatment of Elderly Individuals with Kidney Disease

If kidney disease is identified in an elderly person, the treatment depends on the cause of the problem. If the patient has a bacterial illness, then antibiotics will usually be administered. In other cases, other medications as needed can be given to treat chronic kidney disease. If the kidney disease is very advanced and has already led to kidney failure, then the only therapy that will work is kidney dialysis or a KIDNEY TRANSPLANTATION.

In elderly patients with END-STAGE RENAL DISEASE (kidney failure), the presence or absence of other major diseases (significant comorbidity) is much more important than the chronological age of the patient when the physician chooses the appropriate renal replacement treatment option. For example, the choice between hemodialysis and continuous ambulatory peritoneal dialysis (the two forms of dialysis) is largely dependent on the preferences of the local team and the patient. Patients who are relatively healthy other than their kidney disease may benefit particularly from a kidney transplant, whereas those with significant disease affecting their other organs may not benefit.

The number of octogenarians (people aged 80 to 89) and nonagenarians (people 90 to 99) who are beginning dialysis is increasing rapidly. However, these individuals have a high mortality (death) rate even with normal kidney function, and the risk of death increases with kidney disease. Because hemodialysis can cause substantial fatigue in the 12 to 24 hours following a treatment session and because all types of dialysis involve the need for specialized surgical procedures with their own risks of complications, the decision when and in whom to start dialysis treatments in the elderly is often a difficult decision.

### Kidney Transplantations

A growing number of elderly patients are being evaluated for and receiving a kidney transplant each year. Transplant outcomes in the elderly have significantly improved since 1990; however, concerns about limited life expectancy, other existing chronic diseases, and the relative organ shortage remain unchanged. Only the permanent shortage of suitable kidneys limits the ability of physicians to treat all individuals who, despite their age, could benefit from transplantation. It should be noted, however, that immunosuppression in older patients must often be modified because older age is generally associated with a depressed immune response to infection as well as to organ transplantation.

### Risk Factors for Kidney Failure and Kidney Disease among Elderly Patients

Older African Americans have a higher rate of kidney failure than individuals of other races and ethnicities, which may be because African Americans of all ages have a higher rate of diabetes. Diabetes is the leading cause of kidney failure, followed by hypertension. (It is also true that African Americans in general have a higher rate of kidney failure.) Individuals with hypertension and/or diabetes mellitus also have an increased risk for the development of chronic kidney disease. Researchers have also found that obesity is another factor causing kidney failure, and African Americans also have a higher rate of OBESITY than other races.

Preventive measures for kidney disease include regular screening with urine and laboratory tests so that individuals with any markers that indicate disease can be treated as early as possible.

See also DIABETIC NEPHROPATHY; MEDICATIONS THAT CAN HARM THE KIDNEYS; NEPHROTIC SYNDROME.

Bloembergen, W. E., F. K. Port, E. A. Mauger, and R. A. Wolfe. "A Comparison of Mortality between Patients Treated with Hemodialysis and Peritoneal Dialysis." *Journal of the American Society of Nephrology* 6 (1995): 177–183.

Brugts, Jasper L., et al. "Renal Function and Risk of Myocardial Infarction in an Elderly Population: The Rotterdam Study." *Archives of Internal Medicine* 165 (2005): 2,659–2,665.

Corsonello, Andrea, et al. "Concealed Renal Insufficiency and Adverse Drug Reactions in Elderly Hospitalized Patients." *Archives of Internal Medicine* 165 (2005): 790–795.

Davison, Sara N., M.D. "Chronic Kidney Disease: Psychosocial Impact of Chronic Pain." *Geriatrics* 62, no. 2 (February 2007): 17–23.

Kandel, Joseph, M.D., and Christine Adamec. *The Encyclopedia of Elder Care.* New York: Facts On File, 2008.

Kurella, Manjula, M.D., et al. "Octogenarians and Nonagenarians Starting Dialysis in the United States." *Annals of Internal Medicine* 146 (2007): 177–183.

Macías Núñez, Juan-Florencia, et al. "Biology of the Aging Process and Its Clinical Consequences." In *The Aging Kidney in Health and Disease,* edited by Juan-Florencio Macías Núñez, M.D., J. Stewart Cameron, M.D., and Dimitrios G. Oreopoulos, M.D., 55–91. New York: Springer Science+Business Media, 2008.

Rifken, Dena E., M.D., et al. "Rapid Kidney Function Decline and Mortality Risk in Older Adults." *Archives of Internal Medicine* 168, no. 20 (November 10, 2008): 2,212–2,218.

U.S. Renal Data System. *USRDS 2008 Annual Data Report: Atlas of Chronic Kidney Disease and End-Stage Renal Disease in the United States.* Bethesda, Md.: National Institutes of Health, National Institute of Diabetes and Digestive and Kidney Diseases, 2008.

Zhou, Xin J., Zoltan G. Laszik, and Fred G. Silva. "Anatomical Changes in the Aging Kidney." In *The Aging Kidney in Health and Disease,* edited by Juan F. Macías Núñez, M.D., J. Stewart Cameron, M.D., and Dimitrios G. Oreopoulos, M.D., 39–54. New York: Springer Science+Business Media, 2008.

**electrolytes and electrolyte imbalances** Electrolytes are electrically charged ions and small compounds that are present in the blood and for which accurate regulation of their amount in the blood is necessary for normal health. Examples include POTASSIUM, CALCIUM, MAGNESIUM, and SODIUM. In some cases, the electrolyte balance is affected, such as when a person suffers extreme diarrhea, excessive perspiration, or END-STAGE RENAL DISEASE (kidney failure). In the most serious cases, the person may need to be hospitalized for correction of abnormal electrolyte concentrations. If the individual is not treated, he or she may die.

The substance Gatorade, now a commercially marketed drink, was originally developed at the University of Florida in Gainesville to correct electrolyte imbalances and volume depletion that was caused by physical exertion in healthy individuals.

Sometimes an instability/imbalance of one or more of the electrolytes in the blood occurs, including an imbalance of potassium (the most common form of electrolyte imbalance), and also imbalances of the other key minerals. If one or more electrolytes are out of the normal range (either too low or too high), this then indicates that a problem is present; for example, temporary electrolyte imbalances may be caused by severe diarrhea and/or profuse sweating, as well as by the failure of the individual to drink sufficient fluids. In addition, because the kidneys control the electrolyte levels, kidney failure leads to an electrolyte imbalance, which is remedied by DIALYSIS or by a KIDNEY TRANSPLANTATION.

See also DIURETICS; MEDICATIONS THAT CAN HARM THE KIDNEYS.

**employment** Although not true of everyone, some people with severe kidney disease or even kidney failure continue to work. Some researchers have found some individuals are more likely to continue to work after kidney transplants or when they need dialysis. For example, in a study of 411 individuals who received kidney transplants in the United States, reported in *Social Work and Health Care* in 2007, less than half continued to work after their transplant. Those who continued to work were more likely to be white males who regarded themselves as having a higher level of physical functioning than those who did not continue to work after their transplant. The researchers found that physical factors, such as diabetic status and blood creatinine levels, were not significant predictors of whether individuals worked after a kidney transplant.

Receiving dialysis decreases the rate of work among kidney patients, based on several studies. For example, in a study of 659 patients ages 18–65 in the Netherlands who were in their first year of dialysis, reported in *Peritoneal Dialysis International* in 2001, the researchers found that 31 percent of hemodialysis patients and 48 percent of peritoneal dialysis patients were working at the start of their dialysis, compared to 61 percent of the general population. Within one year, the percentage of patients receiving hemodialysis who worked decreased to 25 percent and the percentage of peritoneal patients who worked decreased to 40 percent. The researchers found that risk factors for job loss within a year were impaired physical and psychological functioning.

In a more recent study on patients receiving dialysis who were employed, published in 2008 in the *Clinical Journal of the American Society of Nephrology,* the researchers studied the employment status of more than 105,000 patients ages 18 to 54 nationwide in the United States. They found that 18.9 percent of the patients were employed but there were very broad variations by facility, and employment rates ranged from the extremes of zero to 100 percent. The

researchers also found that offering a late dialysis shift as well as peritoneal or home hemodialysis training and more frequent hemodialysis were factors that were associated with higher employment rates in patients at dialysis facilities.

### Considering Work Accommodations

Accommodations at work may need to be made but experts say that the common myths about people with kidney disease (or about people with disabilities in general) should be challenged. (See Table 1.) Some people with severe kidney disease may wish to take a leave of absence from work or take a short-term disability to work part time. However, many patients with chronic kidney disease may be completely asymptomatic, and their kidney disease has no impact on their employability or work production.

Individuals with chronic kidney disease who need time off for laboratory tests or to see their

**TABLE 1: MYTHS ABOUT EMPLOYMENT OF PEOPLE WITH DISABILITIES VERSUS REALITIES**

| Employers May Believe . . . | The Department of Labor Says . . . |
|---|---|
| On-the-job safety is a concern when hiring workers with disabilities. | People with disabilities do not have more accidents, so hiring them does not raise worker's compensation costs to employers. |
| Workers with disabilities produce less. | A DuPont study shows that workers with disabilities produce as well or better than other workers. |
| Workers with disabilities are costly to accommodate. | Most workers with disabilities do not need special accommodations. When they do, most accommodations cost less than $50. |
| Workers with disabilities miss too much work. | A DuPont study shows that disabled people do not miss more work than other employees. |

Source: Life Options Rehabilitation Program. *Employment: A Kidney Patient's Guide to Working & Paying for Treatment,* 2003, p. 43. Available online. URL: http://www.lifeoptions.org/catalog/pdfs/booklets/employment.pdf. Accessed November 3, 2010.

doctors can try to schedule their visits to be the least problematic for the employer, such as at lunchtime or other times when they are less needed.

If the person with kidney disease is looking for a new job, the employer may be able to obtain a Work Opportunities tax credit or a Disabled Access tax credit. The state vocational rehabilitation office may be able to assist the individual in obtaining employment. See Appendix II for further information.

See also DAILY LIVING WITH MAJOR KIDNEY DISEASES.

Kutner, Nancy, et al. "Dialysis Facility Characteristics and Variation in Employment Rates: A National Study." *Clinical Journal of the American Society of Nephrology* 3 (2008): 111–116.

Raiz, L., and Monroe, J. "Employment Post-Transplant: A Biopsychosocial Analysis." *Social Work and Health Care* 45, no. 3 (2007): 19–37.

Van Manen, Jeannette G., et al. "Changes in Employment Status in End-Stage Renal Disease Patients during Their First Year of Dialysis." *Peritoneal Dialysis International* 21 (2001): 595–601.

**end-stage renal disease (ESRD)** The most severe stage of CHRONIC KIDNEY DISEASE, at which point the kidneys fail. Chronic kidney disease progresses from Stage 1, which is a very mild form of kidney disease, and Stage 2, also a mild stage, to the moderate and severe Stages 3–5. In Stage 5, which is also ESRD, the patient is either receiving DIALYSIS or will imminently need either dialysis or a KIDNEY TRANSPLANTATION in order to survive. Not everyone with chronic kidney disease progresses to the final stage of kidney disease, and some remain at the earlier stages. Some also die of other diseases before their kidneys deteriorate to the level of Stage 5. The earlier stages of chronic kidney disease usually precede ESRD by at least 10 years, but this can be highly variable, depending on the underlying cause of renal disease. In rare cases, ACUTE KIDNEY INJURY (AKI) may not reverse and may result in ESRD.

Survival rates for individuals with ESRD who receive dialysis are 79 percent after one year, 64 percent after five years, and 10 percent after 10 years, according to the National Center for Health Statistics. The survival rates are significantly better for patients who receive kidney transplants from a live donor: 98 percent of these individuals survive after one year and 77 percent survive after 10 years. If the kidney donor was deceased, patient survival is also better than with dialysis, or a 94 percent survival rate after one year and a 61 percent survival rate after 10 years.

### Individuals Suffering from ESRD: Demographic Data

Among those with ESRD, in considering rates per million, research has revealed that the highest rates in the United States are seen among individuals who are male, elderly, African American, Native American, or Hispanic, as well as among those with DIABETES MELLITUS and/or HYPERTENSION. The absolute numbers of white individuals with ESRD are greater than other races and ethnicities, but when actual rates are considered, the highest rates of ESRD occur among African Americans, followed by Native Americans. See Table 1 for further information on rates and demographic characteristics.

In considering racial and ethnic groups at high risk for ESRD in the United States from 1995–2005, Nilka Rios Barrows and colleagues reported in a 2008 issue of *Advances in Chronic Kidney Disease* that there were much higher age-adjusted incidence (new cases) rates for blacks and other minorities compared to whites; for example, in 2005, the incidence rates of ESRD for whites was 254.8 per million. In contrast, the rate for blacks with ESRD was nearly four times higher, at 936.8 cases per million people. The next highest rate was among Native Americans, or 559.9 per million, followed by a rate of 448.9 for Hispanics and 350.9 for Asians.

More recently (Table 1) in 2007, rates for whites were up to 293.3 per million compared

### TABLE 1: INCIDENT RATES OF REPORTED END-STAGE RENAL DISEASE PER MILLION POPULATION BY AGE, GENDER, RACE, ETHNICITY, AND PRIMARY DIAGNOSIS, 2007

| Characteristic | Rate per Million Population |
| --- | --- |
| **Age** | |
| 0–4 | 10.8 |
| 5–9 | 6.0 |
| 10–14 | 14.6 |
| 15–19 | 28.3 |
| 20–29 | 65.5 |
| 30–39 | 141.0 |
| 40–49 | 269.2 |
| 50–59 | 548.4 |
| 60–64 | 873.8 |
| 65–69 | 1,166.1 |
| 70–79 | 1,538.7 |
| 80–84 | 1,718.5 |
| 85 and older | 1,101.0 |
| **Gender** | |
| Male | 410.3 |
| Female | 313.1 |
| **Race and ethnicity** | |
| White | 293.3 |
| African American | 783.4 |
| Native American | 381.7 |
| Asian | 328.0 |
| **Hispanic status** | |
| Hispanic | 300.6 |
| Non-Hispanic | 371.8 |
| **Primary Diagnosis** | |
| Diabetes | 158.4 |
| Hypertension | 100.8 |
| Glomerulonephritis | 24.7 |
| Cystic kidney | 8.6 |
| Other urologic | 5.0 |
| Other cause | 46.4 |
| Unknown cause | 15.3 |
| Missing disease | 1.9 |
| **All** | 361.0 |

Adapted from United States Renal Data System. *USRDS 2009 Annual Data Report: Atlas of Chronic Kidney Disease and End-Stage Renal Disease in the United States.* Bethesda, Md.: National Institutes of Health, National Institute of Diabetes and Digestive and Kidney Diseases, 2009, p. 433.

Note: The data reported here have been supplied by the United States Renal Data System (USRDS). The interpretation and reporting of these data are the responsibility of the authors and in no way should be seen as an official policy or interpretation of the U.S. government.

to 783.4 per million for African Americans and 381.7 per million for Native Americans.

The high risk for kidney failure among African Americans may be due to a higher rate of diabetes, hypertension, OBESITY, and other factors that are in play among African Americans, although research is ongoing on the causes for the higher rates of ESRD in this racial group. There is also evidence that African Americans have kidneys that are more susceptible to hypertension-induced damage.

In his study of laboratory abnormalities at the onset of treatment for kidney failure, Michael M. Ward, M.D., reported in *Archives of Internal Medicine* in 2007 his findings that black patients and members of other minority groups had significantly more severe laboratory abnormalities when initially starting their treatment for ESRD compared to the white patients. Ward's sample included more than 515,000 people, including white, black, Hispanic, Asian/Pacific Islander, American Indians, and individuals of other races and ethnicities. Their average age was 61.3 years. Ward also found that black patients were 20 percent less likely to be treated with the predialysis use of erythropoietin than were white patients. In addition, Hispanic patients and American Indian patients were also significantly less likely to receive this predialysis treatment.

African Americans with diabetes and hypertension, the two diseases that are the leading causes of ESRD, have an even higher risk for kidney failure than other African Americans with neither diabetes or hypertension. In a study by Chi-yuan Hsu, M.D., and colleagues published in the *Archives of Internal Medicine* in 2009, the researchers analyzed 177,570 individuals starting in 1964–73 and following up with them through December 31, 2000. The researchers were seeking risk factors for the development of ESRD. They found that some factors were predictive for kidney failure, such as male sex, older age, African-American race, proteinuria (the presence of protein in the urine), and a diagnosis of diabetes mellitus.

### Other Factors Predictive for ESRD

Hsu and colleagues found other factors predictive for ESRD, such as a lower educational attainment, higher blood pressure, and a higher body mass index. The two most powerful factors, however, were PROTEINURIA and obesity. In addition, the researchers found other predictive factors for kidney failure, such as lower hemoglobin levels, higher serum uric acid levels, a self-reported history of nocturia (having to urinate frequently at night), and a family history of kidney disease.

**Obesity and the risk for kidney failure** Some experts report that there is a link between obesity and an increased risk for ESRD. In a study of more than 320,000 individuals over the period of 1964–85, researchers Chi-Yuan Hsu and colleagues analyzed ESRD among those with high rates of body mass index (BMI), reporting on their findings in a 2006 issue of the *Annals of Internal Medicine*. The BMI is a derived number that considers both height and weight to determine a specific number. Individuals whose BMI is 30.0 or greater are considered obese, and those with a BMI of 35.0 or greater are extremely obese. Hsu et al. found that a high BMI was both a common and a strong risk factor for ESRD.

**Age and kidney failure** Elderly people have an increased risk for kidney failure. Older people are also increasingly receiving dialysis and kidney transplants. As the large bulk of baby boomers age, there will be greater numbers of people with kidney failure, particularly since many people in this group are obese and hypertensive.

Older patients are more likely than younger patients to have kidney failure that is caused by Type 2 diabetes and/or hypertension rather than by glomerulonephritis or other conditions. Many older patients also have other health problems, complicating their treatment for kidney failure.

Sometimes doctors delay treatment with dialysis for elderly patients because their creatinine levels are misleading. Elderly patients typically have a lower amount of total body muscle than younger patients. Because creatinine, which is used to assess kidney function, results from muscle metabolism, then less muscle mass in elderly patients can result in lower serum creatinine levels than in younger patients. The increasing use of the estimated glomerular filtration rate (eGFR), which takes into account these age-related changes in muscle mass and creatinine production, helps to avoid this problem.

According to Dimkovic and Oreopoulos in their chapter in *The Aging Kidney in Health and Disease,* "An early referral may avoid subclinical uremic manifestations and malnutrition and enable the team to provide better salt and water balance, to better control anemia, and to minimize overall morbidity and mortality."

Moderate to severe malnutrition is a common issue among about 10 percent of all patients who undergo dialysis, but among elderly people the rate of malnutrition is as high as 20 percent, possibly due to social isolation, low income, and gastrointestinal disorders, as well as poor appetite, depression, chronic constipation, and other factors. Malnutrition is also linked to an increased risk for death.

### Patients at High Risk for Kidney Failure

In a study that was published in 2009 in the *Journal of the American Society of Nephrology* by Stein Hallan, M.D., and his colleagues in Norway, the researchers found that it was possible to predict which patients would develop kidney failure based on their glomerular filtration rate (GFR) and their urinary albumin levels. The researchers analyzed data from more than 65,000 patients, identifying 124 patients who developed kidney failure after 10 years of followup. Using the GFR and urinary albumin levels, the researchers were able to predict greater than 65 percent of the patients who ultimately developed kidney failure.

### Causes of ESRD

The most common causes of ESRD are diabetes mellitus and hypertension, and diabetes (including both Type 1 and Type 2 diabetes) is the leading cause. Either diabetes or hypertension is the underlying cause of renal failure in 80–85 percent of patients with ESRD. There are other causes for ESRD, such as GLOMERULONEPHRITIS and autosomal dominant POLYCYSTIC KIDNEY DISEASE.

***Considering diabetes and ESRD***    When diabetes mellitus causes kidney failure, this is referred to as DIABETIC NEPHROPATHY or sometimes as diabetic kidney disease. Up to 40 percent of individuals with both Type 1 and Type 2 diabetes may develop kidney disease, and the disease may progress to kidney failure. It is important to note, however, that most people with diabetes do not develop ESRD. With treatment, in many cases, chronic kidney disease can be arrested so that it never reaches the level of kidney failure. Individuals with diabetes should work with their physicians to keep their glucose levels and their blood pressure as close to normal as possible. Specific medications, such as ANGIOTENSIN-CONVERTING ENZYME INHIBITORS (ACEIs) and ANGIOTENSIN II RECEPTOR BLOCKERS (ARBs), can help to slow the progression of diabetic nephropathy and thereby delay or even prevent the development of ESRD.

According to the United States Renal Data System (USRDS), in the United States in 2007 there were 48,871 new patients with kidney failure and diabetes, with the greatest number in California (6,061) and the least number in American Samoa (12 people). See Table 2 for more information.

***Hypertension and ESRD***    High blood pressure is the second leading cause of kidney failure in the United States after diabetes. Individuals with kidney failure should work with their physicians to try to maintain as normal a blood pressure as possible by taking their medications faithfully, losing weight if they are obese, and getting regular exercise, as well as taking other recommended actions, such as eating a healthy diet, avoiding SMOKING, and avoiding alcohol.

***Glomerulonephritis and kidney failure***    The inflammation of the glomeruli (internal kidney structures), also known as glomerulonephritis, increases the risk for kidney failure. Some disorders are linked to the development of glo-

**TABLE 2: INCIDENCE COUNTS OF REPORTED ESRD PATIENTS WITH DIABETES, BY STATE AND TERRITORY, 2007**

| States | |
|---|---|
| Alabama | 899 |
| Alaska | 59 |
| Arizona | 1,052 |
| Arkansas | 427 |
| California | 6,061 |
| Colorado | 441 |
| Connecticut | 409 |
| Delaware | 146 |
| District of Columbia | 132 |
| Florida | 2,873 |
| Georgia | 1,595 |
| Hawaii | 368 |
| Idaho | 157 |
| Illinois | 1,975 |
| Indiana | 959 |
| Iowa | 313 |
| Kansas | 308 |
| Kentucky | 690 |
| Louisiana | 960 |
| Maine | 119 |
| Maryland | 892 |
| Massachusetts | 686 |
| Michigan | 1,629 |
| Minnesota | 498 |
| Mississippi | 563 |
| Missouri | 917 |
| Montana | 79 |
| Nebraska | 233 |
| Nevada | 361 |
| New Hampshire | 103 |
| New Jersey | 1,585 |
| New Mexico | 373 |
| New York | 3,095 |
| North Carolina | 1,548 |
| North Dakota | 90 |
| Ohio | 2,134 |
| Oklahoma | 638 |
| Oregon | 366 |
| Pennsylvania | 2,149 |
| Rhode Island | 112 |
| South Carolina | 836 |
| South Dakota | 100 |

| | |
|---|---|
| Tennessee | 1,035 |
| Texas | 4,668 |
| Utah | 218 |
| Vermont | 46 |
| Virginia | 1,233 |
| Washington | 660 |
| West Virginia | 385 |
| Wisconsin | 642 |
| Wyoming | 37 |
| **Territories** | |
| American Samoa | 12 |
| Guam | 76 |
| Puerto Rico | 868 |
| Saipan | 21 |
| Virgin Islands | 30 |
| **All** | 48,871 |

Adapted from United States Renal Data System. *USRDS 2009 Annual Data Report: Atlas of Chronic Kidney Disease and End-Stage Renal Disease in the United States.* Bethesda, Md.: National Institutes of Health, National Institute of Diabetes and Digestive and Kidney Diseases, 2009, p. 445.
Note: The data reported here have been supplied by the United States Renal Data System (USRDS). The interpretation and reporting of these data are the responsibility of the authors and in no way should be seen as an official policy or interpretation of the U.S. government.

merulonephritis, such as FOCAL SEGMENTAL GLOMERULOSCLEROSIS, GOODPASTURE SYNDROME, IGA NEPHROPATHY, LUPUS NEPHRITIS, MEMBRANOPROLIFERATIVE GLOMERULONEPHRITIS I, membranoproliferative glomerulonephritis II, poststreptococcal glomerulonephritis, and rapidly progressive glomerulonephritis.

Individuals with kidney failure due to glomerulonephritis have the same symptoms as all people with kidney failure, such as fluid retention and the development of edema, fatigue, itching, and so forth. In addition, they may also experience blood in the urine. The disorder is usually discovered in a routine examination when a urinalysis is ordered and the results are abnormal.

**Cystic kidneys and ESRD** Polycystic kidney disease (PKD) is a genetic disorder which causes the kidneys to fill with thousands of cysts, with the key symptom of cysts forming in the kidneys. There are two forms of PKD, including autosomal dominant PKD (ADPKD), the most common form, and autosomal recessive PKD (ARPKD). ADPKD typically has an onset in adulthood. Asymptomatic cysts may be identified through imaging studies, such as renal ultrasound, at much earlier ages, including the teenage years and sometimes even earlier. ARPKD is a rare disease that typically begins in infancy or even during fetal development.

The most frequent symptoms of autosomal dominant PKD are hypertension, severe flank pain, frequent urinary infections, and blood in the urine (hematuria). Other symptoms may include kidney stones, abnormal heart valves, and cysts in the liver and pancreas. The disease is usually diagnosed with imaging studies such as renal ultrasound, computerized tomography (CT) scans, or magnetic resonance imaging (MRI) scans.

ADPKD frequently causes cysts to develop in other organs, including the liver, pancreas, and the ovaries. In the gastrointestinal tract, ADPKD can cause diverticuli (out-pouchings), particularly in the colon. These can lead to abdominal pain and/or infections. In the heart, ADPKD causes abnormalities in the heart valves. Generally, these effects on the heart valves do not causes symptoms. In the brain, ADPKD can lead to cerebral aneurysms, which can either be asymptomatic or can rupture, leading to severe headaches, permanent neurologic disease, or even death.

### Symptoms of ESRD
Patients with ESRD often have common symptoms, such as an unintentional weight loss, fatigue, nausea with or without vomiting, no urine output (anuria), or a greatly decreased urine output. People who have chronic kidney disease before the initiation of their dialysis therapy should receive annual vaccinations against influenza pneumonia and vaccinations every five years for pneumococcal pneumonia. In addition, immunization against hepatitis B should be performed irrespective of whether patients receive dialysis or a kidney transplant. Flu and pneumonia shots are free for dialysis

patients, and the hepatitis B shot is covered at the 80 percent rate by Medicare.

Patients who have been on dialysis for more than five years are at risk for dialysis-related AMYLOIDOSIS, an arthritis-like disorder than causes stiffness, pain, and fluid in the joints of the body. Dialysis cannot remove all the built-up proteins as well as can a working kidney, which is why many patients develop dialysis-related amyloidosis. These are side effects of ESRD, not of dialysis.

### The Health Care Team for Patients with Kidney Failure

Each person with kidney failure has a health care team. The central members of the health care team are the patient and the NEPHROLOGIST, an expert in treating kidney disease. The patient will also continue to see his or her primary care doctor. Note that if the primary care doctor prescribes any new medications, the patient's nephrologist needs to know right away. Patients with kidney failure also work with nurses and they also often work with a social worker who helps answer questions about kidney failure, family issues, paying for care and medications and related issues. A dietitian helps the patient with ESRD identify which foods to eat and which to avoid.

It is important for patients to talk with their doctors about issues and concerns, and it is also vitally important to take all medications as directed. In addition, it is not recommended that patients with ESRD take any over-the-counter (OTC) drugs, vitamins, or any remedies without first checking with their doctor. Although such remedies may not be harmful to the average person, they can be very harmful or even fatal to the person with kidney failure.

### Patient Rights and Responsibilities

Patients with kidney failure have both rights and responsibilities, according to the Centers for Medicare & Medicaid Services (CMS). Examples of these rights and responsibilities, provided by CMS, are listed below.

*Your rights*    As a person with kidney failure, you have certain rights and responsibilities. When you go to a treatment center, ask for a copy of your rights and responsibilities. This will help you to know what to expect from your health care team and to know what they expect from you. Your center may have a list similar to the following:

- I have the right to be told about my rights and responsibilities.
- I have the right to be treated with respect.
- I have the right to privacy. My medical records cannot be shared with anyone unless I say so.
- I have the right to meet with my whole health care team to plan my treatment.
- I have the right to see the dietitian for help with food planning and the social worker for counseling.
- I have the right to be told about my health in a way that I can understand.
- I have the right to be told about the treatment options that are open to me and to help choose my treatment method.
- I have the right to be told about any tests ordered for me and the test results.
- I have the right to be told about the services offered at the center.
- I have the right to be told about any expenses that will be charged to me if they are not covered by insurance or Medicare.
- I have the right to be told about any financial help that is available to me.
- I have the right to accept or refuse any treatment or medicine that my doctor orders for me.
- I have the right to be told about the rules at the treatment center (for example, rules for visitors, eating, personal conduct, etc.).
- I have the right to choose if I want to be part of any research studies.

*Your responsibilities* The treatment center may provide a list of patient responsibilities that is similar to this list:

- I need to treat other patients and the staff as I would like to be treated, with respect.

- I need to pay my bills on time. If this is hard for me to do, I can ask about making a treatment plan.

- I need to tell my health care team if I refuse any treatment or medicine that my doctor has ordered for me.

- I need to tell my health care team if I do not understand my medical condition or treatment plan.

- I need to be on time for my treatments or when I see my doctor.

- I need to tell the staff at the center if I know that I am going to be late or miss a treatment or an appointment with my doctor.

- I need to tell my health care team if I have medical problems, am going to the dentist, am being treated by another doctor, or have recently been to the hospital.

- I need to follow the rules of the treatment center.

- I need to get to and from the center for my treatments.

- I can talk with my social worker if I need help with doing this. Medicare does not pay for transportation.

### Patients with ESRD Need to Communicate with Their Doctors

According to the Centers for Medicare & Medicaid Services in their book, *You Can Live: Your Guide for Living with Kidney Failure,* patients should write down their questions in advance of an appointment with the doctor. In addition, the following advice is offered by the CMS:

- On a regular basis, talk with your kidney doctor on how your treatment is going and if changes to your treatment plan are needed.

- Every six months, discuss your treatment plan with your kidney doctor and health care team.

- See your family doctor for regular checkups.

- Take a copy of your health records to any doctor that you see. Let all of your doctors know about your treatment and changes to your health.

### Patients Need to Take Their Medications

Many patients fail to comply with the medications that their doctors have prescribed, regardless of the illness that they have. It is very important, however, for the patient with kidney failure to adhere to taking medicines as prescribed. It is also important to avoid some medicines. In addition, alternative remedies and treatments should be avoided unless the doctor specifically states that they may be taken.

*Some reasons why patients with kidney failure need medications* Medications may be ordered for patients with kidney failure for many reasons. Some common reasons include the ordering of medications

- to help the body make red blood cells (to prevent and/or treat ANEMIA)

- to control blood pressure

- to replace vitamins and minerals lost during dialysis or from dietary restrictions

- to keep the bones strong

- to prevent an accumulation of phosphorus, a mineral present in food, particularly food proteins, that the kidneys normally excrete but that patients with ESRD are unable to excrete

- to replace vitamins and minerals that are removed by the dialysis procedure

- to replace vitamins, such as vitamin D, that require chemical activation by the kidneys, but which activation cannot occur in the patient with ESRD

- to treat an infection or illness

It is important for the patient with kidney failure to understand when and how often to take medications; for example, some medicines need to be taken on an empty stomach, while other medicines should be taken with food.

It is best for the patient with kidney failure to write down a list of all medications that he or she takes, as well as why each is taken, when and how (with or without food or with any other restrictions). This list should be kept with the person in the purse or wallet, in the event that a problem occurs when the person is out.

### Some Medications Should Be Avoided

Patients with kidney failure need to avoid some medications that may have been taken safely in the past. Whenever possible, the following medications and remedies should be avoided:

- antacids or constipation-related medications containing aluminum or MAGNESIUM. These substances can build up in the body of the person with kidney failure and cause problems in the brain.
- aspirin at dosages greater than 650 mg twice a day, unless the kidney doctor specifically orders it
- vitamins (unless prescribed), food supplements, or salt substitutes. These items may be high in POTASSIUM or magnesium.
- any "cure-all" remedies, herbs, or over-the-counter (OTC) medicines that the kidney doctor has not specifically approved in advance

### Considering the Hospitalization Rates of Patients with ESRD

Patients with ESRD were somewhat less likely to require hospitalization in 2007 compared to previous years, according to the United States Renal Data System; for example, in 2004, 1,976 patients with ESRD were hospitalized, and this number dropped to 1,825 by 2007. Females with ESRD are more likely to be hospitalized than males with ESRD, and older individuals have a greater risk for hospitalization. African Americans with ESRD in 2007 had the highest risk for hospitalization, and those with diabetes also had the highest risk for hospitalization.

### Patients with ESRD Who Refuse Dialysis or a Transplant

Some patients with kidney failure refuse both dialysis treatment and a kidney transplant. A patient with no remaining kidney function who does so will die, typically within one to two weeks. The patient may have had dialysis for years and may decide to end treatment or the patient may be new to the need for dialysis, having recently received a diagnosis of kidney failure. The individual (or family members acting for the individual) may decide that the side effects of treatment have made or will make the person's quality of life too poor to continue on. It is also possible that the individual who refuses treatment may be suffering from depression, which is a treatable psychiatric condition. As many as one in five deaths of Americans on dialysis nationwide are preceded by withdrawal from dialysis.

According to John M. Bostwick, M.D., and Lewis M. Cohen, M.D., "A demographic profile of patients who discontinue dialysis finds that they are generally elderly, white, diabetic, and severely ill. Between one-third and one-half of the deaths likely occur in situations where patient capacity is impaired and family members or other proxies assist the medical team in arriving at the decision." The authors add that "when symptoms are well-managed and where all participants collaborate and achieve agreement, death is often recalled as being merciful, compassionate, and even uplifting. Families and loved ones may find such deaths to be an epiphany and not a trauma. This stands in stark contrast to descriptions by families after true suicides." The authors report that less than 1 percent of ESRD deaths are classified as true suicides.

Concluded Bostwick and Cohen, "In our society, people may make autonomous choices about how they wish to live and how they prefer to end their lives. Accordingly, such behaviors should not be reflexively opposed by physicians. On the other hand, some patients sabotage, interrupt, or abruptly terminate treatment for psychopathological reasons."

See also CHILDREN AND KIDNEY DISEASE; DEPRESSION; HEMODIALYSIS; HEMOLYTIC UREMIC SYNDROME–THROMBOTIC THROMBOCYTOPENIA PURPURA; MEDICATIONS THAT CAN HARM THE KIDNEYS; NEPHROTIC SYNDROME; PERITONEAL DIALYSIS.

Bostwick, John Michael, M.D., and Lewis M. Cohen, M.D. "Differentiating Suicide from Life-Ending Acts and End-of-Life Decisions: A Model Based on Chronic Kidney Disease and Dialysis." *Psychosomatics* 50, no. 1 (2009): 1–7.

Centers for Medicare & Medicaid Services. *You Can Live: Your Guide for Living with Kidney Failure.* Baltimore, Md.: Centers for Medicare & Medicaid Services, 2007.

Cibulka, R., and J. Racek. "Metabolic Disorders in Patients with Chronic Kidney Failure." *Physiological Research* 56 (2007): 697–705.

Dimkovic, Nada, and Dimitrios G. Oreopoulos. "Substitutive Treatments of End-Stage Renal Diseases in the Elderly: Dialysis." In *The Aging Kidney in Health and Disease,* edited by Juan-Floresco Macías Núñez, M.D., J. Stewart Cameron, M.D., and Dimitrios G. Oreopoulos, M.D., 443–463. New York: Springer Science+Business Media, 2008.

Hsu, Chi-yuan, M.D., et al. "Body Mass Index and Risk for End-Stage Renal Disease." *Annals of Internal Medicine* 144 (2006): 21–28.

Hsu, Chi-yuan, M.D., et al. "Risk Factors for End-Stage Renal Disease." *Archives of Internal Medicine* 169, no. 4 (2009): 342–350.

National Center for Health Statistics. *Health, United States, 2007 with Chartbook on Trends in the Health of Americans.* Hyattsville, Md.: National Center for Health Statistics, 2007.

Rios Burrows, Nilka, Yanfeng Li, and Desmond E. Williams. "Racial and Ethnic Differences in Trends of End-Stage Renal Disease: United States, 1995–2005." *Advances in Chronic Kidney Disease* 15, no. 2 (2008): 147–152.

Tsui, Judith I., M.D., et al. "Association of Hepatitis C Seropositivity with Increased Risk for Developing End-Stage Renal Disease." *Archives of Internal Medicine* 167 (2007): 1,271–1,276.

United States Renal Data System. *USRDS 2009 Annual Data Report: Atlas of Chronic Kidney Disease and End-Stage Renal Disease in the United States.* Bethesda, Md.: National Institutes of Health, National Institute of Diabetes and Digestive and Kidney Diseases, 2009.

Ward, Michael M., M.D. "Laboratory Abnormalities at the Onset of Treatment of End-Stage Renal Disease: Are There Racial or Socioeconomic Disparities in Care?" *Archives of Internal Medicine* 167 (2007): 1,083–1,091.

**estimated glomerular filtration rate (EGFR)**    See GLOMERULAR DISEASES; GLOMERULAR FILTRATION RATE/ESTIMATED GLOMERULAR FILTRATION RATE.

**ethnicity**    See KIDNEYS AND KIDNEY DISEASE.

**Fabry's disease** Fabry's disease is a serious metabolic disorder caused by the lack of or a faulty enzyme needed to metabolize certain lipids. The enzyme is ceramide trihexosidase, also called alpha-galactosidase-A. When there is a mutation in the gene that controls this enzyme, there is insufficient breakdown of lipids, which can accumulate to harmful levels in the eyes, kidneys, autonomic nervous system, and the cardiovascular system. Because the gene that controls this enzyme is located on a mother's X chromosome, each son has a 50 percent chance of inheriting the disorder and each daughter has a 50 percent chance of being a carrier. In general, women with the genetic defect are not symptomatic, but some women may have mild symptoms of the disease.

### Symptoms and Diagnostic Path

Affected individuals typically have symptoms that begin during childhood or adolescence. These symptoms include burning sensations in the hands and small, raised reddish-purple blemishes on the skin. The burning sensation often worsens with exercise and hot weather. Some boys will also have cloudiness of the cornea of their eyes. At later stages, Fabry's disease can lead to impaired arterial circulation and an increased risk of heart attack or stroke. The heart may also become enlarged, and the kidneys may become progressively involved. Other symptoms include decreased sweating, fever, and gastrointestinal difficulties, particularly after eating.

The kidney disease of Fabry's disease most frequently occurs in young adults and presents with mild to moderate proteinuria, sometimes with microscopic hematuria or NEPHROTIC SYNDROME. Specialized urinalysis may reveal oval fat bodies and globules; these are signs of the nephrotic syndrome and are not specific for Fabry's disease.

In the setting of clearly established family history or classic phenotype, it is recommended that levels of leukocyte alpha-Gal A activity should be measured for the diagnosis of the disease. This should be further complemented with genetic mutation analysis for all patients diagnosed with Fabry's disease on the basis of enzyme deficiency (unless the family genotype is known) and for females suspected of being carriers, as the alpha-Gal A activity level may be variable with the latter.

Many others should also be screened for this condition. All male siblings of a diagnosed patient should be screened for Fabry's disease with measurement of alpha-Gal A activity. Female siblings of a diagnosed patient, females with a family history of Fabry's disease, or females with symptoms suggestive of Fabry's disease should also be screened with alpha-Gal A activity measurement. Young men with otherwise unexplained renal failure and individuals with multiple renal sinus cysts should also be screened. In women, genetic testing may be necessary because of variations in enzyme activity that may lead to failure to identify the disease. KIDNEY BIOPSY sometimes leads to the correct diagnosis in patients who may lack other manifestations of the disease or in whom the other manifestations are not recognized at the time of diagnosis. Electron-dense vacuoles in parallel arrays (zebra bodies) in glomerular epithelial cells are easily seen with electron microscopy and are very specific for the diagnosis of this disease.

### Treatment Options and Outlook

Treatment involves administration of recombinant alpha-Gal A enzyme. Treatment may slow the progression of the renal disease and may also reduce the severity of other clinical manifestations. Before the advent of treatment with recombinant alpha-galactosidase, the majority of patients with Fabry's disease developed END-STAGE RENAL DISEASE (ESRD), requiring renal replacement therapy in the form of DIALYSIS or KIDNEY TRANSPLANTATION. Patients who do develop ESRD should be treated with dialysis and/or renal transplantation. Mortality for dialysis patients with Fabry's disease appears to be slightly increased relative to those nondiabetic patients without Fabry's disease. Causes of death for these patients may include stroke, myocardial infarction (heart attack), cardiomyopathy, and pulmonary emboli (blood clots in the lung).

### Risk Factors and Preventive Measures

Fabry's disease is a genetic disorder caused by a gene that is located on a mother's X chromosome. Symptoms related to kidney disease usually develop in more than 50 percent of Fabry's disease-affected patients by the age of 35 years. This incidence increases further with advancing age. There are no known preventive measures.

See also CHILDHOOD NEPHROTIC SYNDROME; PROTEINURIA.

**failure to grow**   See CHILDREN AND KIDNEY DISEASE.

**focal segmental glomerulosclerosis (FSGS)**   A disease characterized by scarring of the loops of the glomeruli of the kidneys. The incidence (annual number of new cases) of this disease is increasing, and it represents up to about one-third of the cases of NEPHROTIC SYNDROME in adults and half of all cases of nephrotic syn-

drome occurring among African Americans. In African Americans, focal segmental glomerulosclerosis (FSGS) is the most common cause of nondiabetic nephrotic syndrome; in Caucasian Americans, it is the second most common cause.

FSGS may also occur as a secondary disorder as a result of other diseases. OBESITY is a very common cause of secondary FSGS, and weight loss can result in reversal of the disease. Another common cause of secondary FSGS is an infection with the human immunodeficiency virus or with HEPATITIS, parvovirus or adenovirus infections. (See HUMAN IMMUNODEFICIENCY VIRUS ASSOCIATED NEPHROPATHY). FSGS can also develop in individuals who abuse drugs intravenously, such as heroin or androgenic steroids.

### Symptoms and Diagnostic Path

The most common sign of FSGS is the development of PROTEINURIA and the clinical features of nephrotic syndrome. FSGS can present with any level of proteinuria or hematuria, (blood in the urine) and may also present with HYPERTENSION or renal insufficiency.

Most patients with FSGS present with the signs and symptoms of the nephrotic syndrome and with concomitant hypertension. They frequently will have peripheral edema, most commonly in the ankles and lower extremities in adults, and around the eyes among children. Sometimes FSGS will be suspected because of screening laboratory studies, often done for other purposes, and which reveal proteinuria, low serum albumin or elevated blood cholesterol levels. The initial evaluation of patients with suspected FSGS typically reveals significant proteinuria, often more than 3 g per 24 hours, as well as a low serum albumin, peripheral edema and elevated serum cholesterol, particularly LDL cholesterol. The diagnosis of FSGS requires a renal biopsy showing the characteristic histologic features of focal and segmental glomerulosclerosis.

Patients with severe obesity may sometimes develop FSGS as a complication of their obesity. In these patients, proteinuria is present, but in most circumstances they do not develop the peripheral edema that is typically present in others with FSGS. Some individuals infected with HIV will develop FSGS. In many of these patients, the disease is a relatively fast progressing course and can lead to renal failure within months.

### Treatment Options and Outlook

Treatment of patients with primary FSGS should include medication inhibitors of the renin-angiotensin system. Corticosteroids may also be used to treat FSGS; however, proteinuria remits in less than half of the patients receiving corticosteroids over six to nine months. Patients who respond to corticosteroids have a much lower risk for developing END-STAGE RENAL DISEASE (ESRD) or kidney failure. Patients who respond to corticosteroids, but whose disease worsens when the dosage is decreased, often benefit from addition of other IMMUNOSUPPRESSIVE DRUGS. If renal function is moderately preserved, such as with an estimated glomerular filtration rate (eGFR) of greater than 40 ml/min/($1.73m^2$), cyclosporine is often added to the medical regimen, and if the eGFR is less than this, then mycophenylate mofetil is often used. Patients who do not respond to corticosteroids will often respond to cyclosporine used in combination with low-dose corticosteroids.

The treatment of secondary FSGS involves treating the underlying cause and also controlling the proteinuria. There is no role for corticosteroids or other immunosuppressive drugs in secondary FSGS.

All patients with FSGS should be treated with ANGIOTENSIN-CONVERTING ENZYME INHIBITOR (ACEI) medication therapy unless there is a contraindication to using this class of medicines. ACEIs have been shown in general to decrease proteinuria and to slow the progression of chronic kidney disease.

### Risk Factors and Preventive Measures

Nephrotic range proteinuria, African-American race, and kidney insufficiency at presentation are all risk factors for kidney failure in patients with FSGS. More than half of these patients will develop ESRD in less than five years.

FSGS recurs in up to two-thirds of patients *after* receiving a KIDNEY TRANSPLANTATION, and this disease could lead to the premature failure of the kidney in such patients.

See also GLOMERULAR DISEASES; GLOMERULO-SCLEROSIS.

**gender, risks for kidney disease**   See KIDNEYS AND KIDNEY DISEASE.

**geriatric population**   See ELDERLY AND CHRONIC KIDNEY DISEASE.

**Gitelman syndrome**   A rare inherited kidney disorder of both hypokalemia (abnormally low potassium blood levels) and hypomagnesia (abnormally low levels of blood magnesium). The disorder is named after H. J. Gitelman, who reported on two sisters with the symptoms of this disorder in 1966. According to authors Nine V. A. M. Knoers and Elena N. Levtchenko in their 2008 article for *Orphanet Journal of Rare Diseases,* this disorder is present in about one of 40,000 people or about 1 percent of Caucasians. Gitelman syndrome is also known as familial hypokalemia-hypomagnesia. The disorder is mapped to the 16q13 gene, according to the genetic database, Online Mendelian Inheritance in Man (OMIM). Experts believe that Gitelman syndrome is a milder form of Bartter's syndrome.

### Symptoms and Diagnostic Path

Most individuals with this disorder have no symptoms until at least the age of six years and in most cases, the diagnosis does not occur until adolescence or adulthood. Patients with Gitelman syndrome may experience periods of muscle weakness and may also have abdominal pain, fever, and vomiting. They may also experience "pins and needles" paresthesias, particularly in the face. However, some patients have no symptoms until adulthood, when they develop joint swelling and pain. The diagnosis is made based on symptoms and Bartter's syndrome, a related syndrome, is ruled out.

### Treatment Options and Outlook

Patients with Gitelman syndrome are treated by NEPHROLOGISTS. They require supplementation of magnesium, and they need to stay on a high potassium and high sodium diet. According to Knoers and Levetchencko, the long-term prognosis is excellent, although patients may suffer from severe bouts of fatigue. However, patients with Gitelman syndrome should be given genetic counseling because the risk of a child having the disorder is 25 percent. Only one patient with Gitelman syndrome has been reported to develop kidney failure.

### Risk Factors and Preventive Measures

Individuals whose parents have Gitelman syndrome are at risk for this disorder. There are no known preventive measures.

See also BARTTER'S SYNDROME.

Knoers, Nine V. A. M., and Elena Levtchenko, "Gitelman Syndrome." *Orphanet Journal of Rare Diseases.* Available online. URL: http://www.ojrd.com/content/3/1/22. Accessed November 8, 2010.

Online Mendelian Inheritance in Man. "Gitelman Syndrome." Available online. URL: http://www.ncbi.nlm.nih.gov/omim/263800. Accessed November 8, 2010.

**glomerular diseases**   An encompassing term that includes all kidney diseases that are linked to the glomeruli, or the tiny looping blood vessels where blood is filtered in the kidney. The most common primary glomerular diseases are

- FOCAL SEGMENTAL GLOMERULOSCLEROSIS (FSGS): Focal segmental glomerulosclerosis is a disorder that scars the loops of the glomeruli of the kidneys. It can result from OBESITY as a secondary cause of FSGS, and weight loss can reverse the problem. Infection with the human immunodeficiency virus or HEPATITIS can also cause FSGS. The disorder may also occur among those who abuse drugs intravenously.

- MEMBRANOUS NEPHROPATHY: Membranous nephropathy is a disorder in which there are harmful deposits and a thickening on the glomerular membrane, the part of the kidneys that filters waste and extra fluid from the blood.

- IGA NEPHROPATHY: IgA nephropathy is caused by the buildup of the protein *immunoglobulin A* (IgA) in the kidneys, which causes inflammation of internal kidney structures.

The most common secondary glomerular disorder, in which the glomerular disorder results from a cause originating outside the kidney, is DIABETIC NEPHROPATHY. This refers to kidney damage that is caused by either Type 1 or Type 2 diabetes.

The first sign of a glomerular disease is often the presence of protein in the urine (PROTEINURIA), although blood in the urine (hematuria) may also indicate the presence of kidney disease. Treatments for glomerular diseases may include the use of steroids to reduce inflammation and proteins in the urine as well as the use of IMMUNOSUPPRESSIVE DRUGS. Different glomerular diseases require different treatment regimens for optimal outcomes. In many cases, a KIDNEY BIOPSY will be necessary in order to identify the specific type of glomerular disease.

**glomerular filtration rate (GFR)/estimated glomerular filtration rate (eGFR)**   The glomerular filtration rate (GFR) is the rate at which the glomeruli, the tiny blood filtering units that lie within the cortex of the kidney, filter waste from the bloodstream. When the glomerular filtration rate decreases, this may mean that kidney damage is present. A normal GFR is 90 or greater, although there may be a tendency for decreased levels with increased age. If the GFR falls to 30–59, this is equivalent to Stage 3 of CHRONIC KIDNEY DISEASE (CKD). When the level drops below 15, this means that the kidneys have failed and the person has END-STAGE RENAL DISEASE.

At present, the preferred measure of the GFR is the estimated glomerular filtration rate (eGFR), which is a different way to calculate the filtration rate to determine kidney function. This measure requires only a blood draw and does not necessitate a 24-hour urine collection or other specialized testing. The eGFR is based on the levels of serum (blood) creatinine, and it also takes into account the age, gender, and race of the individual. The eGFR is accurate at quantifying the degree of kidney impairment if the kidneys are damaged, but is less accurate when assessing normal or "near normal" GFR. If the eGFR calculation reveals a level that is less than 90 but more than 60 ml per min per 1.73 m$^2$, this is not sufficiently accurate to diagnose kidney disease.

Increasing research indicates than the presence or absence of PROTEINURIA is an important factor to consider in conjunction with the eGFR. According to Brenda R. Hemmalgarn, M.D., and colleagues in their 2010 article for the *Journal of the American Medical Association,* a study of more than 920,000 adults in Canada and their eGFR rates and proteinuria rates from 2002–07 revealed that the health outcomes that correlated with different eGFR levels were tied to the presence and severity of proteinuria.

The authors said, "In fact, patients with heavy proteinuria but without overtly abnormal eGFR appeared to have worse clinical outcomes than those with moderately reduced eGFR but without proteinuria. Results were consistent for 2 different measures of proteinuria; consistent for several clinically relevant outcomes, including all-cause mortality myocardial infarction, and the need for renal replacement; and robust to multi-variable adjustment and a variety of sensitivity analyses." Thus, this study indicates that the eGFR should be taken into account along with the presence or absence of proteinuria and the level of the proteinuria, if present.

See also ANEMIA; GLOMERULAR DISEASES; GLOMERULONEPHRITIS.

Hemmelgarn, Brenda R., et al. "Relation Between Kidney Function, Proteinuria, and Adverse Outcomes." *Journal of the American Medical Association* 303, no. 5 (2010): 423–429.

Stevens, Lesley A., M.D., Josef Coresh, M.D., Tome Greene, and Andrew S. Levey, M.D. "Assessing Kidney Function—Measured and Estimated Glomerular Filtration Rate." *New England Journal of Medicine* 3354, no. 3 (June 8, 2006): 2,473–2,483.

**glomerulonephritis** An encompassing term that refers to the inflammation of the glomeruli where the blood is filtered in the kidneys. Sometimes glomerulonephritis is referred to simply as nephritis. This serious medical problem may be caused by an autoimmune disease (as with systemic lupus), in which the body attacks itself, but it may also be caused by an infection. DIABETES MELLITUS, HYPERTENSION, and other kidney diseases may also cause glomerulonephritis. Glomerulonephritis is the third leading cause of kidney failure from END-STAGE RENAL DISEASE (ESRD) in the United States, following the other leading causes of kidney failure, which are diabetes and hypertension. In other countries, such as Australia, glomerular disease is the leading cause of ESRD.

Disorders that are directly linked to the development of glomerulonephritis include FOCAL SEGMENTAL GLOMERULOSCLEROSIS, GOODPASTURE SYNDROME, IGA NEPHROPATHY, LUPUS NEPHRITIS, MEMBRANOPROLIFERATIVE GLOMERULONEPHRITIS Type I, membranoproliferative GN Type II, MINIMAL CHANGE DISEASE, MEMBRANOUS NEPHROPATHY, POSTSTREPTOCOCCAL GLOMERULONEPHRITIS, and rapidly progressive glomerulonephritis. Note that poststreptococcal glomerulonephritis is far more common in developing countries than in industrialized nations such as the United States.

Some INFECTIONS may cause glomerulonephritis, particularly a chronic infection with hepatitis B, HEPATITIS C, or the human immunodeficiency virus. In general, most chronic, unresolved infections, which may include endocarditis or chronic abscesses, can cause glomerulonephritis. In some cases, the body's response to a result of infection, such as streptococcal pharyngitis, can result in glomerulonephritis. In addition, some medications may lead to the development of glomerulonephritis, such as the use of NONSTEROIDAL ANTI-INFLAMMATORY DRUGS (NSAIDs). (See MEDICATIONS THAT CAN HARM THE KIDNEYS.)

### Symptoms and Diagnostic Path

People who experience kidney failure that is caused by glomerulonephritis have the same symptoms as are experienced by all people with kidney failure, such as hypertension, fluid retention, and the development of edema, fatigue, and sometimes severe itching as well. In addition, they may have blood in the urine (hematuria) as well as PROTEINURIA. Because glomerulonephritis is often associated with an underlying etiologic problem, many patients will experience fever or night sweats. The disorder is sometimes discovered in a routine examination when a urinalysis is ordered and the results are abnormal. Because of the number of different conditions that can cause glomerulonephritis, many of which require very different types of treatment, a KIDNEY BIOPSY is often necessary in order to determine the specific type of glomerulonephritis that is present.

### Treatment Options and Outlook

When the kidney fails, the survival options are either DIALYSIS or KIDNEY TRANSPLANTATION. If the kidney has not failed, it is very important for the patient to attain control over any existing hypertension as well as to markedly decrease the level of proteinuria. If the etiology of the glomerulonephritis is determined, then treating the underlying cause is often effective. For example, if a person has hepatitis C virus–associated glomerulonephritis, then treating the hepatitis C with appropriate antiviral agents can result in the reversal and improvement in the glomerulonephritis. Immunologic disorders leading to glomerulonephritis often require the use of IMMUNOSUPPRESSIVE DRUGS. In some cases, treatments that remove the antibodies causing the disease, such as anti-GBM disease, are necessary. The expertise and experience of a nephrologist is often necessary to guide the appropriate therapy.

### Risk Factors and Preventive Measures

Because a chronic infection, particularly a chronic viral infection such as hepatitis C, is often the precipitating cause of glomerulonephritis, treating specific chronic infections is often a preventive measure. Otherwise, there are no specific preventive treatments that prevent the development of glomerulonephritis.

See also CHILDREN AND KIDNEY DISEASE; GLOMERULAR FILTRATION RATE/ESTIMATED GLOMERULAR FILTRATION RATE; GLOMERULOSCLEROSIS; URINE/URINALYSIS/URINE CULTURE.

Isbel, Nicole M. "Glomerulonephritis: Management in General Practice." *Australian Family Physician* 34, no. 11 (2005): 907–913.

**glomerulosclerosis** The scarring of the glomeruli, which are the tiny looping blood vessels that are located where the blood is filtered in the kidney. This scarring may be caused by DIABETES MELLITUS or it may result from deposits in parts of the glomeruli, such as with FOCAL SEGMENTAL GLOMERULOSCLEROSIS (FSGS). Other disorders may cause glomerulosclerosis, including IgA NEPHROPATHY, MEMBRANOPROLIFERATIVE GLOMERULONEPHRITIS (MPGN), and AMYLOIDOSIS.

In the worst case, glomerulosclerosis can lead to kidney failure. One common cause of glomerulosclerosis is DIABETIC NEPHROPATHY (glomerulo-sclerosis that is caused by diabetes), and in many cases, this form of glomerulosclerosis leads to END-STAGE RENAL DISEASE (ESRD), or kidney failure. When it is caused by diabetic nephropathy, the glomerulosclerosis is either a diffuse (widespread) or a more localized and nodular form of glomerulosclerosis.

Some genes have been specifically linked to glomerulosclerosis; for example the MYH9 gene is linked to kidney disease in African Americans that leads to glomerulosclerosis. According to J. Divers and B. Freedman in their 2010 article for *Current Opinion in Nephrology Hypertension,* nearly half (43 percent) of all cases of end-stage renal disease in African Americans in the United States are tied to the MYH9 gene. Other genes such as the ELMO1 and UMOD genes are under study as of this writing for their possible role in causing glomerulosclerosis and resultant ESRD.

### Symptoms and Diagnostic Path

The key signs of glomerulosclerosis are protein in the urine (PROTEINURIA) and swelling in the ankles or the abdomen. However, often there are no signs or symptoms in the early stages of kidney disease. When it is likely that the kidney is damaged based on tests such as the GLOMERULAR FILTRATION RATE, the presence of any form of glomerulosclerosis is made with a KIDNEY BIOPSY. An analysis of the tissue removed for biopsy is made to diagnose the cause of the glomerulosclerosis, so that the most effective and safest treatment regimen for the patient can be devised.

### Treatment Options and Outlook

If the kidneys have completely failed or will fail imminently, then the plan for survival must be either DIALYSIS or KIDNEY TRANSPLANTATION. If the kidneys have not yet failed, then the treatment depends on the cause of the kidney disease. In the case of diabetes as a causal factor, the individual should keep blood glucose levels as close to normal as possible. In all cases, high blood pressure should be aggressively treated in an attempt to bring blood pressure back down to the normal range.

### Risk Factors and Preventive Measures

Individuals with diabetes are at high risk for glomerulosclerosis, as are those with other systemic diseases such as lupus. African Americans with kidney disease are also at a high risk for glomerulosclerosis, particularly if they have a family history of the disease.

See also GLOMERULAR DISEASES.

Alsaad, K. O., and A. M. Herzenberg. "Distinguishing Diabetic Nephropathy from Other Causes of Glomerulosclerosis: An Update." *Journal of Clinical Pathology* 2006. Available online. URL: http://jcp.bmj.com/content/60/1/18.full.pdf. Accessed April 8, 2010.

Divers, J., and B. I. Freedman. "Susceptibility Genes in Common Complex Kidney Disease." *Current Opinion Nephrology Hypertension* 19, no. 1 (2010): 79–84.

**glomerulosclerosis, focal segmental**   See FOCAL SEGMENTAL GLOMERULOSCLEROSIS.

**Goodpasture syndrome**   A rare and potentially life-threatening autoimmune disorder (with an estimated prevalence of one case per million people per year) that severely affects the kidneys and, sometimes, the lungs. Goodpasture syndrome is also known by a variety of other names, such as Goodpasture disease (if it affects the lungs and kidneys) or anti-glomerular basement antibody disease (if it affects only the kidneys). In some cases, Goodpasture syndrome leads to kidney failure within days or weeks; if not identified and treated early the renal failure may be irreversible. The syndrome can also be accompanied by bleeding into the lungs. If excessive, the patient may be unable to breathe because of the bleeding and may die. In most cases, however, the lungs do not any suffer permanent damage. The combination of acute (recent onset) and rapidly progressive renal failure, in association with appropriate kidney biopsy findings, with pulmonary hemorrhage is termed Goodpasture syndrome. If the kidney manifestations are present but not the pulmonary hemorrhage, then it is termed anti-GBM disease.

Goodpasture syndrome was first identified in 1919 by Harvard Medical School professor and pathologist Ernest Goodpasture during an influenza pandemic, based on his autopsy of an 18-year-old male. As a result of his discovery, the syndrome was named after Dr. Goodpasture in 1958 by M. C. Stanton and J. D. Tange, in their discussion of nine patients with the same symptoms and signs. Interestingly, many people now feel that the syndrome Dr. Goodpasture described was not what is now called Goodpasture syndrome, but instead was influenza and its known propensity to cause pneumonia and renal failure.

In most cases, the event that leads to the development of anti-GBM disease and/or Goodpasture syndrome is not known. However, it is known that pulmonary irritants potentially increase the risk of life-threatening pulmonary hemorrhage. These can include cigarette SMOKING, bronchitis, pulmonary edema, and hydrocarbon fume inhalation. The syndrome may last as briefly as a few weeks or as long as two years.

### Symptoms and Diagnostic Path

The initial symptoms of Goodpasture syndrome are typically vague, such as paleness, nausea, and fatigue. Other symptoms may include urine that is typically either red or "tea"-colored. If pulmonary hemorrhage is present then the person may have unexplained shortness of breath or even begin coughing up blood.

To diagnose Goodpasture syndrome, the physician orders a variety of laboratory tests, including a urinalysis (which will show blood and protein in the urine if the syndrome is present) as well as serum creatinine and estimated glomerular filtration rate (eGFR) measurement. Blood tests can reveal the presence of anti-GBM antibody, the protein in the blood that causes the disease. A chest X-ray or chest

CT scan can reveal evidence of pulmonary hemorrhage. A lung biopsy will also detect any damaged alveoli. A KIDNEY BIOPSY will show the presence of damaged glomeruli and will show the presence of the anti-GBM antibody in the kidney. Most specialists believe that the kidney biopsy is necessary in order to diagnose this condition.

### Treatment Options and Outlook

Patients with Goodpasture syndrome are usually treated with drugs that suppress the immune system, such as corticosteroids, particularly prednisone or prednisolone. These medications may be given orally or intravenously, depending on the patient's individual needs and the physician's choice. Another IMMUNOSUPPRESSIVE DRUG frequently given to patients with the syndrome is cyclophosphamide.

Another mainstay of treatment is the process known as plasmapheresis, a procedure that removes proteins from the bloodstream. This is critical in order to remove the anti-GBM antibody, the protein that causes this disease, from the blood as rapidly as possible. With this procedure, the patient's blood is drawn slowly, and a device known as a centrifuge separates the platelets and white and red blood cells from the plasma. The patient's plasma, which contains the anti-GBM antibodies that cause this disease, is discarded. These cells are then mixed with a plasma substitute, and the fluid is subsequently returned to the person's body. Plasmapheresis may be administered on a daily basis for up to two weeks. It is usually performed in conjunction with the administration of immunosuppressant drugs.

If the kidneys fail, the patient will need to undergo either DIALYSIS or a KIDNEY TRANSPLANTATION in order to continue to live.

Individuals who are diagnosed at an early stage of Goodpasture syndrome have the best prognosis. In general, the earlier that the disease is identified the higher the chance of successful treatment. The kidney biopsy often provides important information regarding the likelihood of successful treatment. Complications of Goodpasture syndrome include severe pulmonary hemorrhage (bleeding in the lung), respiratory failure, chronic kidney failure, and end-stage renal disease.

### Risk Factors and Preventive Measures

Goodpasture syndrome is more commonly diagnosed in white males, and it is believed to affect primarily those in their mid-thirties or in their late fifties. It also occurs in women and men who are older than 60 years. It is more often seen among Caucasians than in individuals of other races.

Bergs, Laura. "Goodpasture Syndrome." *Critical Care Nurse* 25, no. 5 (October 2005): 5–58. Available online. URL: http://ccn.aacnjournals.org/cgi/contend/full/25/5/50. Downloaded May 11, 2007.

Hellmark, Thomas, Harald Burkhardt, and Jorgen Wieslander. "Goodpasture Disease." *The Journal of Biological Chemistry* 274, no. 36 (September 3, 1999): 25,862–25,868.

Hudson, Billy G., et al. "Alport's Syndrome, Goodpasture's Syndrome, and Type IV Collagen." *New England Journal of Medicine* 348, no. 25 (June 19, 2003): 2,543–2,556.

**gout**   A common form of arthritis that causes severe joint swelling and pain. In most people, uric acid dissolves in the blood and is then moved by the kidneys into the urine. However, if there is an excessive production of uric acid or if, for whatever reason, the body does not adequately remove the uric acid from the body, then the uric acid levels will increase and accumulate in the blood (HYPERURICEMIA). When uric acid crystals form and accumulate in the joints, then the person has gout.

There are four stages of gout, including the first stage, which is asymptomatic. There are elevated levels of uric acid in the blood at the point of the first stage, but this risk factor will usually not be identified unless the blood is specifically tested for uric acid.

In the second stage, the person has acute gout, also known as gouty arthritis, and at this point, uric acid crystals are deposited in the joint spaces. This can be extremely painful for the affected individual. This circumstance is also known as an acute flare, and acute flares may arise periodically with gout. About half of those patients with an acute flare of gout suffer their pain in their large toe, although the disease may present differently in the elderly, with many potential joints being affected.

In the third stage, the hyperuricemia continues to cause deposits of crystals in the tissues, causing damage.

The fourth stage of the disease is chronic gout, in which there is a chronic aching and soreness of the joints. Some people with gout develop tophi, which are masses of urate crystals that may form in the elbows, finger joints, and other joints of the body.

Increasing evidence suggests that hyperuricemia also has effects unrelated to overt gout. Hyperuricemia has been associated with increased risks of hypertension, metabolic syndrome, obesity, cardiovascular disease such as myocardial infarction or stroke, chronic kidney disease, and renal failure.

### Symptoms and Diagnostic Path

Severe pain, redness, and swelling in a joint are all common indicators of possible gout. Typically, only one joint is involved at a given time. The most common, and classic, joint involved is the big toe. In some cases, the joint that is involved will be so sensitive to any external pressure that the patient will not even be able to tolerate the weight of a bed sheet on the joint.

Physicians often will test the blood to determine if hyperuricemia is present. Sometimes it is necessary to use a sterile needle to remove a small amount of the fluid in the inflamed joint in order to confirm the diagnosis, by identifying the uric acid crystals in the fluid, and to exclude other causes that require different treatments, such as a bacterial infection of the joint fluid. In most cases, men suffer from gout at a greater rate than women, with the exception of postmenopausal women, who have about the same rate of gout as men. Because physicians are aware of this fact, they often rule out the presence of gout in children and premenopausal women.

### Treatment Options and Outlook

Individuals may be treated with colchicine for an acute attack of gout. If the individual has repeated episodes of gout, he or she may be placed on a maintenance dose of allopurinol, a medication that decreases the body's uric acid production. Because allopurinol can also decrease the rate at which the body eliminates uric acid, it should be avoided during an acute gout attack and in the two to three weeks after an attack.

IMMUNOSUPPRESSIVE DRUGS, such as prednisone, ACTH, or related medications, are very effective in rapidly decreasing the patient's symptoms. Physicians also recommend lifestyle changes to reduce the risk of gout, such as weight loss if the individual is overweight or obese and the avoidance of alcohol. If the individual is on a DIURETIC medication, stopping this drug may decrease the risk for flares of gout.

### Risk Factors and Preventive Measures

Individuals with HYPERTENSION have an increased risk for developing gout. Obese individuals have an elevated risk for gout, as do those who consume alcohol and/or a diet that is rich in seafood and meat. Elderly individuals have a greater risk for gout than younger people.

African-American men have a rate of gout that is about twice the rate for white men, or 3.1 per 1,000 person-years for African Americans compared to 1.8 per 1,000 person-years for white men.

Individuals with some diseases have an increased risk for the development of gout, such as those with CHRONIC KIDNEY DISEASE, DIABETES MELLITUS, SICKLE CELL DISEASE, or leukemia and related blood disorders.

Kramer, J. H., et al. "The Association between Gout and Nepholithiasis in Men: The Health Professionals' Follow-up Study." *Kidney International* 64 (2003): 1,022–1,026.

Kutzing, Melinda K., and Bonnie L. Firestein. "Altered Uric Acid Levels and Disease States." *Journal of Pharmacology and Experimental Therapies* 324, no. 1 (2008): 1–7.

Schmucher, H. Ralph, Jr., M.D., and Lan X. Chen, M.D. "The Practical Management of Gout." *Cleveland Journal of Medicine* 75, Supp. 5 (2008): S22–S25.

Weaver, Arthur L., M.D. "Epidemiology of Gout." *Cleveland Clinic Journal of Medicine* 75, Supp. 5 (2008): S9–S12.

**granulomatosis, Wegener's** See WEGENER'S GRANULOMATOSIS.

**growth failure, in children with kidney disease** See CHILDREN AND KIDNEY DISEASE.

**hemodialysis** One of two forms of DIALYSIS commonly used in the United States when the kidneys have failed, and also the most commonly used form of dialysis. The other form of dialysis is PERITONEAL DIALYSIS, a much less frequently used procedure which uses the abdominal cavity as a vehicle for the dialysis chemicals to remove impurities. Dialysis is a mechanical procedure that removes impurities from the blood when a person's kidneys have failed. (See END-STAGE RENAL [ESRD].) Hemodialysis is usually performed three times a week, for three to five hours each time. Most patients receive in-center hemodialysis, but some patients receive home hemodialysis. Increasing attention is being given to hemodialysis treatments that are performed slowly while the patient is sleeping.

Hemodialysis is not a cure for kidney failure, but instead it is a treatment to maintain the individual's life. When the kidneys fail, the only means for survival at that point are either to receive dialysis or KIDNEY TRANSPLANTATION. Hemodialysis helps to maintain the balance of fluid, POTASSIUM, SODIUM, CALCIUM, and bicarbonate. It also helps with controlling the person's blood pressure and removes many of the normal by-products of cellular metabolisms that the kidneys should remove (were they healthy) but they are unable to do so because of the kidney disease.

According to the United States Renal Data System (USRDS), in 2007, there were 333,615 patients in the United States who were receiving hemodialysis. The rates for hemodialysis were highest among African Americans because they also have the greatest risk for kidney failure;

in 2007, 4,050 African Americans per million were receiving hemodialysis. The next greatest rate of hemodialysis was among Native Americans; 2,003 Native Americans per million were receiving hemodialysis in 2006, according to the USRDS. The rate for Hispanics was 1,774 per million, followed by the rate for Asians (1,212 per million) and for whites (702 per million).

*Procedure*

Hemodialysis requires removing blood from the body, passing it through the dialysis machine, and then returning the blood to the patient. In order to do this, the patient needs either to have specially adapted blood vessels that can be used or needs to have a catheter placed into one of the patient's large, central veins. Adapting a patient's blood vessels for hemodialysis involves artificially connecting an artery to a vein. This can be done either using the patient's own blood vessels or using artificial blood vessels. Using the patient's own blood vessels is preferred because of less long-term chance of infection, less clotting of the vessel, and, in general, greater life span of the vessels. This is termed an arteriovenous fistula or AVF. Sometimes the patient's natural blood vessels are too damaged, either from atherosclerosis or from repeated blood drawing, and cannot be used, and consequently, an artificial vessel must be used. This is termed an arteriovenous graft. However, this is generally a less desired option. Multiple attempts to create the adapted vessels using the patient's own vessels are often appropriate in order to minimize the long-term health risks for the patient.

The least desirable option is to use a catheter placed into one of the patient's large, central veins. Because this catheter must exit through the skin, it is associated with a substantially increased rate of infection in the patient. These infections are often serious and generally require hospitalization and intravenous antibiotic treatment. Patients using these catheters have an increased chance of dying.

In order to begin hemodialysis, the patient's blood vessels must be connected to the dialysis machine. If the patient has specially adapted blood vessels, this involves placing two relatively large needles into the blood vessel, one for removing the blood and the other for returning it. The patient may be given a local anesthetic to decrease pain from the needle placement, but many patients do not need this. If the patient uses a catheter, then special care must be taken to minimize the risk of infection during the connection of the catheter to the dialysis machine.

The patient is connected to a dialyzer, which functions as an artificial kidney and cleans the blood. The blood travels through tubes into the dialyzer, and the wastes and extra water are filtered out. Chemicals and other compounds that the kidneys normally make, but that they are unable to make because of the kidney damage, are filtered into the blood in order to replace them. The cleansed blood flows through another set of tubes and into the body.

As a component of the dialysis procedure, the patient may receive certain medications. For example, almost all patients treated with hemodialysis have ANEMIA. This is because the kidneys make a compound named erythropoietin that regulates the bone's ability to make red blood cells and thereby prevent anemia; the patient with ESRD cannot make normal amounts of this compound and he or she becomes anemic. Fortunately, artificially synthesized erythropoietin and related compounds can be given in the dialysis unit, preventing excessive levels of anemia from developing. The dialysis unit must closely monitor the degree of correction of anemia, as an excessive correction can lead to an increased risk of heart attacks and strokes. (See CARDIOVASCULAR DISEASE.)

Another medication that is often given as a component of the dialysis treatment is a special form of VITAMIN D. Vitamin D is a critical vitamin for normal health, and in normal individuals, its generation involves a complex interaction in many tissues, ending with chemical modification in the kidneys, which convert it from an inactive to an active form of vitamin D. In patients with ESRD, this final conversion may not occur. Patients may require treatment with a special form of vitamin D, an "active" vitamin D, which does not require conversion in the kidneys in order to become active. The most commonly used forms of active vitamin D are given as intravenous medications as a component of the hemodialysis procedure, although they can also be given as oral medications.

While receiving hemodialysis treatments, the patient can sleep, read, watch television, or talk to others.

### Risks and Complications

Vascular access problems are common with hemodialysis, and patients may also develop INFECTIONS, as well as blockages from clotting. Both infections and clotting are less common with use of the patient's own blood vessels than if artificial vessels must be used. Catheters are associated with the highest risk of infections. Muscle cramps and hypotension (a sudden drop in the blood pressure) are also common side effects of hemodialysis. These side effects should be reported immediately to the dialysis staff so that they can be treated. Dialysis treatments can be difficult for patients to adjust to, and it often takes several months for the patient to truly adjust to hemodialysis treatments. Although patients may be tempted to end a hemodialysis session early, this can lead to an inadequate amount of dialysis, which can increase the long-term risk from complications.

Patients receiving any form of dialysis are at risk for the development of CHRONIC KIDNEY DISEASE–MINERAL BONE DISORDER (CKD-MBD), a bone disease that results from kidney damage (formerly known as renal osteodystrophy). This is particularly problematic among children with kidney failure because their bones are still growing. CKD-MBD in children may cause deformities of the legs, causing them to bend inwards or outwards. This is often referred to as renal rickets. Children with CKD-MBD often have short stature. The symptoms may occur before the child begins receiving dialysis treatments. (See CHILDREN AND KIDNEY DISEASE.)

Adults with CKD-MBD may have weak, thin bones and may also have joint pain and bone pain. In addition, they also have an increased risk for bone fractures. Some physicians treat individuals with weak bones with BISPHOSPHONATES, but this can be dangerous when patients are undergoing dialysis.

### Outlook and Lifestyle Modifications

Hemodialysis may sustain an individual's life for many years. Individuals on dialysis must make many different lifestyle modifications, such as limiting how much fluid they drink, in order to avoid a fluid buildup. Most individuals are used to their doctors telling them to drink plenty of water, but when the kidneys have failed, the reverse advice is given. The reason for this is that if the patient with kidney failure ingests more fluid than the kidneys can excrete in the urine, then the excess fluid accumulates in their blood vessels, causing worsening high blood pressure, pulmonary edema in their lungs, difficulty breathing, and ankle and leg edema in their legs.

Patients receiving hemodialysis must be particularly careful with their diet; for example, they need to limit the amount of the following foods, which all contain high amounts of PHOSPHORUS:

- milk
- cheese
- nuts
- dried beans
- cola soft drinks

However, even with avoiding these types of foods, the amount of phosphorous absorbed from the diet is generally greater than can be removed by dialysis treatments. If this is not prevented, a progressive accumulation of phosphorous and persistently high blood levels of phosphorous will cause progressive atherosclerosis, progressive renal osteodystrophy, progressive secondary HYPERPARATHYROIDISM, and, most importantly, will substantially increase the risk of dying. Accordingly, patients need to take medications that prevent the absorption of phosphorous from food in the intestinal tract. These medications are called phosphorous binders and must be taken at the time that the patient is eating. They work by chemically binding the phosphorus in the food and thereby preventing its absorption. Multiple types of phosphorus binders are available for the patient and their physician to try in order to identify the optimal treatment regimen for the patient.

Patients receiving hemodialysis also need to be very careful about foods containing potassium, because excessive levels of potassium can be harmful to the heart. As a result, the consumption of the following foods must be very limited among patients receiving hemodialysis:

- some fruits (especially bananas and oranges, which are high in potassium)
- chocolate
- nuts
- vegetables
- salt substitutes

In addition, the patient receiving hemodialysis treatment should also avoid salt because salt increases the individual's thirst and it also causes water retention, which is a problem among patients receiving dialysis.

### Questions Patients Should Ask Prior to Hemodialysis

According to the National Institute of Diabetes and Digestive and Kidney Diseases, individuals should ask their health care team the following questions before agreeing to hemodialysis:

- Is hemodialysis the best treatment choice for me? Why?

- If I am treated at a center, can I go to the center of my choice?

- What should I look for in a dialysis center?

- Will my kidney doctor see me at dialysis?

- What does hemodialysis feel like?

- What is self-care dialysis?

- Is home hemodialysis available in my area? If so, how long does it take to learn? Who will train my partner and me?

- What kind of blood access is best for me?

- As a hemodialysis patient, will I be able to keep working? Can I have treatments at night?

- How much should I exercise?

- Who will be on my health care team?

- How can these people help me?

- With whom can I talk about finances, sexuality, or family concerns?

- How/where can I talk with other people who have faced this decision?

See also DIALYSIS.

**hemolytic uremic syndrome–thrombotic thrombocytopenia purpura (HUS-TTP)**   A blood disorder that is associated with a decrease in the red blood cell count, which causes deposits of a substance known as fibrin in the kidneys. Hemolytic uremic syndrome–thrombotic thrombocytopenic purpura (HUS-TTP) causes ANEMIA, and in the worst case, it can lead to kidney failure requiring either DIALYSIS or a KIDNEY TRANSPLANTATION in order for the individual to survive.

HUS-TTP can result in a mild illness, or it can cause acute kidney failure or even death. Kidney failure occurs in about 12 percent of the cases of HUS-TTP, based on an analysis published in the *Journal of the American Medical Association* in 2003 by Amit X. Garg and colleagues.

According to the National Kidney and Urologic Diseases Information Clearinghouse, most cases of HUS-TTP in children result from a digestive system infection that is caused by the *Escherichia coli (E. coli)* bacterium. This is a common bacterium that is found in contaminated food, such as contaminated meat, dairy products, and juice. In addition, some people develop HUS-TTP after swimming in areas that are contaminated by fecal matter. Most people who are infected are children; they develop gastroenteritis, stomach cramps, and diarrhea, and the infection is subsequently resolved. However, in some children, the bacteria remain in the digestive system and create toxins that destroy the red blood cells. In adults, intestinal symptoms are less common. Instead, adult patients often have associated neurologic disorders such as seizures or coma, as well as fever and decreases in the platelet count.

The majority of cases of HUS-TTP in adults are related to a deficiency of a protein named ADAMTS13. Deficiency of this protein leads, through a progression of steps, to platelet clumping, fibrin deposits, and the development of HUS-TTP.

### Symptoms and Diagnostic Path

The symptoms of HUS-TTP when related to infection with *E. coli* may not appear for about a week after the person has been infected. When symptoms occur, the individual is irritable, tired, and pale. Other symptoms may include unexplained small bruises or bleeding from the nose or mouth because the toxins are destroying platelets that normally enable the blood to clot. The individual's urine output may also decrease and the urine may appear reddish. If the person does not urinate for 12 hours (anuria), then he or she should see a doctor as soon as possible. The most useful laboratory tests that lead to the diagnosis of HUS-TTP show deformed red blood cells and elevated blood levels of lactate dehydrogenase.

Treatment with plasma exchange or plasmapheresis can be life-saving.

Parents and guardians of children should immediately contact the child's physician if the child has the following symptoms and signs:

- unexplained bruises
- unusual bleeding
- swelling of limbs or generalized swelling of the body
- extreme fatigue
- decreased urine output

Adults with HUS-TTP usually do not have a preceding infectious cause. Instead, adults develop unexplained fever, low platelet counts that may lead to unexplained bleeding, new neurologic abnormalities, and otherwise unexplained renal failure. HUS-TTP in adults can result from certain medications, can be an unusual side effect of pregnancy, may be related to an underlying autoimmune condition, or may occur as a result of a bone marrow transplantation. Rarely, it results from infectious causes similar to those that cause the disease in children. Approximately one-third of cases in adults have no identifiable causes.

### Treatment Options and Outlook

The individual with HUS-TTP typically is very ill and requires hospitalization for therapy. If he or she has diarrhea resulting from an intestinal bacterial infection, then intravenous fluids may be needed. If bloody diarrhea has developed, then antibiotics and medications to slow the diarrhea (anti-motility agents) appear *not* to be effective at preventing HUS-TTP and may even increase the risk. Blood transfusions may be necessary to treat the anemia, which may become very severe. Dialysis may be necessary to treat the renal failure. Plasma exchange is the mainstay of therapy in severe cases, and has been associated with dramatic improvements in the prognosis, transforming HUS-TTP from a frequently fatal condition to one with a good prognosis for recovery.

### Risk Factors and Preventive Measures

Since infection is the trigger for the development of HUS-TTP in children and occasionally in adults, it is important to prevent foodborne infections, particularly avoiding a special type of *E. coli* known as *Escherichia coli* O157:H7. This particular bacterium is believed to be responsible for the majority of cases of HUS-TTP in children. This bacterium is transmitted through eating of undercooked meat or unpasteurized fruits or vegetables contaminated with cattle droppings. Very rarely, person-to-person transmission of this bacterium can occur, as in day care centers or long-term care facilities.

In adults, the condition is not generally associated with bacterial infections. If the condition is associated with a specific medication, then repeated exposure to that medication should be avoided. Patients with a previous episode of HUS-TTP are at increased risk for recurrence and should be followed closely for this possibility in the event of a change in their medical health.

See also INFECTIONS.

Garg, Amit X., M.D., et al. "Long-term Renal Prognosis of Diarrhea-Associated Hemolytic Uremic Syndrome: A Systematic Review, Meta-analysis, and Meta-regression." *Journal of the American Medical Association* 290, no. 10 (September 10, 2003): 1,360–1,370.

**Henoch-Schönlein purpura (HSP)** A type of vasculitis that is most common in children but can also rarely occur in adults. In some cases, it leads to kidney disease. Henoch-Schönlein purpura (HSP) causes inflamed small blood vessels on the skin of the legs or buttocks that leak out, causing a rash that looks like the individual has many tiny bruises that are slightly raised above the level of the normal skin. It is the most common type of vasculitis in children. In children, HSP is more commonly associated with abdominal pain. However, when it affects adults, this disease is typically more severe than in children.

This disorder may be an immune response to an infection, such as a cold, but the cause is unknown as of this writing. HSP has also been associated with insect bites or with a vaccination for some diseases, such as measles, cholera, yellow fever, typhoid, or hepatitis B. The disease generally lasts from four to six weeks. According to Brian V. Reamy and colleagues in their 2009 article in *American Family Physician*, "Because Henoch-Schönlein purpura resolves in 94 percent of children and 89 percent of adults, supportive treatment is the primary intervention." In about half of all cases, there is renal involvement and very rarely, HSP can cause kidney failure and a subsequent need for DIALYSIS. However, when the disease is severe, glucocortoicoid medications typically result in the increased rapidity of an improvement in the symptoms.

### Symptoms and Diagnostic Path

HSP causes four primary symptoms, including bruising and rashes, abdominal pain, arthritis, and kidney disease. Arthritis is present in an estimated 80 percent of patients with HSP, and blood in the URINE (hematuria) occurs in about 40 percent. About two-thirds of HSP patients have mild to severe abdominal pain.

HSP is diagnosed with laboratory testing, such as blood tests for elevated levels of creatinine and blood urea nitrogen (BUN). A urinalysis is checked for hematuria and for PROTEINURIA. If the test results are unclear, the physician may order a skin biopsy or a KIDNEY BIOPSY. (A kidney biopsy is rarely needed.)

### Treatment Options and Outlook

The primary treatment goal is to relieve the symptoms; for example, pain symptoms are treated with acetaminophen (Tylenol). If the patient has severe arthritis, corticosteroids such as prednisone may be prescribed, particularly if there is kidney involvement. The doctor will also check kidney and urine functions for at least several months after the main symptoms have disappeared. In general, if it is present, kidney disease starts within three to six months of the initial appearance of the rash.

According to Reamy and colleagues, "Early aggressive therapy with high-dose steroids plus immunosuppressants is recommended for patients with severe renal involvement. Long-term prognosis depends on the severity of renal involvement. End-stage renal disease occurs in 1 to 5 percent of patients."

If symptoms of kidney disease appear, doctors may prescribe immunosuppressant drugs to prevent the kidney from failing. An estimated 20–50 percent of children with HSP develop some kidney disease but about 1 percent will develop kidney failure. The outlook is generally good unless the kidneys become involved. In addition, the presence of proteinuria and HYPERTENSION are risk factors for kidney disease and a poor prognosis.

### Risk Factors and Preventive Measures

There are no known risk factors or preventive measures to HSP. If the disease presents, it should be treated and patients should be carefully watched for an onset of kidney disease.

Ballinger, Susan, M.D. "Henoch-Schönlein Purpura." *Current Opinion in Rheumatology* 15 (2003): 591–594.
Reamy, Brian V., Pamela M. Williams, and Tammy J. Lindsay. "Henoch-Schönlein Purpura." *American Family Physician* 80, no. 7 (2009): 697–704.

**hepatitis C (HCV)** A serious infection that affects the liver and that is transmitted through bodily fluids, as with sexual contact or the sharing of needles that are used to inject illegal drugs intravenously, and exposure to blood from an infected individual that crosses the skin or a mucous membrane. In many patients, the etiology of their hepatitis C is never identified. HCV can cause either acute or chronic hepatitis. With chronic infection, the person is unable to effectively respond to the infection and a persistent infection occurs. Chronic hepatitis C can lead to progressive liver disease and cirrhosis and sometimes to liver cancers. Hepatitis C can also cause CHRONIC KIDNEY DISEASE (CKD), most commonly in the form of MEMBRANOPROLIFERATIVE

GLOMERULONEPHRITIS (MPGN), and may lead to END-STAGE RENAL DISEASE.

According to the Centers for Disease Control and Prevention, there were about 17,000 new infections of HCV in the United States in 2007, the latest information as of this writing. An estimated 15–25 percent of individuals infected with HCV clear the infection from their bodies with no treatment, although the reasons for this are unknown.

### Symptoms and Diagnostic Path

Patients with new cases of HCV usually have no symptoms. If symptoms occur in patients with newly acquired HCV, they usually develop within four to 12 weeks of the time of infection, and may include the following:

- dark urine
- abdominal pain
- fever
- fatigue
- loss of appetite
- nausea and vomiting
- clay-colored stools
- loss of appetite
- joint and muscle pain

About 20–30 percent of individuals with HCV develop the symptoms of acute illness, which includes such symptoms as jaundice, abdominal pain, fatigue, and poor appetite. Otherwise, patients are typically identified because blood tests show low-grade elevations of blood levels of liver injury, such as AST or ALT, or because blood tests show more advanced liver disease, such as elevations in bilirubin levels or an abnormal INR test result.

HCV can be screened for with such tests as the enzyme immunoassay (EIA) and the enhanced chemiluminescence immunoassay (CIA). Another test that may be used is the recombinant immunoblot assay (RIBA). Definitive testing involves direct tests for the HCV virus in the blood, which can quantify the amount of the virus that is present. This test can also determine which HCV genotype is present, which gives important information about the likelihood of the patient of responding to therapy.

Some conditions that are sometimes confused with HCV are alcoholic hepatitis, chronic hepatitis B and D, autoimmune hepatitis, and nonalcoholic steatohepatitis (fatty liver disease). As a result, it is important to obtain a definitive diagnosis.

### Treatment Options and Outlook

Individuals with chronic HCV infection may be treated with combination therapy, including the use of such medications as pegylated interferon and ribavirin. The body's handling of these medications is altered if impaired renal function (either chronic kidney disease or acute kidney injury) is present, and adjustments in dosing may be needed.

Patients with HCV should avoid alcohol altogether, because alcohol likely accelerates the development of liver cirrhosis and liver cancer, and it also decreases the effectiveness of the medications that are used to treat HCV. Patients should also be extremely careful with the use of any prescription medications, particularly acetaminophen, which is present in many over-the-counter (OTC) drugs, such as nonaspirin pain relievers and cold remedies, and is also present in many prescription pain medicines. Any OTC medications that a person with HCV is considering taking should first be discussed with the physician's office, including cold remedies and other OTC drugs. Many cold remedies include a combination of different medications, including pain relievers.

Some patients with HCV should not receive antiviral treatment directed against HCV. Patients who are not compliant with medications are often not treated because the risk of side effects from the medications is likely to exceed the likely benefits. In addition, individuals with psychiatric disorders may need to avoid treatment because prolonged therapy, particularly pegylated interferon, can lead to personality changes, anxiety, DEPRESSION, and even suicidal behavior and psychosis.

Ribavarin is contraindicated in women who are pregnant, thinking about becoming pregnant, or unwilling to assure effective contraception so that they do not become pregnant. Patients with autoimmune diseases, such as systemic lupus erythematosus, may have their autoimmune condition worsened by the interferon component of their therapy.

### Risk Factors and Preventive Measures

Intravenous drug users and those with the human immunodeficiency virus (HIV) have an elevated risk for developing HCV. In addition, those receiving dialysis for end-stage renal disease have an increased risk for HCV. The disease can also be spread by sexual contact in those with many sexual partners. The illegal intranasal use of cocaine increases the risk for the transmission of HCV. Children born to a mother who is infected with HCV have an increased risk for HCV.

See also INFECTIONS; GLOMERULONEPHRITIS; HUMAN IMMUNODEFICIENCY VIRUS ASSOCIATED NEPHROPATHY (HIVAN).

Tsui, Judith I., M.D. "Association of Hepatitis C Seropositivity with Increased Risk for Developing End-Stage Renal Disease." *Archives of Internal Medicine* 167 (June 25, 2007): 1,271–1,276.

**high blood pressure**   See HYPERTENSION.

**Hispanics**   See HEMODIALYSIS: KIDNEYS AND KIDNEY DISEASE.

**human immunodeficiency virus (HIV)**   See HUMAN IMMUNODEFICIENCY VIRUS ASSOCIATED NEPHROPATHY (HIVAN).

**human immunodeficiency virus associated nephropathy (HIVAN)**   The human immunodeficiency virus (HIV) is a serious virus that is often sexually transmitted during unprotected sex, although it may also be transmitted by a mother to a fetus through the placenta; from mother to baby during breastfeeding; or from one drug-using individual to another through the sharing of dirty needles among illegal drug users. HIV may also lead to HIV-associated nephropathy (HIVAN). Eventually, HIV progresses to acquired immune deficiency syndrome (AIDS). HIVAN is not common and represents only about 1 percent of all cases of END-STAGE RENAL DISEASE (ESRD). However, HIVAN is the third leading cause of ESRD among African Americans ages 20–64 years. At least half of this group are believed to be illegal intravenous drug users.

Some children develop HIV as a result of being born to mothers infected with HIV who were not treated with antiretroviral medications, and these children may also develop HIVAN.

### Symptoms and Diagnostic Path

According to Moro O. Salifu in an article for eMedicine on HIV nephropathy in 2009, the following signs and symptoms may be found with HIVAN:

- azotemia (high levels of nitrogen wastes in the blood, such as urea and creatinine)
- FOCAL SEGMENTAL GLOMERULOSCLEROSIS (FSGS), which is identified with a KIDNEY BIOPSY
- normal to enlarged kidneys, particularly enlarged but echogenic kidneys, when imaged with an ultrasound
- PROTEINURIA (protein in the urine) in the nephritic range
- normal blood pressure

Other findings may include IgA NEPHROPATHY and AMYLOIDOSIS, as well as cryoglobulinemia, which is often related to a coexisting infection with HEPATITIS C. Most patients with HIVAN do not have edema, according to Salifu.

Because patients with HIV and proteinuria or other forms of kidney disease can have kidney disease due to causes other than HIVAN, a kidney biopsy may be helpful in order to definitively determine the cause of their kidney disease.

### Treatment Options and Outlook

Patients with HIVAN should be treated by an expert on HIV as well as a nephrologist. In general, patients with HIVAN are treated with combination antiretroviral therapy, referred to as highly active antiretroviral therapy (HAART). The components of HAART change as researchers learn more about what medications work best together. Salifu says some patients with HIVAN also benefit from the short-term use of corticosteroids, and some reports indicate that cyclosporine may reduce proteinuria in children with HIVAN.

Some medications used to treat HIV can lead to other kidney-related problems; for example, didanosine (Videx, Videx EC) can lead to HYPONATREMIA (low blood levels of SODIUM), HYPOKALEMIA (low blood levels of POTASSIUM), hypermagnesia (high blood levels of MAGNESIUM), and HYPERURICEMIA (high blood levels of uric acid), while stavudine (Zerit) can trigger the development of hyperuricemia.

Some medications used to treat common infections among those with HIVAN may cause problems with the kidneys, otherwise known as nephrotoxicity. According to Salifu, medications that may lead to acute renal failure in patients with HIVAN include Bactrim, Amphotericin, Pentamidien, Itraconazol, and Foscarnet. In addition, these drugs may raise or lower the levels of potassium, sodium, calcium, and magnesium; for example, Pentamidine raises potassium levels and lowers the levels of calcium and magnesium, while Bactrim raises potassium levels and lowers the levels of sodium.

If individuals with HIVAN develop kidney failure, then a kidney transplant is not generally recommended. The reason for this is that a mainstay therapy of transplantation is the use of IMMUNOSUPPRESSIVE DRUGS, but the immune system of the person with HIV is already severely compromised. The administration of immunosuppressants often leads to an increased risk of serious opportunistic infections and can lead to worsening of the HIV infection. As a result, kidney transplantation is generally not considered an option for people with HIVAN unless they fit very specific criteria, such as having had no opportunistic infections, having no detectable HIV virus in their blood, and being in very good health other than their end-stage renal disease. However, even under these conditions, a kidney transplant still carries an elevated risk.

Increasing experience with treating HIVAN over the past decade indicates that treatment with highly active antiretroviral therapy (HAART) can change the natural history of HIVAN both by preventing its development and by slowing its progression once developed. In addition, steroids and angiotensin-converting enzyme inhibitor (ACEI) therapy appear to improve kidney function in patients with HIVAN.

### Risk Factors and Preventive Measures

Individuals with HIV are at high risk for the development of HIVAN. There are no known preventive measures, other than avoiding the causes for the development of an HIV infection, such as avoiding illegal intravenous drugs and unprotected sex. Treatment of patients with HIV with HAART therapy, however, appears to reduce the risk of developing HIVAN.

See also GLOMERULONEPHRITIS; INFECTIONS.

Salifu, Moro, M.D., Sidhartha Pani, M.D., and Nilanjana Misra, M.D. "HIV Nephropathy." eMedicine. Available online. URL: www.http://emedicine. medscape.com/article/246031-print. Last updated February 4, 2009. Accessed December 22, 2009.

Wyatt, Christina M., and Paul E. Klotman. "HIV-1 and HIV-Associated Nephropathy 25 Years Later." *Clinical Journal of the American Society of Nephrology* 2 (2007): S20–S24.

**hypercalcemia**  Excessively high levels of CALCIUM in the bloodstream, as measured by laboratory tests. In general, hypercalcemia is defined as a blood calcium level greater than 10.5 mg/deciliter. Levels that are higher than 12.0 mg/dl are a medical emergency, and the individual may need immediate emergency treatment. Chronic hypercalcemia often leads to kidney disease. Hypercalcemia caused by HYPERPARATHYROIDISM, an endocrine disorder, can lead to multiple bone fractures.

Primary hyperparathyroidism is one of the most common causes of hypercalcemia. Some medical students are taught the key aspects of hyperparathyroidism with the phrase, "stones, bones, and groans," which means that hyperparathyroidism may cause kidney stones, osteoporosis, and painful bone fractures. Some types of cancer, especially lung cancers, may also lead to hypercalcemia. In addition, hyperthyroidism, an overactive thyroid, can lead to hypercalcemia. Rarely, patients recovering from RHABDOMYOLYSIS may develop hypercalcemia. In some cases, medications can lead to the development of hypercalcemia, as with certain DIURETICS or with lithium. Excess vitamin D intake is another important cause. Because vitamin D and medications that are analogues of naturally occurring vitamin D are increasingly used in patients with kidney disease, an increasing number of patients with hypercalcemia due to vitamin D are being observed.

### Symptoms and Diagnostic Path

Often there are no symptoms with hypercalcemia, and the high levels of blood calcium are only discovered as part of laboratory testing. However, when blood calcium levels are very high, patients may experience such symptoms as increased urination, decreased alertness, constipation, fatigue, and muscle weakness. If hypercalcemia persists and is not identified or treated, it can lead to the development of KIDNEY STONES.

Calcium is partly bound to proteins in the blood, and the protein-bound calcium does not exert any biologic effect. As a result, diagnosing hypercalcemia requires either measuring the unbound "ionized" calcium or mathematically adjusting the measured serum calcium if the level of the proteins in the blood is low. In the latter case, the adjusted or "corrected" calcium is calculated with the following mathematical formula: $Ca^{+2}_{Corrected} = Ca^{+2}_{Total} + 0.8 \times (4.0-[Albumin])$.

### Treatment Options and Outlook

The physician seeks to find the underlying cause for the hypercalcemia and treat that disorder. If the hypercalcemia is severe, hospitalization and treatment is needed, and patients are treated with normal saline (salt water) given intravenously. Certain DIURETICS commonly known as loop diuretics, such as furosemide and bumetanide, can help in the treatment of hypercalcemia. However, if they cause the person to become dehydrated, these diuretics can actually worsen the hypercalcemia. Other diuretics, thiazide diuretics, block the kidney's ability to excrete calcium in the urine and cause and/or worsen hypercalcemia. In some cases of chronic hypercalcemia, medications such as BISPHOSPHONATES may be helpful. Patients with hypercalcemia due to granulomatous conditions, such as sarcoidosis, can benefit from treatment with corticosteroids, especially prednisone. Calcitonin is another medication that is frequently used to treat hypercalcemia. The outlook depends on the cause of the hypercalcemia and the response to therapy.

### Risk Factors and Preventive Measures

Patients with primary hyperparathyroidism have an elevated risk for hypercalcemia, as do those with hyperthyroidism. Rarely, individuals with Addison's disease, Paget's disease, or sarcoidosis have an elevated risk for developing hypercalcemia. Patients being treated with vitamin D and related medications should be checked regularly for hypercalcemia.

See also HYPOCALCEMIA; HYPOPARATHYROIDISM.

Petit, William A. Jr., M.D., and Christine Adamec. *The Encyclopedia of Endocrine Diseases and Disorders*. New York: Facts On File, 2005.

**hyperlipidemia** See CHOLESTEROL.

**hyperkalemia** Excessively high levels of POTAS-
SIUM in the bloodstream, as measured by laboratory tests. In most cases, hyperkalemia is caused
by disorders that decrease the ability of the kidneys to excrete potassium, including such disorders as ACUTE KIDNEY INJURY, CHRONIC KIDNEY
DISEASE, GLOMERULONEPHRITIS, LUPUS NEPHRITIS,
the rejection of a KIDNEY TRANSPLANTATION, and
specific medications.

In an article by Lisa M. Einhorn and colleagues and reported in *Archives of Internal
Medicine* in 2009, the researchers analyzed
66,259 hyperkalemic events, and they found
that the risk for hyperkalemia was elevated
in those with chronic kidney disease (CKD).
A slight majority of the hyperkalemic events
occurred to hospital inpatients (52.7 percent).
The researchers also found that 2.4 percent of
the hyperkalemic patients died within a day of
their blood draw.

### Symptoms and Diagnostic Path

Often there are no symptoms of hyperkalemia.
When symptoms occur, the individual may have
unexplained weakness, be nauseous, or have a
weakened pulse. There may also be an irregular
heartbeat. When the blood is tested, blood potassium levels will be high. An electrocardiogram
(ECG) will show changes linked to hyperkalemia
and may show dangerous arrhythmias of the
heart. The individual with severe hyperkalemia
is at risk for sudden death and must be hospitalized and closely monitored.

### Treatment Options and Outlook

The treatment of hyperkalemia depends on the
severity of the condition and on the specific
cause. In patients with life-threatening hyperkalemia with evidence of cardiac effects shown
on the ECG, emergent treatment with medications (intravenous calcium) that block the effects
of the high potassium level on the heart are
needed. This is then followed by medications

that cause the cells in the body to take potassium
out of the blood into the cells, thereby decreasing the blood potassium level.

The most common medicine used is intravenous insulin; glucose is given simultaneously to
prevent the insulin from excessively lowering
the blood glucose levels. Inhaled medications
can also be used, but they tend to be associated
with less predictable effects and with increased
risk of side effects, particularly affecting the
heart. Finally, the potassium must be removed
from the body. If the patient has functioning kidneys, then DIURETICS will increase the kidney's
potassium excretion. If the kidneys are not functioning, then an oral medication that absorbs
potassium (sodium polystyrene sulfonate) may
be needed. In rare cases, potassium removal
with hemodialysis is needed.

Patients with CKD often have chronic hyperkalemia. In part this is because many of the
medications used to treat patients with CKD,
such as ACEIs, ARBs, and beta-blockers, increase
the blood potassium level. In many cases these
medications cannot and should not be stopped
because of their beneficial effect on the CKD
and also to prevent cardiovascular events, such
as myocardial infarction or stroke. However,
there are rare patients who have life-threatening
increases in their potassium levels that cannot
be controlled by other mechanisms, and in these
patients these medications are discontinued.

Instruction in a low potassium diet and avoidance of nonessential medications that increase
serum potassium, such as nonsteroidal anti-
inflammatory drugs (NSAIDs) and COX-2 inhibitors, should be routinely considered. Diuretics,
as mentioned above, will increase renal potassium excretion and are often necessary.

Longer-term solutions are needed once the
patient with hyperkalemia is stabilized, such as
identifying all possible causes of the problem and
working on their resolution.

### Risk Factors and Preventive Measures

Individuals taking potassium supplements for
any reason are at risk for hyperkalemia and

they should have their kidney function evaluated on a regular basis. Individuals who have had hyperkalemia should avoid salt substitutes, since potassium is typically used as a substitute for SODIUM.

See also HYPOKALEMIA; MAGNESIUM.

Einhorn, Lisa M., et al. "The Frequency of Hyperkalemia and Its Significance in Chronic Kidney Disease." *Archives of Internal Medicine* 169, no. 12 (2009): 1,156–1,162.

Weiner, I. David, and Charles S. Wingo. "Hyperkalemia: A Potential Silent Killer." *Journal of the American Society of Nephrology,* 9 (1998): 1,535–1,543.

**hypernatremia** Excessively high concentrations of SODIUM in the bloodstream, as measured by laboratory tests. Hypernatremia may be caused by dehydration that may have been developed as a result of an untreated INFECTION. It may also be caused by illnesses such as DIABETES INSIPIDUS or by symptoms such as HYPERCALCEMIA and hyperglycemia (excessive levels of blood glucose), as found with DIABETES MELLITUS.

### Symptoms and Diagnostic Path

Common symptoms of hypernatremia are muscle weakness and confusion, and in severe cases, coma may develop. Somewhat surprisingly, thirst is not always a symptom of hypernatremia, although the individual needs more fluids. In most cases, the absence of the ability to sense increased thirst is a contributing factor leading to the development of hypernatremia.

Hypernatremia is diagnosed based on identifying an elevated level of sodium; the symptoms and the individual's medical history are useful in identifying why the hypernatremia developed. The goal is to identify the cause of the hypernatremia so that the cause can be treated and resolved. Otherwise, recurrence of the hypernatremia is common. If the individual has an infection, then antibiotics are prescribed. If the cause is an illness such as diabetes insipidus, then that illness is treated.

### Treatment Options and Outlook

Treatment depends partly on the cause of the hypernatremia; however, when the hypernatremia is severe, the goal is to reverse it with fluids that are administered intravenously. If the hypernatremia is not severe, then increasing the fluid intake may help resolve the problem until the physician can determine and treat the underlying cause.

### Risk Factors and Preventive Measures

Individuals who are dehydrated and/or suffering from infection and who have either decreased levels of mental alertness or are otherwise unable to seek and obtain fluids to drink are at risk of developing hypernatremia. Adequate fluid intake should prevent hypernatremia.

See also HYPONATREMIA.

**hyperoxaluria** This refers to a condition in which excessive levels of the substance oxalate are present in the urine. Its excessive production can combine with CALCIUM and lead to the development of recurrent KIDNEY STONES. Oxalate is found in many common foods, and in the healthy individual, the oxalate is excreted by the kidneys. Some individuals have primary hyperoxaluria, which is a genetic disorder causing the excessive production of oxalate. This disorder can lead to the development of bladder stones as well as kidney stones. Hyperoxaluria can also affect growth in affected children. Individuals whose bodies are prone to producing oxalate kidney stones are said to have oxalate stone disease.

There are two types of primary hyperoxaluria, Type 1 (PH1) and Type 2 primary hyperoxaluria. PH1 is the more common of the two. They are both rare genetic disorders, although not everyone with hyperoxaluria has a genetic disorder. A nongenetic form of hyperoxaluria is known as enteric hyperoxaluria because it is caused by the excessive absorption of oxalates in the intestinal tract. In addition, some people overeat foods that are high in oxalates (such as chocolate, peanuts, and blueberries, to name a few), and as a result, they may develop hyperoxaluria. In such cases, dietary changes can readily resolve the problem.

With both types of genetic disorders, a liver enzyme malfunctions, but the end-organ which is harmed is the kidney. However, oxalates may also be deposited in other organs, such as in the bones, the heart, and even the eyes. When hyperoxaluria damages the kidneys due to these genetic causes, this can lead to END-STAGE RENAL DISEASE, necessitating either DIALYSIS or a KIDNEY TRANSPLANTATION. If available, a liver transplant raises the possibility of a cure of the underlying condition, by replacing the liver which lacks the appropriate enzyme necessary for oxalate metabolism with a normal liver. Thus, in some cases, a combined kidney and liver transplant may be beneficial.

Some foods that are high in oxalates include the following: fruits, especially berries; vegetables such as spinach, celery, green beans, and parsley. Foods that are high in vitamin C are converted by the body into oxalates.

### Symptoms and Diagnostic Path
There are no specific symptoms of hyperoxaluria in most patients. The most common presenting findings are signs and symptoms related to a kidney stone which results from the hyperoxaluria. With genetic causes of primary hyperoxaluria, a progressive loss of renal function from the deposition of oxalate in the kidneys can occur, and lead to signs and symptoms of progressive chronic kidney disease. In addition, when renal function decreases, the kidney's ability to excrete oxalate also decreases, and this can lead to a massive accumulation of oxalate and other tissues in the body. This can also lead to cardiac conduction defects and arrhythmias, to deposition in the blood vessels leading to gangrene, and to the deposition of oxalate crystals in the retina of the eye and the potential for blindness.

Mild causes of hyperoxaluria can be diagnosed by a 24-hour urine collection to detect the presence of excessive amounts of oxalate in the urine. If very high levels of urinary oxalate are identified, this can suggest the possibility of primary hyperoxaluria. A KIDNEY BIOPSY or liver biopsy can confirm the diagnosis of hyperoxaluria, according to the Oxalosis & Hyperoxaluria Foundation (OHF).

Because of a general lack of awareness of primary hyperoxaluria, often this disorder is not diagnosed until it has caused severe damage to the kidneys or other organs.

### Treatment Options and Outlook
Primary hyperoxaluria is treated with prescription-level doses of vitamin B6 (pyridoxine) to help to reduce the oxalate that is produced by the liver in about half of all patients with primary hyperoxaluria. Patients with healthy kidneys are encouraged to drink as much fluid as possible to increase the kidney's ability to excrete oxalate in the urine without developing kidney stones or oxalate retention in the kidneys. Foods containing oxalates should be avoided or limited. Medications that inhibit calcium oxalate crystallization are recommended, such as potassium citrate.

According to Cochat et al., conventional HEMODIALYSIS will not be effective in patients with PH1 because the constant production of oxalate cannot be overcome with dialysis; however, dialysis may be used if the diagnosis has not been definitively made or if the individual is awaiting kidney transplantation as well as in some other instances. Liver transplantation with kidney transplantation is a good solution because the defective liver will be replaced with a normal one and cannot harm the transplanted kidney.

### Risk Factors and Preventive Measures
Individuals with primary hyperoxaluria are at the greatest risk of suffering from problems with oxalate. Preventive measures may involve limiting the consumption of foods containing oxalates and increasing consumption of fluids if the

kidneys have not failed. Once the disorder has developed, it should be treated.

Cochat, Pierre, et al. "Nephrolithiasis Related to Inborn Metabolic Diseases." *Pediatric Nephrology* 25 (2010): 415–424.

**hyperparathyroidism** Excessively high levels of parathyroid hormone (PTH), a hormone that is produced by the parathyroid glands that are embedded in the thyroid gland. By causing chronic HYPERCALCEMIA, occasionally hyperparathyroidism leads to kidney disease. In addition, kidney disease may itself cause hyperparathyroidism; for example, in the case of individuals with CHRONIC KIDNEY DISEASE (CKD), a secondary form of hyperparathyroidism often may develop. Secondary hyperparathyroidism (SHPT) can lead to the development of some forms of CHRONIC KIDNEY DISEASE–MINERAL BONE DISORDER (CKD-MBD), which is a bone disease that is diagnosed in some individuals with chronic kidney disease or in those patients with END-STAGE RENAL DISEASE, the last stage of CKD.

Secondary hyperparathyroidism is linked to changes, not only to the metabolism of VITAMIN D and to vitamin D deficiencies, but also to the metabolism of CALCIUM and PHOSPHORUS. According to Samina Khan in her article on secondary hyperparathyroidism, SHPT can lead to fragility of the bones and to an increased risk for bone fractures. In addition, poorly controlled secondary hyperparathyroidism in patients who are being treated with dialysis predicts an increased risk of dying.

### Symptoms and Diagnostic Path
With SHPT, the patient may have musculoskeletal pains and aches and may experience bone fractures from very little trauma or even no trauma. Primary hyperparathyroidism can lead to recurrent KIDNEY STONES with their associated symptoms, or to pancreatitis. Pancreatitis often presents with severe abdominal pain associated with nausea and vomiting. Other symptoms may include the following:

- itching skin
- back pain
- fatigue
- upper abdominal pain
- muscle and tongue fasciculations (very tiny and involuntary muscle contractions which cause the muscle to quiver)

The blood level of parathyroid hormone can be measured to determine whether excessive levels of parathyroid hormone are present in the blood. With primary hyperparathyroidism, elevated PTH levels lead to increased calcium levels in the blood. With secondary hyperparathyroidism that is associated with chronic kidney disease, the renal function is abnormal and serum calcium levels are either normal or low, while the serum phosphate levels are often elevated but may also be normal. In some cases, severe and prolonged secondary hyperparathyroidism can transform into a condition termed tertiary hyperparathyroidism. In tertiary hyperparathyroidism, the serum calcium levels are elevated and the serum PTH level is very elevated in the patient who almost always has advanced chronic kidney disease.

### Treatment Options and Outlook
If hyperparathyroidism is caused by kidney disease, which is termed a secondary hyperparathyroidism, treatment often involves diffusive phosphate binders to decrease dietary phosphate absorption and thereby reduce PTH levels. In some cases, prescribing vitamin D to reduce the excessive levels of parathyroid hormone and correct the vitamin D deficiency is beneficial. It is best to identify a vitamin D deficiency in the early stages before SHPT has developed or when it is in the early stages.

Prescribed vitamin D comes in the form of calcitriol, doxercalciferol, alfacalcidol, and paricalcitol, all of which are approved by the Food and Drug Administration (FDA) to treat SHPT.

Paricalcitol may have the least risk of causing hypercalcemia. Patients with very advanced chronic kidney disease may require treatment with calcitriol, doxercalciferol, or paricalcitol; other forms of vitamin D require activation in the kidney before they are effective. This process is likely to be relatively impaired in the patient with advanced chronic kidney disease.

Hyperphosphatemia (excessive levels of phosphorus in the blood) is the most important cause of secondary hyperparathyroidism and must be corrected if present. This is managed with dietary changes and the use of medications that are phosphate binders. Because phosphates are in many foods, management of phosphorus by diet alone can be difficult; for example, phosphorus is present in many processed foods, including those which are high in protein, an important dietary ingredient. Some examples of foods high in phosphorus include roasted soybeans, chicken breast, shrimp, pork, and peanut butter. Phosphorus is also present in cheeses, salad dressings, and many beverages.

Other medications that can be used are calcimimetics. These medications have direct effects on the parathyroid gland to decrease the release of PTH.

When all other treatment measures fail, a parathyroidectomy, or the removal of the parathyroid glands, may be recommended. This is especially true if the individual has bone disease, severe hypercalcemia, and extreme itching (pruritus) and the parathyroid levels are greater than 800 pg/mL. After surgery, the follow-up of calcium blood levels is extremely important. Many patients will have very low levels of calcium in their blood after surgery and require treatment with large amounts of oral calcium and vitamin D in order to avoid HYPOCALCEMIA. This situation will resolve with time and these medications can be decreased eventually.

### Risk Factors and Preventive Measures

Individuals with chronic kidney disease are at risk for secondary hyperparathyroidism. The use of lithium for bipolar disorder can cause primary hyperparathyroidism. Multiple endocrine neoplasia, type I, a rare hereditary disorder, can also cause primary hyperparathyroidism. Otherwise, most cases of primary hyperparathyroidism are spontaneous and not due to an identifiable etiology.

See also HYPOPARATHYROIDISM; LITHIUM AND BIPOLAR DISORDER.

Cibulka, R., and J. Racek. "Metabolic Disorders in Patients with Chronic Kidney Disease." *Physiological Research* 56 (2007): 697–705.

Khan, Samina, M.D. "Vitamin D Deficiency and Secondary Hyperparathyroidism among Patients with Chronic Kidney Disease." *American Journal of the Medical Sciences* 333, no. 4 (2007): 201–207.

Mayo Clinic Staff. "Risk Factors: Hyperparathyroidism." Available online. URL: http://www.mayoclinic.com/health/hyperparathyroidism/DS00396/DSECTION;risk-factors. May 12, 2010. Accessed November 5, 2010.

Petit, William A., Jr., M.D., and Christine Adamec. *The Encyclopedia of Endocrine Diseases and Disorders.* New York: Facts On File, 2005.

Saliba, Wissam, M.D., and Boutros El-Haddad, M.D. "Secondary Hyperparathyroidism: Pathophysiology and Treatment." *Journal of the American Board of Family Medicine* 22 (2009): 574–581.

**hyperphosphatemia**  Excessive levels of the mineral PHOSPHORUS in the bloodstream, which is determined by a blood test of phosphorus levels. The levels of phosphates can build up quickly in damaged or failed kidneys, and this condition necessitates the patient's making DIETARY CHANGES to decrease these blood levels. Many common foods include phosphorus, and these foods must be limited or avoided by individuals with hyperphosphatemia. Individuals with kidney disease who consume foods that are high in phosphorus tend to lose calcium, causing HYPOCALCEMIA, which can cause the bones to become weak and even fracture. In general, however, hyperphosphatemia causes no symptoms.

According to Keith A. Hruska, M.D., and colleagues, hyperphosphatemia is a contributing factor in the high death rates found with CHRONIC KIDNEY DISEASE. It is also a factor in CARDIOVASCULAR DISEASE and in CHRONIC KIDNEY DISEASE—MINERAL BONE DISORDER (CKD-MBD), which was formerly known as renal osteodystrophy.

Hruska et al. say that 1,000–1,200 mg of phosphorus is needed in the average daily diet. Some foods are very high in phosphorus, such as cola drinks, milk, cheese, dried beans, peas, nuts, and peanut butter. Individuals who are on dialysis need to avoid or greatly restrict the consumption of these foods. People with dialysis usually cannot drink more than a half cup of milk per day.

With a normal phosphorus balance, phosphorus is obtained through food; most is absorbed, and some is excreted through the feces. Some of the phosphorus is used for bone formation and resorption. The remaining phosphorus is excreted in the urine. Patients with kidney disease may have an inability to excrete sufficient amounts of phosphorus in the urine, and thereby they develop hyperphosphatemia.

With abnormal phosphorus balance in chronic kidney disease, only about a third as much is used for bone formation and consequently, problems with the bones can occur.

People with hyperphosphatemia may need to take phosphate binders such as calcium carbonate, sevelemer bicarbonate, or lanthanum carbonate to control their phosphorus levels between dialysis sessions.

Hruska, Keith A., M.D., et al. "Hyperphosphatemia of Chronic Kidney Disease." *Kidney International* 74, no. 2 (2008): 148–157.

**hypertension** High blood pressure, or higher than average force of the blood against the wall of the blood vessels. Hypertension is often caused by an excessive level of fluid in the blood vessels or by a narrowing and/or clogging of the vessels. In addition, stress often worsens high blood pressure levels. Chronic hypertension can lead to CHRONIC KIDNEY DISEASE by damaging the blood vessels in the kidneys. According to the Food and Drug Administration, almost one in three adults in the United States has hypertension. Chronic hypertension usually cannot be cured, but it can be controlled effectively with medications, weight loss, effective control of DIABETES MELLITUS, if present, and giving up SMOKING.

Hypertension is the most common diagnosis leading to patients seeing physicians in the United States. Nevertheless, 30 percent of people with hypertension do not know that they have high blood pressure. Of those that do know, only about half have their blood pressure adequately controlled. Effective hypertension control can be achieved in most patients, but the majority of hypertensive individuals require two or more ANTIHYPERTENSIVE DRUGS to achieve that control. Lifestyle modifications are also important (such as weight loss among those who are overweight or obese). When clinicians fail to prescribe lifestyle modifications, adequate antihypertensive drug doses, or appropriate drug combinations, then inadequate blood pressure control may result.

Hypertension is the second leading cause of kidney failure (END-STAGE RENAL DISEASE) in the United States after diabetes mellitus. According to the National Institute of Diabetes and Digestive and Kidney Diseases, hypertension causes about 25,000 new cases of kidney failure every year. When hypertension is combined with diabetes mellitus, the risk for kidney failure is elevated much further. In addition, hypertension is a risk factor in the development of CARDIOVASCULAR DISEASE, such as heart attack (myocardial infarction), heart failure, and stroke.

Blood pressure for an adult is considered normal if it is below 120/80, which refers to a systolic blood pressure of 120 mm Hg and a diastolic pressure of 80 mm Hg. When the systolic pressure is between 120–139 or the diastolic blood pressure is between 80–99, then the person is termed to have prehypertension. If the systolic blood pressure is equal to or greater than 140 or the diastolic blood pressure is equal to or greater than 90, the individual has hypertension and needs to consult with a physician on ways to bring the blood pressure under control.

### Symptoms and Diagnostic Path

In general, hypertension causes no symptoms, which is why hypertension is often called the "silent killer." Once hypertension is more advanced, symptoms and signs may occur. High blood pressure can only be determined by the measurement of the blood pressure with a standard blood pressure cuff. The systolic pressure (the top number on the blood pressure reading) refers to the pressure of the heart beating. The diastolic pressure (the bottom number on the blood pressure reading) is the pressure when the heart is resting.

Symptoms of kidney damage that is caused by high blood pressure can be detected through blood tests; for example, blood levels of creatinine are used to measure the GLOMERULAR FILTRATION RATE, the primary kidney function. PROTEINURIA, or protein in the urine, is another indicator of kidney damage in patients with hypertension.

Rarely, hypertension directly causes symptoms. These may include headaches, shortness of breath, visual changes including blindness, and, in very severe cases, seizures or decreased levels of alertness.

### Treatment Options and Outlook

Individuals who have already been diagnosed with kidney disease should seek to limit their blood pressure to less than 120/80, using medications and lifestyle changes. There are several primary categories of drugs that are used to control hypertension, including ANGIOTENSIN-CONVERTING ENZYME INHIBITORS (ACEIs) and ANGIOTENSIN II RECEPTOR BLOCKERS (ARBs). These medications relax the blood vessels by blocking a hormone that causes the constriction of the vessels. CALCIUM CHANNEL BLOCKERS may also be used to directly relax the vessels. BETA BLOCKERS are another important class of medications that act to decrease blood pressure.

ALPHA BLOCKERS may be used to relax the nerves that tighten the blood vessels. Some individuals also take a DIURETIC medication in addition to other medications to decrease the blood volume and flush out extra salt and water from the body. Some people must take two or more medications to control their hypertension.

Dietary changes can help to decrease blood pressure, as may weight loss among those who are obese. Exercise can often improve hypertension. The avoidance of alcohol and excessive levels of caffeine is also recommended.

### Risk Factors and Preventive Measures

African Americans have a greater than usual risk of having hypertension, and the kidneys of African Americans appear to be at greater risk of developing kidney problems as a result of their high blood pressure. This is true even when the blood pressure of African Americans is only mildly elevated. In addition, African Americans have a four times greater risk of developing hypertension-related kidney failure than Caucasians. The African American Study of Kidney Disease and Hypertension found that an ACE inhibitor medication was the most effective type of drug at preventing hypertensive kidney disease among African Americans. American Indians also have a high rate of hypertension as well as a high rate of diabetes mellitus.

Individuals with a family history of hypertension are at risk for developing high blood pressure. As mentioned, patients who have both diabetes and hypertension have an increased risk for suffering from kidney failure.

Preventive measures of further problems that are caused by or related to hypertension include weight loss among the obese and limiting alcohol and caffeine intake, as well as participating in regular exercise. Men with hypertension should limit their alcohol consumption to no more than two drinks (two 12-ounce servings of beer or two five-ounce servings of wine or two 1.5-ounce servings of distilled liquor). Women with high blood pressure should limit themselves to one drink per day. People with high blood pressure should limit their consumption of sodium (salt) to less than 2,000 milligrams per day, by reading food labels. Increasing the intake of POTASSIUM, a mineral present in many foods, can improve blood pressure.

Periodic blood pressure monitoring at their physician's office should also occur, and the patient with hypertension should be under the care of a physician who is knowledgeable about hypertension. In severe cases, consultation with a hypertension specialist, such as a NEPHROLOGIST, may be helpful. Some patients purchase blood pressure cuffs to measure their own pressure levels, as increasing evidence suggest that using blood pressure measurements taken at home are better than using blood pressure measurements made in the doctor's office to guide therapy.

See also DIALYSIS; MEDICATIONS THAT CAN HARM THE KIDNEYS.

Adrogué, Horacio, M.D., and Nicolaos E. Madias, M.D. "Sodium and Potassium in the Pathogenesis of Hypertension." *New England Journal of Medicine* 356, no. 19 (May 10, 2007): 1,966–1,978.

**hyperuricemia** A clinical condition of excessive levels of uric acid in the bloodstream, which may cause damage to the kidneys. Hyperuricemia may also lead to the development of GOUT, HYPERTENSION, KIDNEY STONES (urolithiasis), or to bladder stones, as well as to heart attack and kidney disease. It is known, however, that abnormal uric acid levels increase with worsening stages of CHRONIC KIDNEY DISEASE (CKD). For example, according to the United States Renal Data System in their 2009 report and based on 1999–2006 data, 5.0 percent of individuals without CKD had abnormal uric acid levels. At Stages 4–5 of the 5 stages of CKD, 41.8 percent had abnormal uric acid levels.

According to authors Melina K. Kutzing and Bonnie L. Firestein in their 2009 article on altered uric acid levels and disease states for the *Journal of Pharmacology and Experimental*

*Therapeutics,* hyperuricemia may stem from such causes as an excessive consumption of alcohol, a diet that is too high in foods with purines (such as shellfish) or too high in proteins, and it may also result from a complication of chemotherapy that is administered for cancer treatment.

In some cases, the uric acid level in the blood is considered too low (hypouricemia), and in such cases, the goal is to elevate it, as when the individual is treated for multiple sclerosis, spinal injury, or stroke. Low levels of uric acid are also linked to such conditions as Parkinson's disease and Alzheimer's disease.

*Hyperuricemia and gout* Many studies have found a link between elevated levels of uric acid in the blood and the presence of gout. As the rate of uric acid concentration increases in the bloodstream in vulnerable individuals, the risk for a gout attack also increases. Kutzing and Firestein report that up to 60 percent of gout patients also have mild to moderate kidney disease, and thus there may be a direct relationship between an increased uric acid level and kidney disease.

*Hyperuricemia and hypertension* According to Kutzing and Firestein, elevated levels of uric acid in the blood are predictive for hypertension if it has not yet developed. Yet it could also be true that hypertension itself leads to microvascular disease resulting in elevated levels of uric acid in the bloodstream. Thus, the cause and effect of hyperuricemia in its relationship to hypertension is still under investigation by researchers.

*Hyperuricemia and cardiovascular disease* Research indicates a correlation between hyperuricemia and CARDIOVASCULAR DISEASE (such as heart attack and stroke), although again, it is not entirely clear which is the driving force: the hyperuricemia or the cardiovascular disease. According to Daniel I. Feig, M.D., and colleagues in their 2008 article for the *New England Journal of Medicine*, whether elevated uric acids actually cause cardiovascular disease is a controversial issue among experts. They also note that high uric acid levels in the blood are often related to other cardiovascular risk factors that may be present in an individual, and they further note that uric acid levels are generally higher in postmenopausal women, who represent a group that is at an elevated risk for cardiovascular disease. Nevertheless, more recent studies examining children with hyperuricemia and hypertension have shown that decreasing uric acid levels with the medication allopurinol decreases blood pressure, suggesting a direct effect of uric acid on blood pressure regulation.

Uric acid levels are often high in individuals with metabolic syndrome, a condition which includes such factors as abdominal OBESITY, insulin resistance (the inability of the body to use the insulin that is produced, but not a high enough level to constitute diabetes), hypertrigylceridemia (high levels of trigylcerides in the blood), a low level of high-density lipoprotein cholesterol (the "good" cholesterol), and an elevated leptin level.

### Treatment of Hyperuricemia

The current indications for treating hyperuricemia are undergoing active investigation as of this writing. Clearly, patients with gout and hyperuricemia benefit from medications such as allopurinol and febuxostat that block uric acid production. For patients with hyperuricemia without a history of gout, it is not clear whether these medications can prevent cardiovascular or renal complications, and, if they do, whether the benefit exceeds the risk of the side effects that they can cause.

Edwards, N. Lawrence, M.D. "The Role of Hyperuricemia and Gout in Kidney and Cardiovascular Disease." *Cleveland Clinic Journal of Medicine* 75, Supp. 5 (2008): S13–S16.

Feig, Daniel I., M.D., Duk-Hee Kang, M.D., and Richard J. Johnson, M.D. "Uric Acid and Cardiovascular Disease." *New England Journal of Medicine* 359 (2008): 1,811–1,821.

Kutzing, Melinda K., and Bonnie L. Firestein. "Altered Uric Acid Levels and Disease States." *Journal of Pharmacology and Experimental Therapies* 324, no. 1 (2008): 1–7.

**hypocalcemia** Below normal levels of the calcium that is circulating in the bloodstream, which may be caused by damage to the parathyroid glands, which causes an output of very low levels of parathyroid hormone. It may also be caused by a VITAMIN D deficiency. Hypocalcemia refers to a total blood calcium level that is less than 8.5 mg/dl. Hypocalcemia can be very serious, if it becomes severe, and if it is not identified and treated, the individual could die.

### Symptoms and Diagnostic Path

Hypocalcemia can cause both acute and chronic complications. Acute, or short-term, complications most classically include paresthesias, which refers to a "pins and needles" sensation, that can occur either in the hands and feet or the area immediately surrounding the mouth. When severe, acute hypocalcemia can lead to bronchospasm and asthma, seizures, heart failure, or cardiac arrhythmias. If present for prolonged periods, as with chronic hypocalcemia, this condition can lead to Parkinson's disease–type symptoms, dementia, abnormal dentition, and dry skin.

In addition to reviewing the medical history and checking the patient, the physician can check for hypocalcemia with the Chvostek sign. (This is a sign which was named after the doctor who first identified this particular indicator of hypocalcemia.) With this test, the doctor taps the patient in about the middle of the cheekbone. If the response is an involuntary sneer-like grimace, this is an indication of hypocalcemia. Another indicator of hypocalcemia is to test for Trousseau's sign (also named after the doctor who created this test). With Trousseau's sign, a blood pressure cuff is inflated on the arm, and if the patient has hypocalcemia, within minutes the arm will spasm and cramp up uncontrollably.

### Treatment Options and Outlook

In an emergency situation, hypocalcemia is treated with calcium that is administered intravenously. If the patient has stabilized but still has hypocalcemia, then oral forms of calcium may be taken, such as calcium carbonate, calcium citrate, and so forth. (See CALCIUM.) Treatment with calcium may cause gastrointestinal upset or constipation. Individuals with hypocalcemia also need to take high levels of vitamin D. If the patient has advanced kidney disease, he or she may need special forms of vitamin D which do not require activation in the kidney; these medications are termed "active" vitamin D.

Individuals who have had hypocalcemia should receive periodic checks of their blood calcium on a schedule that is determined by their physician. This is important because low levels of calcium should be avoided and in contrast, levels that are too high (HYPERCALCEMIA) should also be avoided. If the hypocalcemia was caused by damage to the parathyroid glands, then calcium supplements and vitamin D may need to be continued for the rest of the patient's life.

### Risk Factors and Preventive Measures

Individuals with severe kidney disease or kidney failure are at risk for hypocalcemia. This is because the kidneys are required for the last step in the activation of the vitamin D that either is produced normally by the body or that comes from dietary sources. In the absence of adequate kidney function, inadequate kidney-mediated activation of vitamin D can cause a person to become vitamin D deficient.

Adequate amounts of vitamin D are necessary in order to stimulate intestinal calcium absorption. Accordingly, vitamin D deficiency from inadequate kidney-mediated activation of vitamin D is a very common cause of hypocalcemia in patients with kidney disease. In patients with adequate kidney function, inadequate dietary vitamin D intake and/or sun exposure (which is necessary for one of the steps of activation of vitamin D obtained from dietary sources) are other common causes of hypocalcemia.

In addition, those who are deficient in MAGNESIUM blood levels (hypomagnesemia) are also at risk for the development of hypocalcemia. Those individuals whose parathyroid glands have been damaged by surgery, especially by a thyroidectomy, or by some other form of damage to the parathyroids are at risk for hypocalcemia, although in such cases, the hypocalcemia is temporary in the overwhelming majority of cases, as the parathyroid glands recover in most cases.

The risk for damage to the parathyroids is more common with a total thyroidectomy than with a partial thyroidectomy. The thyroid gland may be removed for hyperthyroidism or for thyroid cancer, among the key reasons for a thyroidectomy. Rarely, patients who undergo subtotal parathyroidectomy, because of severe secondary HYPERPARATHYROIDISM, can become hypoparathyroid. Because the parathyroid gland, through release of parathormone, regulates serum calcium, the inadvertent development of hypoparathyroidism can lead to severe hypocalcemia.

Other individuals at risk for the development of hypocalcemia include the following groups:

- those with pancreatitis
- those with liver disease
- alcoholics
- individuals who have been admitted to an intensive care unit for a severe illness
- those with sepsis (severe bacterial infection)

Petit, William A., Jr., M.D., and Christine Adamec. *The Encyclopedia of Endocrine Diseases and Disorders.* New York: Facts On File, 2005.

**hypokalemia** Low levels of POTASSIUM in the blood, often caused by the use of DIURETICS or which may develop from diarrhea and vomiting that has occurred to an individual. Hypokalemia may also be caused by primary aldosteronism, or a condition of excessive levels of the hormone ALDOSTERONE in the bloodstream (also known as Conn's syndrome). Secondary aldosteronism can be caused by NEPHROTIC SYNDROME or by HYPERTENSION and can also lead to hypokalemia.

Chronic hypokalemia is harmful to the kidneys. It also can increase blood pressure, increase the risk of abnormal heart rhythms and the risk of death from a myocardial infarction (heart attack), and can worsen the control of blood sugar in patients with DIABETES MELLITUS.

### Symptoms and Diagnostic Path

If hypokalemia is caused by primary or secondary aldosteronism, the patient may have no symptoms or may have such symptoms as headaches, muscle weakness, muscle cramps, and frequent urination. The blood pressure may also be high. The individual may have below normal levels of magnesium. Hypokalemia is diagnosed with laboratory testing for potassium.

### Treatment Options and Outlook

The treatment depends upon the cause. If the hypokalemia is caused by dehydration, the administration of potassium and other ELECTROLYTES as needed should resolve the problem. If hypokalemia is caused by diuretics, then instructing the patient to eat a higher potassium diet, or go on a lower sodium chloride (salt) diet, or adding a potassium-sparing diuretic can be beneficial. If the hypokalemia is caused by primary hyperaldosteronism, then addition of medications that block aldosterone's action, such as spironolactone or eplerenone, can be effective at treating the hypokalemia and also improving the severe hypertension which is frequently associated with primary hyperaldosteronism. If the primary hyperaldosteronism is due to an aldosterone-producing adenoma, then surgical removal of the adenoma may cure the condition.

### Risk Factors and Preventive Measures

Patients with chronic kidney disease have an elevated risk for hypokalemia, as do those with hypertension and cirrhosis of the liver. If the condition is identified, it should be treated.

See also HYPERKALEMIA; HYPOCALCEMIA.

**hyponatremia**   Below normal levels of sodium in the bloodstream, which may be caused by a variety of conditions, including dehydration.

Hyponatremia may also occur as a temporary but serious condition that has resulted from an ELECTROLYTE imbalance that was caused by extended and severe nausea and vomiting. The nausea and vomiting may have occurred as a result of a gastrointestinal infection or other type of infection that affected the gastrointestinal system. Rarely, women who are pregnant have such excessive vomiting that they can throw off the normal balance of their electrolytes. In most cases, after intravenous treatment they will recover.

### Symptoms and Diagnostic Path

Signs and symptoms differ, depending on whether the hyponatremia is acute, i.e., lasting only a few hours or days, or chronic, i.e., present for several days, weeks or even months.

Acute hyponatremia causes the following:

- nausea and vomiting
- headache
- seizures
- respiratory failure
- coma
- death

With chronic hyponatremia, there are typically no symptoms other than those due to the underlying condition.

If acute hyponatremia is not diagnosed and treated, then the patient may worsen to develop seizures, coma, and death. Treatment is complicated by the physician's knowledge that correcting the hyponatremia too quickly can cause the development of a possibly irreversible and/or fatal neurologic condition that is known as central pontine myelinolyis (CPM). The problem of an overly rapid correction is particularly of concern for patients with chronic hyponatremia.

Hyponatremia is diagnosed from the results of a blood test of sodium concentration.

### Treatment Options and Outlook

The treatment of hyponatremia takes into account the duration of the hyponatremia (acute versus chronic) as well as any associated symptoms in the patient with acute hyponatremia and the underlying cause. Patients with acute hyponatremia, particularly if they have related symptoms, frequently need to be treated with concentrated sodium chloride solutions that are administered intravenously. The sodium chloride solution used is 3 percent NaCl, which is more than three times more concentrated than the usual sodium chloride solution, or 0.9% NaCl, also known as "normal saline."

Patients with acute hyponatremia who do not have symptoms can be treated either with 3 percent NaCl or, if the hyponatremia is not severe, with the simultaneous administration of potent diuretics, such as furosemide or bumetanide in concentration with intravenous solution of normal saline. In either case, frequent measurements of the blood sodium concentration should be made to ensure that overly rapid correction does not occur.

Individuals with chronic hyponatremia should be treated with diagnosis and correction of the underlying condition. Dehydrated patients should have their dehydration corrected. Patients with congestive heart failure or liver failure should have these conditions treated. Patients without either of these conditions should be evaluated for a cancer that might be causing their hyponatremia. If the patient is receiving medications that can cause hyponatremia, such as thiazide-type DIURETICS, these medications should be discontinued. Rarely, endocrine disorders, such as thyroid or adrenal insufficiency, can be the cause of hyponatremia.

Patients with chronic hyponatremia who have edema, such as those seen with congestive heart failure, liver disease, or nephritic syndrome, should be instructed to minimize their fluid intake.

Finally, a new class of medications, termed aquaretics, have direct effects in the kidneys that can result in improvement in hyponatremia. Unfortunately, once these medications are stopped, the hyponatremia typically returns unless the underlying etiology is effectively treated.

### Risk Factors and Preventive Measures

Individuals with hypothyroidism, an endocrine disorder, may develop hyponatremia. An insufficiency of the adrenal glands may also lead to hyponatremia in rare cases. There are no known measures to avoid hyponatremia, and individuals identified with this disorder need to be diagnosed and treated.

See also HYPERNATREMIA; HYPOCALCEMIA; HYPOKALEMIA.

Petit, William A., Jr., M.D., and Christine Adamec. *The Encyclopedia of Endocrine Diseases and Disorders.* New York: Facts On File, 2005.

**hypoparathyroidism** Below normal levels of parathyroid hormone, also known as parathormone, a hormone that is produced by the parathyroid glands which are embedded in the thyroid gland. The individual may also develop HYPOCALCEMIA, a condition of low calcium levels in the bloodstream, and this condition may lead to seizures and death if it is not diagnosed and treated.

### Symptoms and Diagnostic Path

Individuals with hypoparathyroidism have similar symptoms to those with hypocalcemia, such as experiencing the sensation of pins and needles in the face, hands, and feet and also the development of painful muscle cramps. In addition, the patient may have abdominal pain and muscle spasms in the hands and/or the feet. In the worst case, the patient may experience seizures and develop tetany, a condition which means the calcium blood levels are so low that if the person is not diagnosed and treated, he or she is at risk for death.

The diagnosis is based on the medical history and the current symptoms as well as the results of blood tests of the calcium level and the levels of parathyroid hormone. As with hypocalcemia, the physician may test for the Chvostek sign, which involves tapping the patient at the mid-cheekbone. If the involuntary response is a grimace, then hypocalcemia is likely to be present. Another test for hypocalcemia is Trousseau's sign, which involves inflating a blood pressure cuff on the patient's arm to a level above their systolic blood pressure for at least three minutes. If the hand or forearm develops uncontrollable spasms, this can be an indicator of hypocalcemia, which may be caused by hypoparathyroidism. (Hypocalcemia also has other causes.)

### Treatment Options and Outlook

Hypoparathyroidism is treated with the administration of calcium. In an emergency, the calcium must be administered intravenously. After the patient begins to recover, oral calcium may be sufficient. Calcitriol (a synthetic form of vitamin D) is often prescribed to increase absorption of the calcium in the intestinal tract. This is a prescribed medication because oral supplements of vitamin D are insufficient.

### Risk Factors and Preventive Measures

Thyroid surgery can temporarily or permanently damage the parathyroid glands embedded in the thyroid gland. Another cause is the self-destruction of the parathyroid glands because of an autoimmune disorder. Very rarely, hypoparathyroidism may be caused by treatment with radioactive iodine that was administered to treat hyperparathyroidism, or a condition characterized by excessively *high* levels of parathyroid hormone. Sometimes hypomagnesia, a condition of very low blood levels of MAGNESIUM, may rarely lead to hypoparathyroidism. Individuals at risk for hypomagnesia include those who are alcoholics and/or those who are malnourished.

Rarely, patients with END-STAGE RENAL DISEASE with severe hyperparathyroidism require surgical therapy to treat their hyperparathyroidism. This involves removing three of the four parathyroid glands and part of the fourth gland. In the event that there is damage to the remaining parathyroid gland, the patient may inadvertently develop hypoparathyroidism as a result of the surgery.

There are no specific measures known to prevent hypoparathyroidism. If the condition develops, it must be treated, preferably by an endocrinologist. If the patient also has kidney disease, the expertise of a nephrologist is needed. Patients undergoing parathyroid surgery should use a surgeon who has extensive expertise in this type of surgery.

Marx, Stephen J., M.D. "Hyperparathyroid and Hypoparathyroid Disorders." *New England Journal of Medicine* 343, no. 25 (2000): 1,863–1,875.

Petit, William A., Jr., M.D., and Christine Adamec. *The Encyclopedia of Endocrine Diseases and Disorders.* New York: Facts On File, 2005.

Shoback, Dolores, M.D. "Hypoparathyroidism." *New England Journal of Medicine* 359, no. 4 (2008): 391–403.

# I

**IgA nephropathy** A kidney disease that is caused by the inflammation of internal kidney structures as a result of the buildup of the protein immunoglobulin A (IgA) in the kidneys. It is also known as Berger's disease.

### Symptoms and Diagnostic Path
IgA nephropathy almost always presents with hematuria, or red blood cells in the urine. In some cases the number of red blood cells in the urine is so large as to color the urine either frankly red or give it a cola-colored or tea-colored appearance. In other cases, the number of red blood cells is lower, and is detectable only with microscopic and/or a dipstick analysis of the urine. PROTEINURIA may be present, but NEPHROTIC SYNDROME is relatively rare. In some cases, IgA nephropathy is recognized only when screening blood tests identify CHRONIC KIDNEY DISEASE, leading to further studies of the urine and, often, to a KIDNEY BIOPSY which reveals the diagnostic finding of IgA nephropathy.

A urinalysis is used to help with diagnosis, but there are no definitive diagnostic tests by either URINE or blood analysis for IgA nephropathy. Only a kidney biopsy can confirm the diagnosis of IgA nephropathy by showing the presence of IgA deposits in the glomerular mesangium.

### Treatment Options and Outlook
As with many diseases and disorders, IgA nephropathy cannot be cured, but it can be treated so that the condition can be stabilized. To achieve this goal, medications are used, such as ANGIOTENSIN-CONVERTING ENZYME (ACE) inhibitor medications as well as ANGIOTENSIN II RECEPTOR BLOCKERS (ARBs). These medications

work to protect kidney function by lowering the individual's blood pressure and decreasing the protein loss into the urine (proteinuria). Medications are also prescribed to protect against high cholesterol, which can also help preserve the individual's kidney function as long as possible. Sometimes cortiocosteroids such as prednisone are used to treat IgA nephropathy.

Some patients with IgA nephropathy are also treated with IMMUNOSUPPRESSIVE drugs, such as mycophenolate mofetil (MMF).

If the kidneys fail completely, the individual must have either DIALYSIS or a KIDNEY TRANSPLANTATION in order to survive.

### Risk Factors and Preventive Measures
Men are more likely than women to have IgA nephropathy, according to the National Kidney and Urologic Diseases Information Clearinghouse (NKUDIC). It is also a disorder that is more commonly found among whites and Asians. It is possible that IgA nephropathy may be related to respiratory infections. There may also be a hereditary link in some individuals.

Age is another risk factor for IgA nephropathy. In contrast with many diseases, IgA nephropathy is typically a disease of younger adults. Approximately 80 percent of patients with this disease are 16–35 years old when they are diagnosed. IgA nephropathy is often found in conjunction with HENOCH SCHÖNLEIN PURPURA, a form of vasculitis that can affect many different parts of the body.

**immunosuppressive drugs** Medications that are taken to suppress the immune system so that a

## TABLE 1: IMMUNOSUPPRESSIVE MEDICATIONS USED IN SOLID ORGAN TRANSPLANTS

| Immunosuppressive Group | Examples |
| --- | --- |
| Calcineurin inhibitors | Cyclosporine and tacrolimus (Prograf) |
| Corticosteroids | Prednisone and methylprednisone |
| Anti-metabolite agents | Azathioprine, mycophenolate mofetil, enteric-coated mycophenolic acid |
| Anti-proliferative agents | Sirolimus and everolimus |
| T-cell depleting agents | OKT3, Polyclonal antilymphocyte or antithymocyte antibodies, Campath-1H |
| Anti-CD25 antibodies | Basiliximab and Daclizumab |
| Anti-B-cell antibodies | Rituximab |

transplanted organ, such as a transplanted kidney or other organ, or multiple simultaneously transplanted organs, will not be rejected by the body. Without the use of immunosuppressants, transplanted organs are viewed as invaders by the immune system, which seeks to attack and destroy them. Only in the case of identical twins, where both are genetically the same, are immunosuppressants not needed, as with the first transplants that were performed in the 20th century.

In addition to their use with patients who receive transplanted organs, immunosuppressants are given to individuals who are diagnosed with some diseases and disorders, such as GOODPASTURE SYNDROME or IGA NEPHROPATHY. Immunosuppressants may also be used to treat some forms of cancer.

A key disadvantage of the use of immunosuppressant medications is that with a suppressed immune system, the individual becomes more prone to contracting infectious diseases, and the risk for developing cancer is also increased. Thus, individuals taking immunosuppressants must be closely monitored by their physicians with regular examinations as well as with frequent laboratory tests. Any fever, even a low-grade fever, should be rapidly evaluated and treated to minimize the chance of a severe and possibly life-threatening infection from developing.

See also KIDNEY TRANSPLANTATION.

**infection, bladder**  See CYSTITIS.

**infection, kidney**  See PYELONEPHRITIS.

**infections**  Usually refers to an overgrowth of bacteria which causes symptoms in the individual. An infection in the kidneys is known as PYELONEPHRITIS, while an infection in the bladder is termed CYSTITIS. Often the physician can determine the type of infection (or at least, the most likely cause) through blood tests or urine cultures and then can prescribe the appropriate antibiotics to kill these bacteria. Recurrent infections can weaken an individual and increase the probability that more infections will occur. It is also true that individuals who are already weak from disease are more prone to infections.

The body can suffer from many other types of bacterial or viral infections, and frequent infections can weaken the individual and make it difficult to fight off new invading microbes. This is particularly true for viral infections, which can directly weaken the immune system; even a single viral infection can predispose the infected individual to a subsequent bacterial infection.

### Symptoms and Diagnostic Path

Infections may cause fever, dehydration, nausea and vomiting, weight loss, and other symptoms. In extreme cases, a severe infection may be life-threatening. An infection is diagnosed by a physical examination and by laboratory tests. In the case of kidney or bladder diseases, a urinalysis or urine culture can detect most forms of infections. Viral infections are usually diagnosed through blood testing that tests for the body's response to the infection. Bacterial infections usually are diagnosed through identification of the bacteria by culturing the infected fluid. Fungal infections are typically diagnosed through either testing for the body's response to the infection, identification of the fungus in the infected tissue through a microscopic examination of specially stained body fluids or tissues, or by culturing the infected body fluid or tissue and subsequent identification of the fungus.

### Treatment Options and Outlook

The individual with a bacterial infection is usually treated with antibiotics for 10–14 days, depending on the type of antibiotic, the severity of the infection, and the patient's past responsiveness to the drug, if known. Some infections, such as bacterial infection of heart valves (endocarditis) or of bone (osteomyelitis) may require as much as six weeks of therapy. Many viral infections will resolve spontaneously and do not require specific therapy. Others, such as hepatitis C and HIV (human immunodeficiency virus) may need treatment for six months or for the remainder of the patient's life, respectively. The chosen antibiotic and the length of treatment depend on the type of virus, bacteria, or fungus as well as the patient's medical history.

### Risk Factors and Preventive Measures

Individuals who take IMMUNOSUPPRESSIVE DRUGS to prevent the rejection of a kidney transplant (or to prevent the rejection of another transplanted organ) have an increased risk for infection. Individuals who are not on immunosuppressants but who develop frequent bladder or kidney infections should consult with their physician to determine what measures they can take to decrease the number of infections, such as drinking more water and urinating more frequently. Further investigation may indicate a problem with the immune system.

See also ANTIBIOTICS; MEDICATIONS THAT CAN HARM THE KIDNEYS.

**injury, acute kidney**  See ACUTE KIDNEY INJURY.

**interstitial nephritis**  A kidney disorder that is caused by inflamed spaces between the kidney tubules, which may affect the ability of the kidneys to filter wastes from the blood. It is also known as tubulointerstitial nephritis, nephritis, and acute interstitial (allergic) nephritis.

The following conditions can lead to interstitial nephritis:

- an allergic reaction to a drug (as with acute interstitial allergic nephritis)
- ANALGESIC NEPHROPATHY (a reaction to painkillers that caused kidney disease, particularly narcotic painkillers)
- a reaction to the use of some medications, such as NONSTEROIDAL ANTI-INFLAMMATORY DRUGS (NSAIDs) or thiazide diuretics

According to R. John and A. M. Herzenberg in their 2009 article for the *Journal of Clinical Pathology,* more than two-thirds of the cases of acute interstitial nephritis (AIN) are drug-induced, and the patient's symptoms may start from two to three weeks after starting the medication.

### Symptoms and Diagnostic Path

Symptoms of interstitial nephritis may include the following:

- fever
- blood in the urine (hematuria)
- an increased or decreased urinary output
- mental changes (confusion, drowsiness or even coma)
- nausea and vomiting
- swelling of the body, anywhere
- weight gain from fluid retention (edema)

If the physician suspects that interstitial nephritis is the problem, he or she may order the following diagnostic tests:

- blood urea nitrogen (BUN) and creatinine blood levels
- complete blood count with differential
- examination of the urine for eosinophils
- KIDNEY BIOPSY
- urinalysis
- white blood cell count

### Treatment Options and Outlook

The treatment of interstitial nephritis depends on the cause. If it is believed that the cause is a medication, then the medication must be stopped. It may also be necessary to start steroid therapy to hasten improvement. There are many medications that may cause acute interstitial nephritis, including antibiotics such as cephalosporins, fluoroquinolones, penicillins, rifampicin, and sulfonamides. Proton pump inhibitors, medications that are used to treat acid reflux, may also cause acute interstitial nephritis. Other drugs that may cause AIN include thiazides, protease inhibitors, NSAIDs, phenytoin, 5-aminosalicylates, and allopurinol (used to treat chronic GOUT). Drugs that may cause chronic interstitial nephritis include lithium and phenacetin.

### Risk Factors and Preventive Measures

Individuals taking medications that can cause interstitial nephritis are at risk, but in the absence of a history of interstitial nephritis to a specific agent, it is not possible to predict who will develop a reaction.

See also CHRONIC KIDNEY DISEASE.

John, R., and A. M. Herzenberg. "Renal Toxicity of Therapeutic Drugs." *Journal of Clinical Pathology* 62 (2009): 505–515.

**K**

**kidney biopsy** A procedure in which tissue from the kidneys is removed for the purpose of examination by a pathologist, who will then determine the etiology of the kidney dysfunction, either decreased GLOMERULAR FILTRATION RATE (GFR), PROTEINURIA, or both, that the person is experiencing. This biopsy can be used either to test the individual's native kidneys or it can be used to examine a transplanted kidney.

### Procedure

There are several different ways to perform a kidney biopsy, but many doctors rely upon ultrasound guidance to localize the kidney for the biopsy, while others use computerized tomography (CT) scan guidance during the procedure. This biopsy must be performed in a hospital, and the procedure takes about 30 minutes for the physician.

If a biopsy is being done on the person's native (natural) kidneys, he or she will typically lie face down, whereas the individual will lie face up if it is a transplanted kidney that is being biopsied. The skin will be sterilized, and a local anesthetic is used at the site in the skin where the needle used for the biopsy is to be inserted. Frequently, a tiny incision, 2–3 mm, is then made, into which the biopsy needle is inserted and then advanced to the kidney surface. Because the kidney typically is only about 10 cm below the skin surface, the needle is advanced slowly and carefully.

The typical biopsy device is an automated device which, when activated by the physician, will cut and remove a small piece (about 1–2 mm diameter by 15–20 mm length) of kidney tissue. In most cases the physician will biopsy two pieces of kidney to have sufficient tissue for all of the testing which will need to be performed. When the needle is withdrawn, pressure is applied to stop the bleeding. The doctor may need to reinsert the needle several times to obtain sufficient tissue for the biopsy.

The patient will stay in the hospital in bed for about six hours after the biopsy in order to carefully observe the patient for any evident complications. If none are observed, the patient is usually discharged home. In particular, the initial observation includes careful observation of the patient's blood pressure and heart rate, blood counts, and evidence of blood in the urine (hematuria).

### Risks and Complications

Some risks of the kidney biopsy include infection and bleeding from the kidney, although these problems happen rarely. Much more commonly, the area that was biopsied may feel tender to the individual for several days after the procedure. Rarely, bleeding may be persistent, and may require blood transfusions, procedures to stop the bleeding, or even the surgical removal of the kidney if the bleeding cannot be controlled. These latter complications are very rare.

### Outlook and Lifestyle Modifications

After the test, the individual should avoid any heavy lifting or strenuous activities for at least two weeks, depending on the advice of the physician. After that time, the individual can usually resume all normal activities.

See also GLOMERULONEPHRITIS; KIDNEY TRANSPLANTATION.

**kidney cancer**   A malignant tumor that is located in the kidneys or that has spread to other organs but originated in the kidneys. Renal cell carcinoma is one form of kidney cancer. According to the National Cancer Institute, there were an estimated 58,240 new cases of cancers of the kidney and renal pelvis in 2010. An estimated 13,040 people died of kidney cancer in 2009.

### Symptoms and Diagnostic Path

Symptoms of kidney cancer may be minimal, but some symptoms that may appear, particularly as the disease progresses are:

- blood in the urine (hematuria) that causes rusty-looking or red urine
- a continuous pain in the side
- a mass or lump in the side or the abdomen
- an unintended weight loss
- fever
- extreme fatigue

These symptoms may also occur in people who do *not* have kidney cancer; however, anyone with any of these symptoms should be sure to see their physician for diagnosis and treatment. The doctor will check the patient for general health signs and for the presence of HYPERTENSION (high blood pressure). The physician will also examine the abdomen and side for possible signs of tumors. Urine tests to detect the presence of blood in the urine and other indicators of disease are usually performed.

A computerized tomography (CT) scan or an ultrasound test may provide important information by showing the presence of a mass or abnormal growth in the kidney. A KIDNEY BIOPSY is generally not performed. Instead, if imaging tests, such as a magnetic resonance imaging (MRI) scan or CT scan, show characteristic findings of cancer, then treatment should begin.

### Treatment Options and Outlook

Treatment for kidney cancer may include the following options:

- surgical removal of the kidney (nephrectomy)
- arterial embolization
- radiation therapy
- biological therapy
- chemotherapy
- a combination of treatments

*Surgery and kidney cancer*   The most common form of treatment for kidney cancer is surgery, such as a radical nephrectomy in which the entire kidney is removed along with the adrenal glands, as well as some of the tissue surrounding the kidney. Alternatively, a simple nephrectomy, in which only the kidney is removed, may be performed if the physician feels this is best. Another option is a partial nephrectomy, in which only the part of the kidney with the tumor is removed. This procedure may be chosen when the person has only one remaining functional kidney or when cancer is affecting both kidneys. Individuals with small kidney tumors may also have a partial nephrectomy.

According to the National Cancer Institute, people with kidney cancer may wish to ask their physician the following questions before making their decision either for or against surgery:

- What kind of operation do you recommend for me?
- What are the risks of surgery? Will I have any long-term effects? Will I need DIALYSIS?
- Should I store some of my own blood in case I need a transfusion?
- How will I feel after the operation?
- How long will I need to stay in the hospital?
- When can I get back to my normal activities?
- How often will I need checkups?
- Would a clinical trial be appropriate for me?

*Arterial embolization*   An arterial embolization is a procedure that shrinks the cancerous kidney tumor, and it may be performed before surgery occurs. The doctor inserts a catheter into

TABLE 1: INCIDENCE RATES OF KIDNEY CANCER BY GENDER, RACE, AND ETHNICITY PER YEAR,
BASED ON DATA FROM 2002–2006

| Race/Ethnicity | Male | Female |
| --- | --- | --- |
| All races | 18.6 per 100,000 men | 9.5 per 100,000 women |
| White | 19.2 per 100,000 men | 9.9 per 100,000 women |
| Black | 21.3 per 100,000 men | 10.3 per 100,000 women |
| Asian/Pacific Islander | 9.6 per 100,000 men | 4.8 per 100,000 women |
| American Indian/Alaska Native | 21.7 per 100,000 men | 14.1 per 100,000 women |
| Hispanic | 17.6 per 100,000 men | 9.6 per 100,000 women |

a blood vessel in the leg, moving the catheter up to the renal artery, which is the main blood vessel supplying blood to the kidney. The doctor then injects a substance to block the blood flow to the kidney in order to prevent the tumor from receiving any oxygen that would help it to grow more. Some patients who have this procedure will experience back pain or nausea or vomiting.

*Radiation therapy* Radiation therapy may be used to treat kidney cancer, and sometimes it is also used before surgery in order to help shrink the tumor and make the later removal of the tumor easier. Radiation therapy can also be used to relieve cancer pain. However, radiation therapy for kidney cancer can cause nausea and vomiting, diarrhea, and urinary discomfort. Radiation therapy will not generally result in a cure if used alone.

*Biological therapy* Biological therapy is another form of therapy for kidney cancer. If patients have cancer that has spread to other parts of the body, the doctor may suggest that specific substances, such as interferon alpha or interleukin-2, be administered. Biological therapy may induce flu-like symptoms, such as fever, chills, and muscle aches. These side effects will end when the treatment ends. Biological therapy is more commonly available in large medical centers or university medical schools.

*Chemotherapy* Chemotherapy is the use of anticancer drugs to destroy the cancer cells. These drugs may cause hair loss, poor appetite, nausea and vomiting, bruising or easy bleeding, and extreme fatigue. However, many side effects can be controlled with other drugs. Chemo-therapy does not typically result in cure when used alone.

### *Risk Factors and Preventive Measures*
Men have about twice the risk of women for developing kidney cancer in the United States based on data for 2002–06 from the federal Surveillance Epidemiology and End Results administered by the National Cancer Institute of the National Institutes of Health. The rate for men of all races was 18.6 per 100,000 men compared to 9.5 women per 100,000 women who developed kidney cancer. There were some variations in incidences by race and ethnicity; for example, American Indian/Alaska Native males had the highest rate or 21.7 per 100,000 men, followed by black men at 21.3 per 100,000 men. Among women, the highest rates were also found among American Indian/Alaska Native women, or 14.1 per 100,000 women. (See Table 1.)

In considering death rates by age, the highest death rates from kidney cancer were found among American Indian or Alaska Native males, or 9.0 per 100,000 men. Among women, American Indians/Alaska Natives also had the highest rates of all women, or 4.2 per 100,000 women. (See Table 2.)

Cigarette SMOKING increases the risk for developing kidney cancer by approximately two-fold. People who are obese also have an increased risk for developing kidney cancer. High blood pressure increases the risk for kidney cancer. Individuals on long-term dialysis also have an increased risk for kidney cancer.

**TABLE 2: DEATH RATES FROM KIDNEY CANCER BY GENDER, RACE, AND ETHNICITY, BASED ON DATA FROM 2002–2006**

| Race/Ethnicity | Male | Female |
| --- | --- | --- |
| All races | 6.0 per 100,000 men | 2.7 per 100,000 women |
| White | 6.1 per 100,000 men | 2.8 per 100,000 women |
| Black | 6.0 per 100,000 men | 2.7 per 100,000 women |
| Asian/Pacific Islander | 2.4 per 100,000 men | 1.2 per 100,000 women |
| American Indian/Alaska Native | 9.0 per 100,000 men | 4.2 per 100,000 women |
| Hispanic | 5.2 per 100,000 men | 2.4 per 100,000 women |

With regard to preventing kidney cancer, the best means to avoid this disease is to never smoke or to end a smoking habit which has already begun. Obese individuals should lose weight, and individuals with hypertension should work to decrease their blood pressure to as close to normal levels as possible.

See also BLADDER CANCER; MYELOMA KIDNEY.

Wallen, Eric M., Geoffrey F. Joyce, and Matthew Wise. "Kidney Cancer." In *Urologic Diseases in America*, edited by M. S. Litwin and C. S. Saigal, 335–378. Bethesda, Md.: National Institute of Diabetes and Digestive and Kidney Diseases, 2007.

**kidney disease, chronic**   See CHRONIC KIDNEY DISEASE.

**kidney disease, in children**   See CHILDREN AND KIDNEY DISEASE.

**kidney dysplasia**   See RENAL DYSPLASIA.

**kidney failure**   See ACUTE KIDNEY INJURY; END-STAGE RENAL DISEASE.

**kidney infection**   See PYELONEPHRITIS.

**kidney injury, acute**   See ACUTE KIDNEY INJURY.

**kidneys and kidney disease**   The kidneys are two bean-shaped organs that lie in about the middle of the back, each only about 4 inches high and weighing about 4 ounces in the average 180-pound male. They filter an estimated 170 quarts of blood every 24 hours, removing impurities and excreting excess water. The filtering of this blood is performed by the glomeruli, and then the nephrons determine the final amount of impurities and other excess compounds, as well as the total volume of urine that is excreted. There are approximately 1 million glomeruli and nephrons in each kidney.

The kidneys work constantly in a 24/7 operation to cleanse the human bloodstream of accumulated impurities, medications, and excess fluid, while simultaneously generating several critical vitamins and hormones necessary for normal health and for the normal response to challenges faced on a regular basis. The kidneys are essential to life itself, and kidney disease is the ninth leading cause of death in the United States, according to the Centers for Disease Control and Prevention.

An estimated 500,000 people in the United States experience kidney failure each year, and slightly less than 6 percent of the total Medicare budget, or $24 billion per year in 2007, was spent to treat individuals with end-stage renal disease.

As seen in Figure 1, the kidneys are connected to the bladder by the ureters, small tubes through which the urine travels. The image of the man and his kidneys shows the location of the kidneys in the body.

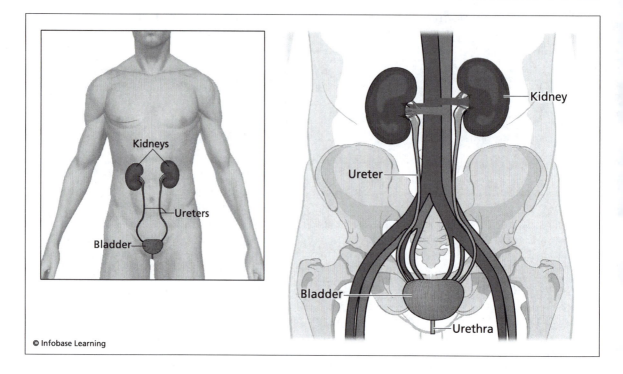

© Infobase Learning

The kidneys have other functions in addition to filtering out waste products and excess fluid; for example, they help to maintain normal blood pressure and they also regulate the levels of important substances in the blood, such as POTASSIUM, PHOSPHORUS, and SODIUM, as well as CALCIUM and MAGNESIUM. In addition, the kidneys convert VITAMIN D from an inactive form to an active form, a process which is necessary for healthy bones in children and adults; increasing evidence also suggest this process is important in cancer protection, cardiovascular health, and immune system function.

Many people have no problems with their kidneys and they work well from before birth until death. If the smooth functioning of the kidneys becomes threatened, either temporarily or more permanently, the threat can enter from outside the body, as when infectious microbes find entry to the kidneys and the kidneys become infected, a condition that is known as PYELONEPHRITIS. Once diagnosed and treated, in most cases, the infection resolves and harmony is restored to the body. Rarely, however, infection can cause serious damage to the kidneys, particularly if the infection is untreated, if the individual is elderly, or if the immune system response to the infection itself causes damage to the kidneys, as can occur with chronic HEPATITIS C infection or POSTSTREPTOCOCCAL GLOMERULONEPHRITIS.

The threat can also come from within the body itself, as when KIDNEY STONES develop, and the kidneys cannot excrete these extremely painful impediments unless or until medical treatment is received. Anyone who has ever experienced a kidney stone can attest to the excruciating physical pain of this disorder, which some have compared to the hard labor of childbirth. The threat can also be a slow and insidious process, as with CHRONIC KIDNEY DISEASE (CKD), which may take years to steadily harm the kidneys, usually with no symptoms until the harm is substantial. It is known that more than 8 million people in the United States have chronic kidney disease, and another 11 million have persistent microalbuminuria, which is a common early sign of incipient chronic kidney disease. CKD can progress to kidney failure, necessitating either DIALYSIS or a KIDNEY TRANSPLANTATION for the individual to survive. In some cases, genetic disorders harm the kidneys. In other cases, toxic medications or physical injuries lead to ACUTE KIDNEY INJURY and may cause the kidneys to fail. In addition, there are inherited kidney diseases, such as BARTTER'S SYNDROME or GITELMAN SYNDROME.

### A History of Past Means to Treat Kidney Disease

In the recent past and prior to the advent of dialysis and kidney transplantation, most people with serious kidney disease worsened until their kidneys failed altogether, and then the patient always died. It was only in the 20th century that the first method of kidney dialysis was devised, and it was later in the 20th century that it became possible to transplant working kidneys from either deceased donors or live donors into the person with kidney failure, using immunosuppressive medications to prevent the body from rejecting the organ of another person.

In the past, the kidney disease that is now known as edema was referred to as "dropsy," and the afflicted person often was severely bloated with the fluid that the kidneys could not remove. (Sometimes the primary problem of the person with dropsy could have been either heart failure or liver failure.) Said author Steven J. Peitzman in his historical account of the treatment of failed kidneys: "Enormous extra work is involved in carrying the weight of the dropsy, often easily fifty pounds or more. The muscles can barely move the legs, and the effort triggers the breathlessness. The unused muscles wither, even if the underlying disease has not directly injured them." The great general and former president Andrew Jackson died of massive dropsy, and Jackson said before his death, "I am a blubber of water."

According to Peitz, doctors in ancient Greece tapped the abdomen to drain out the fluid, as did the great Greek physician Hippocrates and doctors who followed. Other remedies were sweating the patient as well as treating the patient with drugs to induce vomiting or diarrhea, which sometimes did have a temporary apparent effect in reducing the excessive water level of the patient. Some physicians recommended a warmer climate.

In 1827, British physician Richard Bright discovered that deceased patients with dropsy often had severely damaged kidneys upon autopsy. The disease was named after him; Bright's disease may be the first disease to be named after its discoverer. Bright discovered albumin in the urine of his patients with kidney disease, and he wrote that he had detected proteinuria by placing urine in a spoon over a lighted candle and looking for coagulated material. He wrote that in the patients in whom he detected proteinuria, kidney damage would often be present after death in an autopsy. When Bright's disease was diagnosed, it was considered incurable and fatal, along with diagnoses for cancer and tuberculosis.

The famous and reclusive poet Emily Dickinson was diagnosed with Bright's disease, from which she died at home in 1886. (Bright's disease is now known to be a nonspecific term and not diagnostic of a specific type of kidney disease.)

What Bright had discovered in his patients' urine was proteinuria, which is primarily the protein albumin and which is also present in patients with kidney disease. Bright treated the disease with bloodlettings that were induced by "cuppings" applied to the chest and low back. He also treated with the drug calomel (considered an anti-inflammatory drug and a DIURETIC) and with remedies that contained camphor, magnesium sulphate and potassium supertartrate. Sometimes ipecac was used, a drug that induces vomiting. Some patients were advised to wear only flannel. These treatments were continued by physicians until the early 20th century.

Back to the future, physicians in the 21st century use sophisticated equipment and high technology imaging to diagnose and treat people with kidney disease. Unfortunately, if patients are not diagnosed with kidney disease until they are in an advanced stage, and also if they are not referred to NEPHROLOGISTS (doctors who specialize in kidney disease), then often there is little that can be done for them. Yet simple laboratory tests of kidney function can provide early markers of kidney disease that should be followed up. In addition, individuals with diabetes and hypertension, the leading causes of kidney failure, should be even more closely followed.

In fact, diabetes is the number one cause of kidney failure, followed by hypertension. Yet according to the United States Renal Data System, the rate of referral to a nephrologist among Medicare patients with diabetes or hypertension is no higher than about 16 percent, despite their greater risk for kidney disease and kidney failure.

In an analysis of patients with chronic kidney disease receiving a late referral to nephrologists, researchers found clear patterns. A late referral was defined by the researchers as individuals who were referred to a nephrologist in the period ranging from one month prior to the initiation of dialysis to less than six months after dialysis started. Another definition that was used was the definition of the National Kidney Foundation for late-stage chronic kidney disease. This research was published in 2008 in *BMC Nephrology*.

The researchers found that in general, older age, membership in a minority group, lower education, lack of health insurance, multiple diseases, and a lack of communication between primary care physicians and nephrologists were all significant factors in a late referral to a nephrologist. This is important information because patients who see nephrologists early in the disease are more likely to have a better outcome.

### Chronic Kidney Disease and Demographic Differences

It is known that more than 8 million people in the United States have chronic kidney dis-

ease, and another 11 million have persistent microalbuminuria, which is a common early sign of incipient chronic kidney disease. Current estimates suggest that anywhere from 9–11 percent of adult Americans have some degree of renal damage. Unfortunately, according to the National Center for Health Statistics, in 2006, only an estimated 3.35 million adults in the United States knew that they had kidney disease, out of more than 8 million people. Most were white, although kidney disease is increasingly problematic among nonwhite populations, who suffer kidney disorders at a higher rate than Caucasians. (See Tables 1 and 2.)

Some groups of adults are particularly prone to the development of kidney disease, such as individuals who are African Americans and Native Americans. As a result, blacks or Native Americans should have their kidney health carefully monitored.

Age is a risk factor for kidney disease, and older individuals are more likely to develop chronic kidney disease and kidney failure than younger people. According to the United States Renal Data System, the prevalence of CKD among Medicare patients ages 65 years and older was 7.6 percent in 2008, which was nearly five times greater than the rate seen in 1995. With the continuously aging population, this rate is likely to increase.

Gender is another significant factor, and in general, males are more likely than females to have kidney disease and kidney failure.

As can be seen from Table 1, there were a total of 220,267,000 adults age 18 and older living in the United States in 2006. Of these individuals, 3,347,000 reported being diagnosed with kidney disease. The table further breaks down the total population as well as the number of people with kidney disease by different characteristics, such as age, race, education, marital status, and so forth. For example, there were 110,391,000 people ages 18–44 years old living in the United States in 2006. Of this number, 797,000 adults had been diagnosed with kidney disease. Table 2

**TABLE 1. FREQUENCY OF KIDNEY DISEASE AMONG PERSONS AGES 18 AND OLDER, BY SELECTED CHARACTERISTICS, UNITED STATES, 2006**

| Selected Characteristic | All Persons Age 18 and Older (in thousands) | Number Knowing That They Have Kidney Disease[1] (in thousands) |
|---|---|---|
| Total | 220,267 | 3,347 |
| **Gender** | | |
| Male | 106,252 | 1,621 |
| Female | 114,014 | 1,726 |
| **Age** | | |
| 18–44 years | 110,391 | 797 |
| 45–64 years | 74,203 | 1,339 |
| 65–74 years | 19,081 | 464 |
| 75 years and older | 16,593 | 747 |
| **Race** | | |
| 1 race | 217,760 | 3,292 |
| White | 179,456 | 2,691 |
| Black or African American | 26,223 | 476 |
| American Indian or Alaska Native | 1,784 | Not available |
| Asian | 10,066 | 105 |
| Native Hawaiian or Other Pacific Islander | 231 | Not available |
| **Hispanic or Latino origin and race** | | |
| Hispanic or Latino | 28,664 | 370 |
| Mexican or Mexican American | 18,116 | 221 |
| Not Hispanic or Latino | 191,603 | 2,976 |
| White, single race | 153,235 | 2,361 |
| Black or African American, single race | 25,145 | 446 |
| **Education** | | |
| Less than a high school diploma | 31,750 | 1,025 |
| High school diploma or GED | 54,586 | 877 |
| Some college | 51,159 | 756 |
| Bachelor's degree or higher | 51,863 | 518 |
| **Family income** | | |
| Less than $20,000 | 38,472 | 1,056 |
| $20,000 or more | 169,172 | 2,092 |
| $20,000–$34,999 | 30,921 | 621 |
| $35,000–54,999 | 33,488 | 501 |
| $55,000–74,999 | 23,782 | 159 |
| $75,000 or more | 49,556 | 441 |
| **Poverty status*** | | |
| Poor | 20,299 | 485 |
| Near poor | 31,738 | 783 |
| Not poor | 115,519 | 1,296 |

*(table continued)*

TABLE 1. *(continued)*

| Selected Characteristic | All Persons Age 18 and Older (in thousands) | Number Knowing That They Have Kidney Disease[1] (in thousands) |
|---|---|---|
| **Health insurance coverage** | | |
| Under age 65 years: | | |
| Private | 125,610 | 885 |
| Medicaid | 14,080 | 556 |
| Other | 6,564 | 322 |
| Uninsured | 37,409 | 348 |
| Age 65 years and older: | | |
| Private | 20,731 | 753 |
| Medicaid and Medicare | 2,322 | 89 |
| Medicare only | 9,827 | 239 |
| Other | 2,449 | 129 |
| Uninsured | 283 | Not available |
| **Marital Status** | | |
| Married | 124,727 | 1,922 |
| Widowed | 13,182 | 460 |
| Divorced or separated | 24,244 | 511 |
| Never married | 44,415 | 285 |
| Living with a partner | 12,860 | 168 |
| **Place of residence** | | |
| Large metropolitan statistical area (MSA) | 110,233 | 1,533 |
| Small MSA | 70,790 | 1,075 |
| Not in MSA | 39,243 | 739 |
| **Region** | | |
| Northeast | 39,033 | 678 |
| Midwest | 51,565 | 600 |
| South | 83,511 | 1,402 |
| West | 46,157 | 667 |
| **Sex and ethnicity** | | |
| Hispanic or Latino, male | 14,739 | 126 |
| Hispanic or Latina, female | 13,925 | 245 |
| **Not Hispanic or Latino:** | | |
| White, single race, male | 73,951 | 1,240 |
| White, single race, female | 79,285 | 1,121 |
| Black or African American, single race, male | 11,208 | 178 |
| Black or African American, single race, female | 13,937 | 268 |

[1] Respondents were asked if they had been told in the last 12 months by a doctor or other health professional that they had weak or failing kidneys (excluding kidney stone, bladder infections or incontinence).

*Poor persons are defined as below the poverty threshold. Near poor persons have incomes of 100 percent to less than 200 percent of the poverty threshold. Not poor persons have incomes that are 200 percent of the poverty threshold or greater. Poverty status is based on family income and family size using the U.S. Census Bureau's poverty threshold for the previous calendar year.

Adapted from Pleis, J. R., and M. Lethbridge-Çejku. "Frequencies of Selected Diseases and Conditions among Persons 18 Years of Age and Over, by Selected Characteristics, United States, 2006." *Summary Health Statistics for U.S. Adults: National Health Interview Survey, 2006.* December 2007, p. 28–29.

**TABLE 2: PERCENTAGE OF INDIVIDUALS WITH KIDNEY DISEASE IN INDIVIDUALS AGE 18 AND OLDER, BY SELECTED CHARACTERISTICS, UNITED STATES, 2006**

| Selected Characteristic | Percent of Population Reporting a Known Diagnosis of Kidney Disease[1] | Selected Characteristic | Percent of Population Reporting a Known Diagnosis of Kidney Disease[1] |
|---|---|---|---|
| Total | 1.5 | **Health insurance coverage** | |
| **Gender** | | Under age 65 years: | |
| Male | 1.6 | Private | 0.7 |
| Female | 1.5 | Medicaid | 4.2 |
| **Age** | | Other | 3.7 |
| 18–44 years | 0.7 | Uninsured | 1.0 |
| 45–64 years | 1.8 | Age 65 years and older: | |
| 65–74 years | 2.4 | Private | 3.7 |
| 75 years and older | 4.5 | Medicaid and Medicare | 3.9 |
| **Race** | | Medicare only | 2.5 |
| White | 1.5 | Other | 5.3 |
| Black or African American | 2.0 | Uninsured | Unknown |
| American Indian or Alaska Native | Unknown | **Marital Status** | |
| Asian | 1.2 | Married | 1.5 |
| **Hispanic or Latino origin and race** | | Widowed | 2.8 |
| Hispanic or Latino | 1.5 | Divorced or separated | 2.1 |
| Mexican or Mexican American | 1.7 | Never married | 1.1 |
| Not Hispanic or Latino | 1.5 | Living with a partner | 1.6 |
| White, single race | 1.4 | **Place of residence** | |
| Black or African American, single race | 1.9 | Large metropolitan statistical area (MSA) | 1.4 |
| **Education** | | Small MSA | 1.5 |
| Less than a high school diploma | 2.9 | Not in MSA | 1.8 |
| High school diploma or GED | 1.5 | **Region** | |
| Some college | 1.5 | Northeast | 1.7 |
| Bachelor's degree or higher | 1.2 | Midwest | 1.1 |
| **Family income** | | South | 1.7 |
| Less than $20,000 | 2.7 | West | 1.4 |
| $20,000 or more | 1.3 | **Sex and ethnicity** | |
| $20,000–$34,999 | 1.9 | Hispanic or Latino, male | 1.1 |
| $35,000–54,999 | 1.6 | Hispanic or Latina, female | 2.0 |
| $55,000–74,999 | 1.0 | Not Hispanic or Latino: | |
| $75,000 or more | 1.2 | White, single race, male | 1.6 |
| **Poverty status*** | | White, single race, female | 1.3 |
| Poor | 2.7 | Black or African American, single race, male | 1.8 |
| Near poor | 2.4 | Black or African American, single race, female | 2.0 |
| Not poor | 1.2 | | |

[1] Respondents were asked if they had been told in the last 12 months by a doctor or other health professional that they had weak or failing kidneys (excluding kidney stone, bladder infections, or incontinence).

*Poor persons are defined as below the poverty threshold. Near poor persons have incomes of 100 percent to less than 200 percent of the poverty threshold. Not poor persons have incomes that are 200 percent of the poverty threshold or greater. Poverty status is based on family income and family size using the U.S. Census Bureau's poverty threshold for the previous calendar year.

Adapted from Pleis, J. R., and M. Lethbridge-Çejku. "Frequencies of Selected Diseases and Conditions among Persons 18 Years of Age and Over, by Selected Characteristics, United States, 2006." *Summary Health Statistics for U.S. Adults: National Health Interview Survey, 2006.* December 2007. pp. 30–31.

offers a percentage breakdown so that it can be seen what percentage of a particular population had kidney disease in 2006. For example, of all adults in the United States, an estimated 1.5 percent reported having been diagnosed with kidney disease. In looking at age alone, the highest percentage of people with kidney disease were those ages 75 years and older. In this group, 4.5 percent had kidney disease. Other factors were also relevant. For example, in taking gender alone into account, males were slightly more likely (1.6 percent) to have kidney disease than females (1.5 percent).

### Race and Ethnicity and Kidney Disease and Disparities

Race and ethnicity are significant factors that are directly related to chronic kidney disease, and nonwhites have a significantly higher rate of kidney disease and kidney failure. Recent studies have begun to identify the genetic risk factors for an increased susceptibility to developing kidney disease in specific racial groups, most notably in African Americans.

*American Indians and Alaska Natives* In looking at race alone and percentages, the National Center for Health Statistics found that the highest percentages of diagnosed kidney disease were seen among American Indians/Alaska Natives, or 2 percent, and also those individuals who were both African American and white, or mixed race. Native Americans have a high risk of death from KIDNEY CANCER, and they also have a high prevalence of end-stage renal disease, as do African Americans.

In a study of Navajo Indians reported in *Kidney International* in 2007, the researchers found that the age-adjusted prevalence of end-stage renal disease was nearly four times the average for adults in the United States, or 0.63 percent compared to 0.19 percent in the United States.

*African Americans* Considerable research has been performed on kidney disease and kidney failure among African Americans in the United States. African Americans have a significantly increased risk for the development of chronic kidney disease (CKD) compared to individuals of other races in the United States. For example, African Americans have nearly a four times higher risk of developing CKD than Caucasians (whites), and they also have a greater risk for the development of END-STAGE RENAL DISEASE, (ESRD) requiring either dialysis or kidney transplantation for survival.

According to the National Kidney Disease Education Program, African Americans comprise about 12 percent of the population in the United States, but they represent 32 percent of all people with kidney failure in the United States. The underlying reasons for this high risk of kidney failure may be linked to the higher risk for HYPERTENSION and DIABETES MELLITUS among African Americans; however, the high rate of these illnesses alone does not fully explain the high level of kidney failure among African Americans.

Even when African Americans with hypertension are treated with recommended therapies (as often they are not), many continue to suffer from increasingly debilitating kidney disease. For example, a study published in 2008 in *Archives of Internal Medicine* revealed that although renin-angiotensin system–blocking therapy was beneficial in treating African Americans with chronic kidney disease, in about 25 percent of the subjects, despite this treatment and tight control of their hypertension, many African Americans continued to develop increasingly progressive disease.

African-American men ages 20 to 29 years old have a 10 times greater risk of developing kidney failure from hypertension than do Caucasian men in the United States of the same age. In addition, African-American men ages 30 to 39 years old have a 14 times greater risk of developing kidney failure that is caused by hypertension than is faced by Caucasian men in the same age group.

Despite the high risk that adult African-American males (and females) have for developing chronic kidney disease and kidney failure, most are unaware of the problem; for example, a survey of 1,017 African Americans from seven states, published in 2007 in the *American Journal of Kidney Disease,* revealed that only 23.5 percent were screened for kidney disease in the past year. The researchers found that 43.7 percent of all the subjects were at risk for chronic kidney disease, but only 2.8 percent of the subjects said that they believed kidney disease was a major health concern.

**Research on African Americans and kidney disease**   Researchers have studied many aspects of African Americans and kidney disease, such as their awareness of kidney disease (which is poor) and their risk for kidney disease (which is high).

Research shows that most African Americans are not aware of the risks for disease nor do they know there are simple tests to detect kidney disease. For example, a study of 2,017 African Americans from Georgia, Louisiana, Maryland, Mississippi, Missouri, Ohio, and Tennessee, published in the *American Journal of Kidney Disease* in 2008, revealed that nearly half (43.7 percent) of the subjects had a risk factor for kidney disease but only 2.8 percent said that chronic kidney disease was a major health concern, and only 18.1 percent were aware that African Americans were at a significantly greater risk for developing kidney disease compared to other races.

Many studies have demonstrated that African American men and women with hypertension are at high risk for both serious kidney disease and kidney failure. For example, a study that was published in 2001 found that African Americans comprised 12 percent of the population at the time, but they represented 33 percent of all dialysis patients. An estimated one in three African-American adults has high blood pressure.

**The African American Study of Kidney Disease and Hypertension**   The African American Study of Kidney Disease and Hypertension (AASK) is a major clinical study that was initially launched in 1995 to determine if more aggressive treatment of hypertension or if specific antihypertensive medications would decrease the risk of African Americans developing ESRD. In 2001, a major finding of this study was released, showing that it was possible to slow down kidney disease caused by hypertension in the African-American patients enrolled in this study. In this study, ANGIOTENSIN-CONVERTING ENZYME (ACE) INHIBITOR medications, compared with other medications in the category of CALCIUM CHANNEL BLOCKERS, were proven to slow the progression of kidney disease by 36 percent. The AASK study researchers recommend prescribing ACE inhibitors to African Americans with chronic kidney disease and hypertension to help protect the kidneys from the damaging effects of hypertension.

**Asians and Pacific Islanders**   Individuals of Asian or Pacific Islander race and ethnicity have a lower rate of kidney disease and kidney failure than Native Americans or African Americans but their rates still exceed those among whites/Caucasians. For example, in 2006, 1,559.9 per million population of Asians and Pacific Islanders had end-stage renal disease, compared to 1,252.9 among whites. (Whites had the lowest rates.)

**Hispanics**   According to the American Society of Nephrology, chronic kidney disease is 17 percent more prevalent in Hispanics and Latinos than in whites, and Hispanics/Latinos are twice as likely to die from kidney failure as are whites. It is also known that Hispanics and Latinos have a higher prevalence of diabetes than whites. This may be because of a higher rate of obesity in these racial groups than among whites, but it is likely that other genetic or environmental factors contribute to this increased risk.

**Whites/Caucasians**   For the most part, whites generally have a lower risk for kidney diseases and disorders than individuals of other races. However, research by the Centers for Disease Control and Prevention (CDC) has shown that white women have an elevated risk for high CHOLESTEROL levels compared to women of other races and ethnicities.

**Comparing racial and ethnic groups and risks for kidney disease**   As can be seen from Table 3, blacks have the highest incidence of end-stage renal disease (ESRD) for the period 1995–2005, or 936.8 per million, followed by Native Americans, whose incidence rate was 559.9 per million. In looking at those with ESRD caused by diabetes, as illustrated in Table 3, blacks still led with an incidence rate of 412.9 but were followed closely by Native Americans, with a rate of 384.7 per million. Interestingly, however, when considering ESRD caused by hypertension, Native Americans had the lowest rate of ESRD, or 61.1 per million.

As Table 3 also illustrates, the rates of ESRD caused by diabetes are lowest among whites, followed by Asians and then Hispanics. It should also be noted that in nearly all cases, the rates of ESRD increased markedly from 1995 to 2005, with one exception: Native Americans had a very high rate (the highest rate in 1995) of 400.1 cases per million (ESRD-HT) and this rate dropped somewhat by 2005 to 384.7 per million. However, in all other cases, the rates increased, sometimes by a great deal; for example, the rate of ESRD caused by diabetes rose from 315.9 in 1995 among blacks to 412.9 by 2005. This rate may have coincided with an elevated rate of obesity among blacks (and other racial groups) over this period.

*Other factors relating to chronic kidney disease: education and family income* As can be seen from Table 2, those with the lowest levels of education, or those individuals with less than a high school diploma, are also the most likely to have diagnosed kidney disease, or 2.9 percent, compared to only 1.2 percent of those with a bachelor's degree or higher. Family income is also directly linked to kidney disease, among families with an annual income of less than $20,000, the rate was 2.7 percent. Poverty status was also linked to diagnosed kidney disease, and 2.7 percent of the poor had kidney disease, followed by 2.4 percent of the near poor and 1.2 percent of the "not poor" category. It may be that individuals who are more educated or who have a higher income are also more likely to receive medical treatment and avoid kidney problems.

**TABLE 3: AGE-ADJUSTED INCIDENCE RATES± OF ESRD, ESRD-DM, ESRD-HT, BY RACE AND ETHNICITY, UNITED STATES, 1995–2005**

| Race/Ethnicity* | 1995 | 2005 | Period |
|---|---|---|---|
| **ESRD** | | | |
| Whites | 181.7 | 254.8 | 1995–1998 |
| | | | 1998–2001 |
| | | | 2001–2005 |
| Blacks | 759.6 | 936.8 | 1995–1998 |
| | | | 1998–2005 |
| Native Americans | 541.2 | 559.9 | 1995–1999 |
| | | | 1999–2005 |
| Asians | 309.6 | 333.4 | 1995–1999 |
| | | | 1999–2005 |
| Hispanics | 395.0 | 448.9 | 1995–2000 |
| | | | 2000–2005 |
| All | 260.7 | 350.9 | 1995–1998 |
| | | | 1998–2001 |
| | | | 2001–2005 |
| **ESRD-DM** | | | |
| Whites | 71.6 | 103.5 | 1995–1997 |
| | | | 1997–2001 |
| | | | 2001–2005 |
| Blacks | 315.9 | 412.9 | 1995–1998 |
| | | | 1998–2005 |
| Native Americans | 400.1 | 384.7 | 1995–1999 |
| | | | 1999–2005 |
| Asians | 141.6 | 161.4 | 1995–1999 |
| | | | 1999–2005 |
| Hispanics | 228.8 | 274.7 | 1995–2000 |
| | | | 2000–2005 |
| All | 108.2 | 153.6 | 1995–1997 |
| | | | 1997–2001 |
| | | | 2001–2005 |
| **ESRD-HT** | | | |
| Whites | 44.3 | 63.2 | 1995–1999 |
| | | | 1999–2005 |
| Blacks | 263.1 | 325.6 | 1995–1998 |
| | | | 1998–2003 |
| Native Americans | 47.9 | 61.1 | 1995–2005 |
| Asians | 70.1 | 80.8 | 1995–1999 |
| | | | 1999–2005 |

| Race/Ethnicity* | 1995 | 2005 | Period |
|---|---|---|---|
| **ESRD-HT** | | | |
| Hispanics | 78.2 | 87.7 | 1995–1997 |
| | | | 1997–2000 |
| | | | 2000–2005 |
| All | 70.0 | 94.8 | 1995–1998 |
| | | | 1998–2003 |
| | | | 2003–2005 |

Abbreviations: ESRD-DM, end stage renal disease therapy with diabetes listed as the primary diagnosis; ESRD-HT, end-stage renal disease therapy with hypertension listed as the primary diagnosis.
*Racial groups include persons of non-Hispanic origin only; Hispanics may be of any race.
±Per million population, age-adjusted based on the 2000 U.S. standard population.

Reprinted from *Advances in Chronic Kidney Disease*, Volume 15, Number 2, Nilka Rios Burrows, Yanfeng Li, and Desmond E. Williams. "Racial and Ethnic Differences in Trends of End-Stage Renal Disease: United States, 1995–2005." Page 149, Copyright 2008, with permission from the National Kidney Foundation.

### Chronic Kidney Disease and Key Issues

Many have no idea that they have chronic kidney disease because the symptoms of early chronic kidney disease are very mild or they are altogether nonexistent. Yet there *are* markers for chronic kidney disease when an individual is asymptomatic, such as tests for serum creatinine and assessment of either the urine protein-to-creatinine ratio or urinary albumin-to-creatinine ratio. Physicians can order these simple and relatively inexpensive blood and urine tests which will reveal early on that there may be a problem that should be followed up. This is important, because if the disease is not treated early on, it could progress through the five stages of chronic kidney disease, with the last stage of kidney failure. Not everyone with chronic kidney disease develops kidney failure, but few people would wish to take the chance that they will not (or will) suffer from kidney failure. In addition, even early chronic kidney disease increases the risk of cardiovascular disease, making recognizing this condition important in order to optimize overall health maintenance.

Laboratory tests for checking markers of kidney disease are increasingly being used by physicians to screen for kidney disease, just as the mammogram is now an accepted screening test for breast cancer in women, and the colonoscopy is an accepted test for the presence of colorectal cancer in both men and women.

*A growing problem linked to diabetes and hypertension* Disturbingly, chronic kidney disease is a rapidly growing problem in the United States; for example, the number of individuals who are directly affected by kidney diseases and disorders is anticipated to increase exponentially with the aging population in the United States, including among the huge bulge of baby boomers (born from 1946–64) as well as among their parents, aunts, uncles, and other relatives who already are or soon will be impacted by the ravages of kidney disease.

Chronic kidney disease is also directly linked with many other common chronic diseases, particularly with diabetes and hypertension, which are also diseases whose numbers are rapidly increasing along with the aging population. In addition, the modern problem of OBESITY is also associated with kidney disease, and the United States and many other countries face an increasingly obese adult population. Also, many children and adolescents in the United States are obese, and consequently their risk for childhood kidney diseases is elevated.

### Other Risk Factors for Chronic Kidney Disease

There are also personal risk factors for the development of chronic kidney disease; for example, people who engage in SMOKING substantially increase their risk for developing kidney disease. Individuals who are obese have a greater risk for kidney diseases than those who are not obese. Many people have multiple risk factors: they smoke and they are obese, and the obesity may cause Type 2 diabetes mellitus. They are in serious danger of developing kidney disease.

*Genetic risks* Researchers have found that genetic variations of the MYH9 gene are associated with much of the extra risk for kidney disease that is present in African Americans with hypertension. The study was performed by the Family Investigation of Nephropathy and Diabetes consortium, a group that studied over 2,100 participants. This research was combined with research from the National Institutes of Health of a scan of the human genome of 190 African Americans who had FOCAL SEGMENTAL GLOMERULOSCLEROSIS (FSGS) (some of whom also had HIV) and 222 African Americans who did not have FSGS.

The researchers did not find a link between the gene and kidney failure related to diabetes. Researchers also reported that the risk conferred by the MYH9 gene was greater than genetic risks seen for other risk factors for disease, including the genetic risk for diabetes, prostate cancer, breast cancer, cardiovascular disease and hypertension—clearly a dramatic risk. Interestingly, the MYH9 gene was not associated with an increased risk of end-stage renal disease in patients with diabetes, suggesting the different genetic factors predispose to progressive kidney disease in patients who have diabetes more than in patients who do not have diabetes.

**Personal lifestyle risk factors**   There are some modifiable lifestyle factors that increase the risk for the development of kidney disease. Obesity may increase the risk for kidney disease, based on recent findings. Dietary habits also increase the risk of chronic kidney disease. In particular, excess dietary salt intake increases the risk for PROTEINURIA and can also worsen hypertension control in patients with chronic kidney disease and thereby predispose to an increased risk of progressive renal damage. In contrast, a diet high in foods enriched in potassium, typically fruits and vegetables, can decrease blood pressure and decrease sensitivity to sodium intake, and thereby help to protect the kidneys. However, patients need to be carefully monitored with regard to their potassium intake, because excess potassium levels can accumulate in the blood in patients with chronic kidney disease and may also have adverse cardiovascular effects.

**Multiple risk factors**   Many individuals have two or more risk factors for serious kidney dis-

ease; for example, an individual may have both hypertension and diabetes, greatly increasing the risk for ultimate kidney failure. In addition, the individual may have personal lifestyle risk factors, such as being obese and smoking. The individual may have other factors that he or she has no control over, such as being African American or Native American. The greater the number of risks that are present, the more likely the person is to suffer from kidney disease, although the risk is not 100 percent.

### Most People with Chronic Kidney Disease Are Unaware of Their Illness

Although about 3.35 million people in the United States know that they have kidney disease, according to National Kidney and Urologic Diseases Information Clearinghouse (NKUDIC), there are millions more in the United States who have kidney disease but do not know it, and as a result, the kidney disease continues its relentless damaging assault on the body. In Canada, there are an estimated 1.9 to 2.3 million people with chronic kidney disease. People with undetected kidney disease are likely to have the early stages of the five stages of chronic kidney disease, either Stage 1, 2, or 3, but even patients with Stage 4 chronic kidney disease can have no symptoms from this condition.

The reason for unawareness of kidney disease is that very often, there are few or no symptoms of chronic kidney disease until the disease has progressed to a dangerous level. The symptoms, even when present, can be vague, such as mild fatigue, SLEEP PROBLEMS, and mild intestinal upset. As a result, individuals with chronic kidney diseases usually obtain no treatment for their unknown illness, nor will they take any preventive actions which could stave off further harm to their kidneys. The reality is that if chronic kidney disease is not detected and treated, it will ultimately worsen and accelerate. Moreover, because chronic kidney disease increases the risk for heart attacks, strokes, and other forms of cardiovascular disease, many patients with chronic kidney disease can have complications due to chronic kidney disease, such as a heart attack or stroke, without having to develop renal failure. Yet simple laboratory tests, such as simple urine tests for protein in the urine (proteinuria), measurement of the serum creatinine, and calculation of the estimated glomerular filtration rate (eGFR) can detect chronic kidney disease at early and asymptomatic stages.

With more advanced kidney disease, the signs and symptoms of disease are more apparent, including such signs as edema (excess fluid retention), increasingly difficult-to-control hypertension, worsening anemia, worsening cholesterol control, persistent nausea and vomiting (particularly in the morning), and extreme fatigue. These symptoms rarely occur within a short period and instead usually occur after years of damage to the kidneys.

According to the NKUDIC, only about 12 percent of the men and 6 percent of the women in the United States who have moderate kidney disease actually realize that they have chronic kidney disease. The awareness levels of their disease state steadily increase among those who have severe kidney disease (Stage 4 kidney disease), largely because the symptoms increase and are more likely to send them to see a physician. However, even in the cases of individuals with Stage 4 kidney disease, only 42 percent of such individuals realize that they are ill, versus the majority (58 percent) who are unaware that they are sick and that they urgently need to be treated to decrease or delay the likelihood of needing either dialysis or kidney transplantation in the future.

**Causes of Kidney Diseases**   There are many potential causes of kidney disease. The kidneys may be harmed by other disorders, most prominently diabetes and hypertension. They may also be harmed by medications that are toxic to the kidneys, either over time or in a short period. Some people inherit diseases that cause harm to the kidneys. In addition, some individuals suffer from acute kidney injury (AKI), which may be caused by medications, infections, drug abuse, physical injury, and other causes.

***Endocrine disorders and the kidneys***   A number of endocrine disorders, in addition to their effects on the other organ systems, can damage the kidneys, sometimes irreversibly. The most common endocrine disorder that can cause kidney disease is diabetes mellitus. Here, the abnormal glucose levels directly damage the kidneys. Approximately 20 percent of all people with diabetes will develop kidney damage. This damage can cause kidney failure and a need for either dialysis or kidney transplantation to remain alive. It may also cause partial kidney damage, which can have a number of systemic effects, such as predisposing an individual to hypertension, heart attacks, strokes, and bone disease. According to the National Kidney and Urologic Diseases Information Clearinghouse, in 2007, there were nearly 50,000 new beneficiaries of treatment for kidney failure whose disease stemmed from diabetes.

There are also a number of less common endocrine disorders which may damage the kidneys. For example, primary hyperaldosteronism can cause severe hypertension, which can directly damage the kidneys. It can also cause abnormal blood glucose regulation, and in susceptible individuals, can lead to diabetes mellitus, which as described above can damage the kidneys. Hyperaldosteronism can also lead to HYPOKALEMIA, and chronic hypokalemia through a variety of mechanisms can cause chronic kidney damage. (See ALDOSTERONE AND ALDOSTERONISM.)

Of course, there are many other diseases that may develop within the kidneys; for example, the kidneys may fill with cysts, as with POLYCYSTIC KIDNEY DISEASE (PKD), which by compressing normal kidney tissue can lead to kidney failure. As with all other organs in the body, the kidneys may also develop cancer, and treatment for kidney cancer is urgently needed. The primary treatment for kidney cancer is the surgical removal of the affected kidney. In addition, one of the most common sites of recurrence of kidney cancer is in the opposite kidney. If the other kidney has to be removed, the patient will need either dialysis or renal transplantation.

*Acute kidney injury (AKI)*    Acute kidney injury (AKI) is associated with an elevated risk for kidney failure. The United States Renal Data System reports that 28 percent of patients who survive a hospitalization for AKI will die within a year.

According to the United States Renal Data System, AKI in Medicare patients is directly associated with age, and increasing age brings increasing risk. For example, among Medicare patients ages 65–69 years, the rate of AKI in 2008 was 10.3 per 1,000 patient years. (The term patient years is a statistical device used to illustrate trends and is based on the number of patients in a study and the number of years that they are studied.) The rate increased to 19.2 per 1,000 patient years for individuals ages 75–79 years and further to 34.7 per 1,000 patient years among those ages 85 years and older.

Researchers have also found that the risk for hospitalization for AKI is significantly higher for African Americans who are Medicare members compared to their white cohorts. For example, the rate is 2.1 times higher for AKI among African Americans compared to white Americans, and the rate of dialysis is 1.9 times greater for African Americans.

In considering race alone, the incidence of AKI is 34.2 per 1,000 patient years for African Americans compared to the rate of 18.4 per 1,000 patient years for whites and 18.6 for individuals of other races.

The United States Renal Data System also noted that among those hospitalized for AKI, 26 percent will be rehospitalized within the next year. The risk of rehospitalization is higher for African Americans than whites.

*Genetic disorders*    Some genetic diseases may lead to kidney disease; for example, SICKLE CELL DISEASE (also known as sickle cell anemia) may lead to multiple organ failure. In the kidneys, sickle cell disease can lead to abnormal filtering and loss of proteins, which can lead to edema, cholesterol disorders, and malnutrition.

Sickle cell disease and its effects on the kidneys can also impair the kidney's ability to regulate how much urine is formed, leading to the excretion of large amounts of urine and an increased predisposition to becoming volume depleted. Finally, sickle cell disease can lead to renal failure and the need for dialysis or renal transplantation. There is also an array of rare genetic syndromes of the kidney, such as ALPORT SYNDROME, a genetic disorder which is particularly problematic for the kidneys among males who inherit this disease. An estimated 80 percent of men with Alport syndrome received the gene from their mothers.

*Multiple interactions of the kidneys with the body may lead to kidney disease*    The kidneys interact daily with the body in the process of filtering the blood, and multiple processes that impinge from without and within the body can lead to kidney disease. Sometimes the exact cause of the disease cannot be pinpointed, and it is only known that kidney disease is present and needs to be treated. For example, a medication that was formerly taken may have been toxic to the individual and harmed the kidneys but this medication is no longer in use.

Sometimes individuals take multiple forms of vitamin or mineral supplements or a combination of minerals, vitamins, or herbs, and they may fail to tell their physician that they take these drugs because they do not regard them as "drugs." Many people mistakenly assume that because a substance is "natural," this also means that it is good for the body. This is an erroneous generalization; for example, snake venom and poison ivy are natural substances but most people realize that they are harmful. It is very important for patients to tell their doctors about every drug, vitamin, herbal supplement, or other medication that they take, to avoid dangerous interactions with other medications or overall harm to the body.

Excessive or insufficient levels of vitamins and/or minerals may result from endocrine disorders or other illnesses, and this excess or insufficiency may escalate and cause damage to the kidneys.

Because of the very high blood flow to the kidneys, approximately 15 gallons per hour, and because of the filtration and subsequent concentration of many compounds in the kidney, the kidneys are highly susceptible to harm.

*Medications can harm the kidneys* Some medications or an excess of some medications may lead to problems with the kidneys. (See MEDICATIONS THAT CAN HARM THE KIDNEYS.) Medications as well as illegal drugs are often filtered by the kidneys rather than the liver, and if the medication is used excessively or abused, as with ANALGESIC NEPHROPATHY, then the risk for damage is further escalated.

### Kidney Disease Causes Other Medical Problems

Kidney disease can also lead to serious complications throughout the body; for example, kidney disease can cause hypertension (high blood pressure), nerve damage (neuropathy), ANEMIA, and other diseases and disorders. It also raises the risk for the development of CARDIOVASCULAR DISEASE. According to the American Society of Nephrology, 50 percent of patients with kidney failure die from heart disease rather than kidney failure.

In some cases, kidney disease leads to problems with the abilities of the kidneys to normally regulate body fluid contents. For example, genetic conditions such as Bartter's syndrome and Gitelman syndrome can lead to persistent hypotension (low blood pressure) and severe hypokalemia; the hypokalemia can lead to skeletal muscle disorders, cardiac arrhythmias, and severe weakness and fatigue.

### When the Kidneys Fail

The kidneys fail either because of end-stage renal disease, the final stage of chronic kidney disease, or because of acute kidney injury. ESRD is a slower and more insidious form of kidney failure than the sudden failure of AKI; however, some AKI patients may regain kidney function, while those with ESRD cannot regain the use of their kidneys because the damage is permanent.

When the kidneys fail, the individual will need to receive dialysis or kidney transplantation to survive. With ESRD, kidney function is less than 10–15 percent of its normal rate.

Almost 30 million people in the United States, most of them adults, have some form of chronic kidney disease, although most do not realize they have it because they have few or no symptoms. About a half million people in the United States have had kidney failure and they require either dialysis or a kidney transplant.

Kidneys do not usually fail catastrophically and at once, although such a condition can occur in a car crash or other serious accident or when serious medical problems cause an acute kidney injury. In general, the kidneys fail slowly and over a period of years. But at some point, they can no longer function. When the kidneys completely fail, for whatever reason, the only treatments that can continue a person's life are either dialysis, which is an artificial cleansing of the toxins from the kidneys, or a kidney transplant that has been "harvested" (very carefully removed and preserved) from another person. Most people have two working kidneys, so it is possible for an individual to donate a kidney to another person and still survive. Considerable evidence shows that in carefully screened individuals, donating a kidney is safe and has no long-term health consequences. Such a procedure is usually performed only on behalf of a genetically related family member, but it is possible for one spouse to donate a kidney to their other spouse, and donations to friends or other completely unrelated individuals are becoming increasingly common.

By 2030, an estimated 2 million people in the United States are expected to be receiving treatment for kidney failure. Unfortunately, there are not enough donors to provide kidney transplants to all the people who need them; for example, according to the National Kidney Foundation in 2010, 4,573 kidney patients died waiting for an organ transplant in 2008. Potential donors may not realize the costs of organ donation are almost always paid for by the recipient's insurance.

In 2007, there were an estimated 74,000 people awaiting a kidney for transplantation, according to the National Kidney and Urologic Disease Information Clearinghouse (NKUDIC).

Of those who did receive a transplant then from a deceased person, 94.9 percent survived at least one year, in contrast to the much lower survival rate of 59.4 percent in 1995. If the transplant was received from a living donor, the survival rate for at least one year was 98.4 percent.

Nearly 107,000 people each year develop new onset ESRD, and the largest proportion of these cases, about 47,000, are caused by diabetes, followed by hypertension (about 29,000 cases). Both the incidence and prevalence of ESRD in the United States have risen steadily from 1980 to the current data available in 2006. (Incidence is the number or percentage of new cases per year, while prevalence refers to the entire population that has the disease.) For example, the prevalence of ESRD among those under age 20 years (the age group least likely to have ESRD), increased from 32.7 per million in this group in 1980 to 86.1 per million in 2006.

The prevalence of ESRD among blacks or African Americans, the racial group most likely to have ESRD, increased 6.5-fold, from 608.7 per million in 1980 to 4,004.0 in 2006. In addition, the numbers of people whose kidneys failed because of diabetes was 24.4 per million in 1980 and it increased to 610.6 by 2006, 25 times greater than the 1980 figure. (See Table 4.) A large portion of this increase in diabetes leading to kidney failure can be attributed to the increased frequency of obesity and subsequent diabetes mellitus in westernized countries, including the United States; an aging population; and increased effectiveness at treating the complications of early chronic kidney disease, such as heart attacks and strokes, which enables people to live longer, and thus be more likely to develop other complications of chronic kidney disease, in this case end-stage renal disease.

**Dialysis**    Dialysis is a procedure that is used with individuals whose kidneys have failed. It is necessary for their survival; their only other survival option is kidney transplantation. There are two primary types of dialysis: HEMODIALYSIS and PERITONEAL DIALYSIS. Hemodialysis uses a dialysis machine to remove the blood from the body in order to remove the wastes from the blood and then returns the cleaned blood back into the body. Peritoneal dialysis uses a special catheter in the abdominal cavity to fill the abdomen with dialysis solution and then empty the solution.

Hemodialysis is more commonly used in the United States. Dialysis can be an arduous process for the patient, although it is typically not painful. It may also be emotionally difficult for the family.

Physician decisions about recommending dialysis often depend on demographic factors, according to an analysis by Kellier Hunter Campbell, M.D., and colleagues in their 2008 article for the *Journal of General Internal Medicine.* The researchers analyzed the decision for or against dialysis among older adults with chronic kidney disease based on more than 100 articles on this topic. They found that increasing age was associated with a lower likelihood for recommending dialysis (or kidney transplantation). They also found that women were less likely to receive dialysis than men. African Americans were more likely to receive dialysis than whites but they were less likely to receive kidney transplantation than whites. One study found that socially isolated patients were less likely to be recommended for dialysis, as were those with functional impairments. The underlying reasons for these findings are unknown but appear worthy of further research.

Although dialysis provides short-term replacement of kidney function, it does not completely reproduce normal kidney function. As a result, many patients experience a shortened life expectancy despite their dialysis treatments. According to the *American Society of Nephrology,* two-thirds of dialysis patients die at some point within five years after starting dialysis, which is a lower survival rate than for many patients diagnosed with cancer. The damage to the kidneys may also be of a shorter duration, as with acute kidney injury that may lead to temporary or permanent kidney failure.

**Kidney transplantation**    The kidney transplant is an amazing means for an individual's life to be sustained and an opportunity to avoid the often difficult process of dialysis. The vast majority of those receiving transplants survive for at least one year and many survive for five years or longer. As shown in Figure 2, the diseased kidneys remain in place, and the transplanted kidney is placed into the abdomen and is directly hooked into both an artery and a vein. In addition, a direct connection is also made from the transplanted kidney into the bladder.

However, transplants of the kidneys, as with transplants of any major organ, come with risks. Individuals who have had a kidney transplant must stay on IMMUNOSUPPRESSIVE DRUGS for the rest of their lives, even if the transplant came from a close relative such as a parent or a sibling. The only exception is a transplant from an identical twin. Except in that case, these medications are necessary to avoid the rejection of the organ by the person's immune system. Yet suppressing the immune system increases the risk for the development of infections as well as other serious diseases, including cancer.

Since the kidney transplant patient cannot live in a bubble, he or she will be exposed to pathogens. These patients can, however, use good judgment, avoiding individuals with colds or other communicable infections. Patients with a transplanted kidney need to work closely with specialized physicians known as transplant nephrologists in order to optimize their use of immunosuppressive drugs. There is a continuing and ongoing balance for the patient in providing sufficient levels of immunosuppressive medications to decrease the risk of rejection of the transplanted kidney while at the same time minimizing the amount of the medications in order to minimize the risk of infection, cancer, and medication-associated complications.

Researcher Emmanuel Morelon and colleagues found that a kidney transplant significantly improves the outlook of not only the

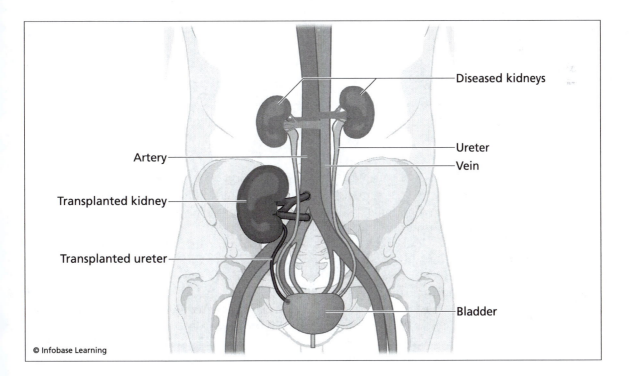

Artery

Transplanted kidney

Transplanted ureter

Diseased kidneys

Ureter

Vein

Bladder

© Infobase Learning

TABLE 4: PREVALENCE OF END-STAGE RENAL DISEASE, BY SELECTED CHARACTERISTICS: UNITED STATES, SELECTED YEARS, 1980–2006 (RATE PER MILLION POPULATION)

| | 1980 | 1990 | 2000 | 2005 | 2006 |
|---|---|---|---|---|---|
| Patients alive on December 31 per million population | 254.8 | 726.1 | 1,351.3 | 1,589.1 | 1,640.8 |
| **Age** | | | | | |
| Under 20 years | 32.7 | 62.1 | 78.0 | 85.3 | 86.1 |
| 20–44 years | 236.0 | 565.1 | 840.4 | 877.6 | 889.2 |
| 45–64 years | 530.5 | 1,439.1 | 2,468.4 | 2,798.0 | 2,868.2 |
| 65–74 years | 83.5 | 1,953.0 | 4,149.5 | 4,912.2 | 5,101.9 |
| 75 years and over | 273.5 | 1,372.8 | 3,361.6 | 4,128.6 | 4,235.2 |
| **Sex** | | | | | |
| Male | 289.5 | 802.6 | 1,502.5 | 1,795.7 | 1,861.7 |
| Female | 221.9 | 653.3 | 1,205.5 | 1,388.6 | 1,426.1 |
| **Race[1]** | | | | | |
| White | 209.2 | 562.6 | 1,021.9 | 1,212.5 | 1,252.9 |
| Black or African American | 608.7 | 1,851.7 | 3,410.3 | 3,900.0 | 4,004.0 |
| American Indian or Alaska Native | 255.7 | 1,037.8 | 1,800.0 | 2,035.9 | 2,075.9 |
| Asian or Pacific Islander | 99.4 | 583.9 | 1,253.8 | 1,487.5 | 1,559.9 |
| **Hispanic origin[1]** | | | | | |
| Hispanic | n/a | n/a | 1,164.0 | 1,374.12 | 1,432.3 |
| Not Hispanic | n/a | n/a | 1,378.8 | 1,625.9 | 1,677.5 |
| **Primary diagnosis** | | | | | |
| Diabetes | 24.4 | 186.7 | 478.9 | 587.7 | 610.6 |
| Hypertension | 41.2 | 187.8 | 332.9 | 389.5 | 399.9 |
| Glomerulonephritis | 58.4 | 157.9 | 238.1 | 257.0 | 259.7 |
| Cystic kidney | 15.9 | 39.7 | 62.9 | 74.3 | 77.5 |
| Other urologic | 7.0 | 24.3 | 41.2 | 44.6 | 43.4 |
| Other cause | 28.5 | 84.8 | 137.7 | 163.6 | 173.3 |
| Unknown cause | 25.7 | 32.9 | 49.8 | 60.7 | 64.0 |
| Missing disease | 53.7 | 12.1 | 9.8 | 11.7 | 12.3 |

Source: *Health, United States, 2009,* p. 259.

[1] The race groups, white, black or African American, American Indian or Alaska Native, and Asian or Pacific Islander, include persons of Hispanic and non-Hispanic origin. Persons of Hispanic origin may be of any race.

transplant recipient but also his or her family; for example, a study of 1,815 respondents who were partners of individuals with kidney failure revealed that two of three partners of individuals with partners on dialysis said that the overall impact of the disease on their life was major, compared to only one in four partners of individuals who received kidney transplants.

The researchers said, "Partners of patients on dialysis devote more time to the patient, are more likely to experience negative practical, relational, social, psychological and professional consequences and they judge their own quality of life as significantly lower than do the partners of transplanted patients."

The researchers also found that 87 percent of the dialysis partners regarded themselves as indispensable to the person with kidney failure (which can be a huge emotional burden), compared to 61 percent of the partners of kidney transplant patients. Clearly a kidney transplant alleviates much of the emotional and psychological burden of many partners of individuals whose kidneys have failed.

Agoda, L. Y., et al. "Effect of Ramipril vs. Amlodipine on Renal Outcomes in Hypertensive Nephrosclerosis: A Randomized Controlled Trial." *Journal of the American Medical Association* 285, no. 21 (2001): 2,719–2,728.

Alpern, Robert J., and Steven C. Hebert. *Seldin and Giebisch's The Kidney: Physiology and Pathophysiology. Volume 1.* Burlington, Mass.: Academic Press, 2008.

Appel, Lawrence J., M.D., et al. "Long-term Effects of Renin-Angiotensin System–Blocking Therapy and a Low Blood Pressure Goal on Progression of Hypertensive Chronic Kidney Disease in African Americans." *Archives of Internal Medicine* 168, no. 8 (April 28, 2008): 832–839.

Aronson, Jeff. "Dropsy." *British Medical Journal* 326, no. 7387 (2003): 491.

Cameron, J. S. "Bright's Disease Today: The Pathogenesis and Treatment of Glomerulonephritis-I." *British Medical Journal* 4 (1972): 87–90.

Coresh, Josef, M.D., et al. "Prevalence of Chronic Kidney Disease in the United States." *Journal of the American Medical Association* 298, no. 17 (November 7, 2007): 2,038–2,047.

Crumbley, Paul. "Emily Dickinson's Life." Modern American Poetry. Available online. URL: http://www.english.uiuc.edu/maps/poets/a_f/dickinson/bio.htm. Accessed January 13, 2009.

Ferri, C. V., and R. A. Pruchno. "Quality of Life in End-Stage Renal Disease Patients: Differences in Patient and Spouse Perceptions." *Aging Mental Health* 13, no. 5 (2009): 708–714.

Gassman, Jennifer, et al. "Design and Statistical Aspects of the African American Study of Kidney Disease and Hypertension (AASK)." *Journal of the American Society of Nephrology* 14 (2003): S154–S165.

Hochman, M. E., et al. "The Prevalence and Incidence of End-Stage Renal Disease in Native American Adults on the Navajo Reservation." *Kidney International* 71 (2007): 931–937.

Levin, Adeera, M.D., et al. "Guidelines for the Management of Chronic Kidney Disease." *Canadian Medical Association Journal* 179, no. 11 (November 18, 2008): 1,154–1,162.

Macías Núñez, Juan F., M.D., J. Stewart Cameron, M.D., and Dimitrios G. Oreopoulos, M.D., eds. *The Aging Kidney in Health and Disease.* New York: Springer Science+Business Media, 2008.

Morelon, Emmanuel, et al. "Partners' Concerns, Needs and Expectations in ESRD: Results of the CODIT Study." *Nephrology Dialysis Transplantation* 20 (2005): 1,670–1,675.

National Kidney Foundation. "25 Facts About Organ Donation and Transplantation." Available online. URL: http://www.kidney.or/news/newsroom/fs_new/25fatsorgdon&trans.cfm. 2010. Accessed March 22, 2010.

Peitzman, Steven J. *Dropsy, Dialysis, Transplant: A Short History of Failing Kidneys.* Baltimore, Md.: Johns Hopkins University Press, 2007.

Petit, William, Jr., and Christine Adamec. *The Encyclopedia of Diabetes.* New York: Facts On File, 2002.

———. *The Encyclopedia of Endocrine Diseases and Disorders.* New York: Facts On File, 2005.

Pleis, J. R., and M. Lethbridge-Çejku. "Frequencies of Selected Diseases and Conditions among Persons 18 Years of Age and Over, by Selected Characteristics, United States, 2006." *Summary Health Statistics for U.S. Adults: National Health Interview Survey, 2006.* December 2007.

Schoolwerth, Anton C., M.D., et al. "Chronic Kidney Disease: A Public Health Problem that Needs a Public Health Action Plan." *Preventing Chronic Disease* 3, no. 2 (April 2006): 1–6.

U.S. Renal Data System. *USRDS 2008 Annual Data Report: Atlas of Chronic Kidney Disease and End-Stage Renal Disease in the United States.* Bethesda, Md.: National Institutes of Health, National Institute of Diabetes and Digestive and Kidney Diseases, 2008.

———. *USRDS 2010 Annual Data Report: Atlas of Chronic Kidney Disease and End-Stage Renal Disease in the United States.* Bethesda, Md.: National Institutes of Health, National Institute of Diabetes and Digestive and Kidney Diseases, 2010.

Waterman, A. D., et al. "Attitudes and Behaviors of African Americans Regarding Early Detection of Kidney Disease." *American Journal of Kidney Disease* 51, no. 4 (2008): 554–562.

**kidneys**   See KIDNEYS AND KIDNEY DISEASE.

**kidneys, ectopic**   See ECTOPIC KIDNEY.

**kidney stones**   Tiny and hard crystalline substances that can develop within the kidney. (Stones may also develop in the bladder.) The condition of having kidney stones is also known as nephrolithiasis or urolithiasis. Individuals who develop kidney stones are often otherwise healthy, while those who develop bladder stones are more likely to have anatomic abnormalities in their bladder. Individuals who have had gall-stones do *not* have an increased risk of developing kidney stones.

Kidney stones can be as tiny as particles of sand or they can be as large as a lightbulb. They also present in many different shapes and colors, based on the composition of the stone. Most kidney stones are comprised of calcium oxalate, uric acid, or calcium phosphate, while some are composed of cystine. Struvite stones may also develop in the presence of an underlying tendency for stone formation, as well as in the case of repeated urinary tract infections

Uric stones usually result from a diet that is very high in animal protein. These stones may pass into the urine by themselves or physicians may need to use other means, such as LITHO-TRIPSY (shock waves), to break up these kidney stones so that they may be more easily passed by the patient.

Cystine stones develop from a rare genetic disorder that causes cystine, which is an amino acid which leaks through the kidneys and into the urine, forming the crystals/kidney stones.

### Symptoms and Diagnostic Path

Kidney stones often cause excruciating pain. Some women have compared the pain of a kidney stone to the pain of childbirth, and they may present at the hospital emergency room in agony. Many males with kidney stones report that it is the worst pain that they have ever experienced. In most individuals, the first episode of a kidney stone is associated with such substantial pain that the person feels nauseated and vomits.

In addition to severe pain and nausea and vomiting, other symptoms of kidney stones may include

- blood in the urine, which is clearly visible
- urine that looks cloudy or smells foul

- a burning feeling during urination
- fever and chills

Gross hematuria (blood in the urine that is evident by visual inspection) occurs in approximately 90 percent of patients; however, the absence of hematuria does not rule out the possibility of stones. At times, the stone may obstruct the flow of urine into the bladder and the patient will develop kidney distention (hydronephrosis). Sometimes hydronephrosis will develop into PYELONEPHRITIS (kidney infection), which is also an urgent indication to remove the stone and relieve the obstruction.

According to Margaret Pearle and colleagues in *Urologic Diseases in America*, published by the National Institute of Diabetes and Digestive and Kidney Diseases (NIDDK) in 2007, the most sensitive method for detecting stones in the kidneys, ureters, or bladder is the helical computerized tomogram (CT) scan. This scan can identify nearly all stones, including stones as small as 1 millimeter in diameter. When a CT scan confirms the presence of a stone, a plain abdominal X-ray should also be obtained in order to assess whether the stone is radioopaque. If a CT is not an available option, then plain abdominal X-rays should be used, since 75–90 percent of urinary calculi are radioopaque.

Another diagnostic technique and one which is noninvasive and does not involve any exposure to radiation is an ultrasound of the kidneys and the bladder. It is the diagnostic imaging choice in pregnant patients with a possible kidney stone.

An ultrasound examination of the kidney is very effective at determining whether the kidney stone is obstructing the flow of urine out of the kidney, resulting in the development of hydronephrosis. The early diagnosis and treatment, with removal of the stone, is quite critical in such patients to prevent long-term damage to the kidney.

### Treatment Options and Outlook

The severe pain of a kidney stone typically requires treatment with narcotic pain medications. Fluids are needed to maintain the affected person's hydration and to assist in passing the kidney stone. Certain medications, such as tamsulosin (Flomax), may be helpful in relaxing the affected tissues and allowing the stone to pass. If an infection is present, then ANTIBIOTICS are needed.

The most commonly used option to treat kidney stones as well as the stones that are associated with the obstruction of the bladder is shock wave lithotripsy (SWL). This is a procedure that breaks up the stones nonsurgically. Other treatment options are the ureteroscopy, the percutaneous nephrostolithotomy, and the surgical open or laparoscopic removal of the stones.

The ureteroscopy is used to treat kidney stones in cases where SWL has either failed or it is inadvisable. Percutaneous nephrosolithotomy is used for very large kidney stones and stones that are associated with anatomic abnormalities. Open and laparoscopic surgery, used in less than 2 percent of the patients diagnosed with urolithiasis, is used either when less invasive treatment options have failed or when major anatomic abnormalities require the physician to make repairs at the same time as the removal of the kidney stones.

### Risk Factors and Preventive Measures

More than 55 percent of those with kidney stones may have a family history of kidney stones, either in their first degree relatives or other relatives. Kidney stone disease is more common in white men, followed in order of highest frequency by white women, black women, and black men.

The primary risk factors for hospitalization with kidney stones are gender, age, race, and the geographic country where the patient resides. Men have a risk of developing kidney stones that is about one to three per 1,000 men, while women have a much lower risk of 0.6 to 1.0 per 1,000 women.

The risk for developing kidney stones among males peaks in those who are ages 40–59 years, then decreases after that age, while the risk for kidney stones among women is not dependent on age, and it is about the same at any age group.

Whites have the greatest risk for inpatient hospital stays that are caused by kidney stones; in 2000, the rate for whites was 55 per 100,000 individuals, followed by Hispanics, with a rate of 36 per 100,000 individuals. Asian/Pacific Islanders had the lowest risk for being hospitalized for kidney stones, or 17 per 100,000 people. The risk for blacks was 19 per 100,000 people.

In sheer numbers, research has shown that individuals in the southeastern part of the United States have the highest risk of developing kidney stones; this area is sometimes termed the "stone belt." For unknown reasons, rates were low in the Midwest. (For more information, see Table 1.) Since most people with kidney stones are treated in an outpatient setting, the hospitalization rates may not accurately reflect the occurrence rate of this condition.

Among children who were hospitalized for urolithiasis in 2001, the length of stay (an average of 6.2 days) was highest among those children ages zero (newborns) to two years old, followed by those who were ages 11–17 years (3.1 days) and children who were ages 3–10 years (2.9 days). Clearly, babies and toddlers are more fragile than older children suffering from kidney stones.

### Prevention of nephrolithiasis (development of renal stones)

According to John S. Rodman et al. in their book, *No More Kidney Stones,* chronic dehydration is one cause that may lead to the development of kidney stones. As a result, one simple preventive measure is to drink a sufficient amount of fluid each day. At least eight glasses per day should be consumed, and water is preferable to other beverages, such as caffeinated drinks, because of its lack of unneeded chemicals and caffeine.

Some medical conditions, such as GOUT, significantly increase the risk of the development of kidney stones. Gout causes a high level of uric acid in the blood stream, escalating the likelihood of a stone that is formed by uric acid. Controlling gout will also help to limit the risk of the development of kidney stones that are linked to gout.

**TABLE 1: INPATIENT HOSPITAL STAYS BY INDIVIDUALS WITH UPPER TRACT UROLITHIASIS LISTED AS THE PRIMARY DIAGNOSIS, BY NUMBER AND BY RATE PER 100,000, IN 2000**

| | Count | Rate per 100,000 |
|---|---|---|
| **Total** | 170,316 | 62 |
| **Age** | | |
| Under 18 | 3,419 | 4.7 |
| 18–24 Years | 9,478 | 36 |
| 25–34 Years | 25,511 | 68 |
| 35–44 Years | 36,956 | 83 |
| 45–54 Years | 36,935 | 101 |
| 55–64 Years | 26,138 | 112 |
| 65–74 Years | 18,955 | 107 |
| 75–84 Years | 10,684 | 91 |
| 85+ Years | 2,236 | 72 |
| **Race/ethnicity** | | |
| White | 107,087 | 55 |
| Black | 6,497 | 19 |
| Asian/Pacific Islander | 1,804 | 17 |
| Hispanic | 11,855 | 36 |
| **Gender** | | |
| Male | 99,214 | 74 |
| Female | 71,087 | 51 |
| **Region of U.S.** | | |
| Midwest | 43,700 | 69 |
| Northeast | 36,149 | 70 |
| South | 66,628 | 70 |
| West | 23,828 | 38 |
| **Metropolitan statistical area (MSA)** | | |
| Rural | 39,373 | 65 |
| Urban | 130,651 | 61 |

Source: Adapted from Pearle, Margaret S., M.D., Elizabeth A. Calhoun, and Gary C. Curhan, M.D., "Urolithiasis." In *Urologic Diseases in America,* edited by Litwin, M. S. and C. S. Saigal. Bethesda, Md.: National Institute of Diabetes and Digestive and Kidney Diseases (NIDDK), 2007, p. 291.

***Dietary modifications in patients with recurrent stone disease*** The consumption of animal protein is a major dietary constituent that is responsible for the relatively high prevalence of stones in the populations of developed countries. An increased intake of animal proteins increases the risk for uric acid and for calcium-containing kidney stones. Hence, excessive animal protein intake (as is found in meat) can predispose to the development of calcium stones among individuals belonging to a susceptible population.

Another dietary risk factor for the development of kidney stones is sodium ingestion, although to date, no controlled studies have shown that sodium (salt) restriction prevents stone formation. Higher sodium excretion rates also increase uric acid excretion. Therefore, patients should be warned about the risks of using excessive amounts of table salt and cautioned to be aware of the salt content of processed meats, cheese, canned foods, soy sauce, baked goods, and restaurant food. Certainly individuals should at least taste their food before deciding that it needs to be salted.

Stones that are comprised of uric acid form from a diet that is rich in meats, fish, and shellfish, all of which contain animal proteins and purines. Individuals who have produced uric acid kidney stones should avoid consuming liver altogether, and they should also limit their meat consumption to no more than six ounces per day, according to the NIDDK.

Individuals who have formed calcium oxalate stones should not avoid calcium but instead should include at least 800 mg of calcium every day, to prevent kidney stone formation as well as to help maintain their bone density. Individuals who have lactose intolerance can drink orange juice that is fortified with calcium.

Individuals who have formed oxalate stones should limit their consumption of nuts, spinach, rhubarb, and wheat bran. Other foods that are high in oxalate are beets, wheat germ, peanuts, okra, chocolate, and sweet potatoes. Foods that have a moderate level of oxalate include grits, grapes, celery, green pepper, red raspberries, strawberries, marmalade, and liver. In addition, individuals with a history of oxalate stone formation should consult their physicians before taking vitamin supplements of vitamin C or D, which could increase their risk for stones. Calcium supplements should be taken with meals so that the calcium will bind with the oxalate in food.

After a first kidney stone episode, up to 50 percent of patients have at least a second stone within 10 years, and up to 80 percent develop more stones within 20 to 30 years. These data, combined with the memory of the pain, inconvenience, and the high cost of the first acute stone episode, may help motivate patients to comply with suggested modifications in their diet and fluid intake.

The most important aspect of stone prevention is to increase the daily urine volume to dilute the urine. To achieve this, the individual should drink as much fluid as he or she can tolerate. Fluid intake should also be increased when the individual's level of perspiration is increased (as with exercise and/or heat). Note that thirst alone is *not* a sufficient indicator of adequate hydration.

The pharmacologic treatment to prevent recurrence of calcium stones involves lowering urinary calcium excretion with thiazide medications. Medications such as hydrochlorothiazide and chlorthalidone (Clorpres, Tenoretic, and Thalitone) may successfully lower urinary calcium levels. HYPOKALEMIA (low potassium blood levels) is a major side effect of thiazides. Therefore, thiazide therapy is usually accompanied by potassium citrate supplementation to replace potassium and replenish urinary citrate. It is also important to limit salt consumption. Potassium citrate comes in oral tablets and liquid forms (with various flavors to improve palatability).

Uric acid stones are usually treated with potassium citrate, which causes an increase in the urinary pH and thereby results in an increase in uric acid solubility. The medication allopurinol is generally limited for use in patients with hyperuricosuria (high urinary levels of uric acid).

Children with kidney stones may have an underlying genetic condition that is causing their kidney stones. They may be at high risk of developing multiple recurrent stones or of having disease in other parts of their body resulting from this genetic condition. An evaluation by a specialist in kidney stones is often particularly helpful in these individuals who need specialized therapies. In rare conditions, even combined kidney and liver transplantation may be needed.

Individuals who have had kidney stones should ask their physicians the following questions:

- What kind of kidney stone do I have?
- How much fluid should I drink every day?
- How much protein and what type of protein should I eat every day?
- Am I getting enough calcium in my diet?
- Can you recommend a dietitian who specializes in kidney stone prevention or renal nutrition?
- Do I need to take medication to prevent kidney stones?

See also BACK PAIN AND KIDNEY DISEASE; MEDICATIONS THAT CAN HARM THE KIDNEYS; MEDULLARY SPONGE KIDNEYS.

Lemann, J., Jr. "Composition of the Diet and Calcium Kidney Stones." *New England Journal of Medicine* 328 (1993): 880–882.

Pearle, Margaret S., M.D., Elizabeth A. Calhoun, and Gary C. Curhan, M.D. "Urolithiasis." In *Urologic Diseases in America,* edited by M. S. Litwin and C. S. Saigal. Bethesda, Md.: National Institute of Diabetes and Digestive and Kidney Diseases, 2007.

Rodman, John S., M.D., et al. *No More Kidney Stones: The Experts Tell You All You Need to Know about Prevention and Treatment.* New York: John Wiley & Sons, 2007.

**kidney transplantation**   The removal of a functioning kidney from one human and then placing it (with the use of special surgical techniques) into another human with either END-STAGE RENAL DISEASE (kidney failure) or ACUTE KIDNEY INJURY (AKI). When a patient who is not yet on DIALYSIS is treated with kidney transplantation, it is called a preemptive kidney transplantation. Preemptive transplantation may be used with children or with others who would find dialysis very hard to tolerate. Increasing evidence shows that preemptive kidney transplantation may provide better long-term health than starting dialysis and then obtaining a kidney transplant at a later time.

The person from whom the kidney is removed is the kidney donor, and the one who receives the kidney is the kidney recipient. Some patients receive multiple transplants at the same time, such as a kidney-pancreas transplant, a kidney-liver transplant, or even a kidney-heart transplant. At most, three organs have been transplanted within the same procedure, as of 2010.

Prior to receiving a kidney transplant, it is important that the potential recipient undergo a thorough medical evaluation. The surgical procedure is major surgery for the recipient, and the medications that are used to prevent rejection of the transplanted kidney have their associated side effects. It is important to ensure that the person is healthy enough to undergo the procedure and receive these medications. In addition, the person is usually already receiving dialysis or has established or advanced kidney disease, typically with a GLOMERULAR FILTRATION RATE (GFR) of less than 20 mL per minute per 1.73 m$^2$.

Some individuals receive donations from a living person, and as a result, they do not need to go on the waiting list. There are multiple advantages to receiving a kidney donation from a living person. These include not having to wait on a waiting list, being able to schedule the transplant at the convenience of the donor and the recipient, an increased likelihood of the kidney transplant working immediately after the transplant occurs, and overall, a better expectancy for the life span of the transplanted kidney.

### Historical Background

The first attempt at a temporary kidney transplant of a cadaver kidney (a kidney from a deceased person) occurred in 1945 and was performed by Dr. Joseph E. Murray at Peter Bent Brigham Hospital in Boston, Massachusetts. The attempt failed. The first successful kidney transplant in the United States occurred in 1954, when an identical twin donated his kidney to his brother. One of the doctors who performed this transplant was Dr. Joseph E. Murray, the same doctor who had first tried the procedure in 1945. No antirejection drugs were given to the patient. Because the donor and recipient were identical twins, and thus immunologically identical, antirejection medications were not needed. The kidney recipient lived for eight years, getting married and fathering a child before dying of a heart attack. Other kidney transplants were performed in the same time frame, but only between identical twins.

In the period 1962–63, the first donations of kidneys from deceased donors were made; however, these donations failed because highly effective immunosuppressive medications were still not available. In 1983, the Food and Drug Administration (FDA) approved cyclosporine, the first highly effective immunosuppressive medication used for recipients of transplanted organs. In 1984, the National Organ Transplant Act was passed, which banned the selling of organs and established the Organ Procurement and Transplantation Act.

The National Organ Transplant Act of 1984 allowed for the development of uniform national policies to provide for the equitable distribution of available deceased donor kidneys to individuals needing kidney transplants across the nation. This act was developed to ensure that patients awaiting a kidney transplant anywhere in the United States would be transplanted in an established order.

In 1986, the United Network for Organ Sharing (UNOS) was established to provide for the fair access of organs to individuals needing transplants. This organization still exists and is funded through the Department of Health and Human Services.

### Financial Assistance for a Kidney Transplant

Among eligible individuals, Medicare pays for the transplant procedure and aftercare and for 80 percent of the cost of medications needed by transplant recipients for the first three years after the transplant. (See Table 1 for some basic services covered by Medicare.)

**TABLE 1: KIDNEY TRANSPLANT SERVICES COVERED BY MEDICARE**

| Service or Supply | Medicare Part A | Medicare Part B |
|---|:---:|:---:|
| Inpatient services in an approved hospital | √ | |
| Kidney Registry Fee | √ | |
| Laboratory and other tests needed to evaluate your medical condition * | √ | |
| Laboratory and other tests needed to evaluate the medical condition of potential kidney donors* | √ | |
| The costs of finding the proper kidney for your transplant surgery (if there is no kidney donor) | √ | |
| The full cost of care for your kidney donor (including care before surgery, the actual surgery, and care after surgery | √ | |
| Any additional inpatient hospital care for your donor in case of problems due to the surgery | √ | |
| Doctors' services for kidney transplant surgery (including care before surgery, the actual surgery, and care after surgery) | | √ |
| Doctors' services for your kidney donor during their hospital stay | | √ |
| Immunosuppressive drugs | | √ |
| Blood (whole or units of packed red blood cells, blood components, and the cost of processing and giving you blood) | √ | |

Source: Adapted from Centers for Medicare & Medicaid Services. Medicare Coverage of Kidney Dialysis and Kidney Transplant Services. Baltimore, Md.: Centers for Medicare & Medicaid Services, May 2008, p. 30.
* These services are covered whether they are done by the Medicare-approved hospital where you will get your transplant, or by another hospital that participates in Medicare.

Individuals must apply for Medicare and be accepted in order to receive benefits. Applications can be made at the nearest Social Security Administration office, where officials can explain whether benefits are available to a person and what forms are needed to apply for these benefits.

If individuals are not eligible for Medicare benefits, they may be eligible for state Medicaid benefits. In addition, if patients *are* eligible for Medicare, some states will use state Medicaid to pay for the 20 percent copayment that Medicare does not cover. Medicaid applications must be made through the state social services office, often through the state health department. (Appendix II B offers a listing of state health departments for each state.)

If the patient is a military veteran, he or she may be eligible for veterans' benefits to pay for their kidney transplant. Veterans should contact their local Veterans Administration (VA) Office to learn more. Sometimes veterans may gain assistance with their application for VA benefits through service organizations, such as the American Legion or the Disabled American Veterans.

Many individuals receiving Medicare cannot afford the 20 percent copayment that is not covered by Medicare, but there are other means to cover these fees in addition to Medicaid or self-payment. In addition, many people are not eligible for Medicare nor do they have other means to pay for kidney transplantation and/or needed medications, and they must use other resources. For example, the Pharmaceutical Research and Manufacturers of America provides a *Directory of Prescription Drug Patient Assistance Programs* for those who need financial assistance to pay for medications. (Contact them at www.pparx.org or write to them at 1100 Fifteenth Street NW, Washington, D.C.). Another program called The Medicine Program offers assistance in finding free medications. (Contact them at www.themedicineprogram.com or write to them at P.O. Box 1089, Poplar Bluff, Mo. 63902.) The State Health Insurance Assistance Program (SHIP) also offers financial assistance.

State programs are listed at www.shiptalk.org and are also provided in Appendix II A.

Every hospital has a social worker, and in the case of individuals who will receive a kidney transplant, many programs have a nephrology social worker. This individual should be knowledgeable about programs that can help patients to pay for their kidney transplant.

### Statistics on Kidney Transplants

From July 1, 2008 to June 30, 2009, there were 10,589 donor transplant procedures using deceased donors and 6,232 kidney transplants from live donors, for a total of 16,821 transplants, according to the Scientific Registry of Transplant Recipients, an organization that tracks transplant statistics. At the beginning of this period, there were 78,417 people waiting for a kidney transplant, there were 32,987 new patient registrations during the year, and at the end of the year there were 83,053 people waiting for a kidney.

Some patients receive more than one transplanted kidney, and as of June 30, 2009, 14.1 percent of those receiving a kidney transplant from a deceased donor were repeat recipients, as were 12.1 percent of those receiving their donated kidneys from a live donor. See Tables 2 and 3 for more information; Table 2 covers the key characteristics of recipients who received a transplant from a deceased person and Table 3 covers characteristics of those who received their transplant from a living person, such as a parent, sibling, or other person.

### Kidney Donors

Kidney transplant recipients may receive their kidneys from live or deceased donors, although there are more kidneys donated from deceased individuals. Some donated kidneys cannot be used for various reasons, thus, the number of people who receive transplantations is less than rather than equal to the number of kidneys donated.

*Live donors have a normal life span*  As was known in the past and has been confirmed by

**TABLE 2: TRANSPLANT RECIPIENT CHARACTERISTICS: DECEASED DONOR TRANSPLANTS, PATIENTS TRANSPLANTED WITH KIDNEY BETWEEN JULY 1, 2008 AND JUNE 30, 2009**

| Characteristic | Percentage in Each Category, U.S. (n=10,589) |
|---|---|
| **Ethnicity/Race (%)** | |
| White | 45.9 |
| African American | 31.9 |
| Hispanic/Latino | 14.9 |
| Asian | 5.8 |
| Other | 1.4 |
| **Age (%)** | |
| <2 years | 0.2 |
| 2–11 years | 1.8 |
| 12–17 years | 2.8 |
| 18–34 years | 10.0 |
| 35–49 years | 25.3 |
| 50–64 years | 42.2 |
| 65 years+ | 17.7 |
| **Gender (%)** | |
| Male | 60.6 |
| Female | 39.4 |
| **Blood Type (%)** | |
| O | 45.0 |
| A | 36.9 |
| B | 13.2 |
| AB | 5.0 |
| **Previous Transplant (%)** | |
| Yes | 14.1 |
| No | 85.9 |
| **Primary Disease (%)** | |
| Glomerular Disease | 22.0 |
| Tubular and Interstitial Disease | 5.0 |
| Polycystic Kidneys | 8.3 |
| Congenital, Familial, Metabolic | 2.8 |
| Diabetes | 24.7 |
| Renovascular & Vascular Diseases | 0.2 |
| Neoplasms (cancers) | 0.4 |
| Hypertensive Nephrosclerosis | 27.0 |
| Other Kidney Disease | 9.0 |
| Missing Data | 0.5 |

Source: Adapted from Scientific Registry of Transplant Recipients. *Organ Summary: National Report. Organ: KI: Kidney. Activity: 7/1/2008–6/30/2009.* Available online. URL: http://www.ustransplant.org/csr/current/nats.aspx. Accessed March 12, 2010.

the long-term follow-up of kidney donors (such as research published by Hassan N. Ibrahim, M.D., and colleagues in 2009 in the *New England Journal of Medicine*), kidney donation from living donors is safe, and it does not portend major risks for the long-term health and well-being of the donor. In addition, more recent data published in the *Journal of the American Medical Association* in 2010 on kidney donor survival analyzed data from 80,347 live donors of kidneys in the United States from 1994–2009, and found that there were only 25 deaths within 90 days of donation.

Researchers Dorry L. Segev, M.D., and colleagues also found that compared to a healthy matched cohort of non–kidney donors, the death rate was not increased after a median of 6.3 years (3.2–9.8 years). The researchers also analyzed demographic data on the kidney donors and found that the majority (62 percent) were well educated, ranging from those with some college to those who were postcollege in education. Most kidney donors were females (58.5 percent) and white (73.1 percent). See Table 4 for more information on kidney donors. Of the donors for whom body mass index (BMI) was provided, 22.6 percent were obese (equal to or greater than a BMI of 30), thus, most were not obese.

*Characteristics of live donors* The living donor of a kidney can be an individual who is a blood relative, which is often referred to as a living related kidney transplant, or it may be from an unrelated person, which is called a living unrelated kidney transplant. In general, the survival rate is higher for patients receiving their kidney from a live donor compared to a deceased donor. Further, the survival rate is slightly higher for a kidney obtained from a living related donor than from a living unrelated donor, but both donations are associated with better outcomes than with kidneys that were obtained from deceased donors. For example, according to the Scientific Registry of Transplant Recipients, 77.0 percent of individuals who

**TABLE 3: TRANSPLANT RECIPIENT CHARACTERISTICS: LIVING DONOR TRANSPLANTS, PATIENTS TRANSPLANTED WITH KIDNEY BETWEEN JULY 1, 2008 AND JUNE 30, 2009**

| Characteristic | Percentage in Each Category, U.S. (n=6,232) |
|---|---|
| **Ethnicity/Race (%)** | |
| White | 66.6 |
| African American | 13.6 |
| Hispanic/Latino | 14.3 |
| Asian | 4.3 |
| Other | 1.41 |
| **Age (%)** | |
| <2 years | 0.3 |
| 2–11 years | 2.2 |
| 12–17 years | 2.5 |
| 18–34 years | 19.7 |
| 35–49 years | 29.4 |
| 50–64 years | 34.6 |
| 65 years+ | 11.3 |
| **Gender (%)** | |
| Male | 61.2 |
| Female | 38.8 |
| **Blood Type (%)** | |
| O | 43.9 |
| A | 38.3 |
| B | 13.6 |
| AB | 4.2 |
| **Previous Transplant (%)** | |
| Yes | 12.1 |
| No | 87.9 |
| **Primary Disease (%)** | |
| Glomerular Disease | 29.6 |
| Tubular and Interstitial Disease | 5.7 |
| Polycystic Kidneys | 11.0 |
| Congenital, Familial, Metabolic | 4.1 |
| Diabetes | 21.2 |
| Renovascular & Vascular Diseases | 0.3 |
| Neoplasms (cancers) | 0.4 |
| Hypertensive Nephrosclerosis | 18.3 |
| Other Kidney Disease | 9.0 |
| Missing Data | 0.4 |

Source: Adapted from Scientific Registry of Transplant Recipients. *Organ Summary: National Report. Organ: KI: Kidney. Activity: 7/1/2008–6/30/2009.* Available online. URL: http://www.ustransplant.org/csr/current/nats.aspx. Accessed March 12, 2010.

TABLE 4: DEMOGRAPHIC AND PREDONATION CHARACTERISTICS OF LIVE KIDNEY DONORS[a]

| Characteristics | No. (%) of Donors | Characteristics | No. (%) of Donors |
|---|---|---|---|
| **Age** | **39,516 (49.2)** | **BMI** | |
| 18–39 | 24,375 (30.3) | 15–24 | 7,343 (37.0) |
| 40–49 | 13,349 (16.7) | 25–29 | 8,016 (40.4) |
| 50–59 | 13,439 (16.7) | ≥30 | 4,473 (22.6) |
| ≥60 | 3,017 (3.8) | **SBP, mm Hg** | |
| **Sex** | | <120 | 25,713 (53.3) |
| Men | 33,380 (41.5) | 120–139 | 19,114 (39.6) |
| Women | 46,967 (58.5) | ≥140 | 3,430 (7.1) |
| **Race/ethnicity** | | **Hypertension** | |
| White | 58,683 (73.1) | No | 29,848 (98.2) |
| Black | 10,505 (13.1) | Yes | 545 (1.8) |
| Hispanic | 9,846 (12.3) | **Smoking (ever)** | |
| Other | 1,252 (1.6) | No | 19,391 (76.0) |
| **Education** | | Yes | 6,114 (24.0) |
| Grade school | 910 (2.3) | Creatinine values, mean (SD) [b] | 0.9 (0.2) |
| High school | 14,497 (36.1) | Serum creatinine, mg/dL | |
| Some college | 11,259 (28.0) | Creatinine clearance, mL/min | 117 (36) |
| Bachelor degree | 9,660 (24.1) | | |
| Postcollege | 3,820 (9.5) | | |

Abbreviations: BMI, body mass index (calculated as weight in kilograms divided by height in meters squared); SBP, systolic blood pressure
SI conversions: To convert serum creatinine to μmol/L, multiply by 88.4; and creatinine clearance to mL/S, multiply by 0.0167.
[a] Characteristics of age, sex, and race/ethnicity were available throughout the study period. For race/ethnicity, other included American Indian, Native Hawaiian, Alaskan Native, Pacific Islander, and multiracial. Education was only available after 1998 (46% missing between 1999–2004; 24% missing between 2005–09). BMI was only available after 2003 (49% missing between 1999–2004; 31% missing between 2007–09). SBP was only available after 1999 (22% missing between 2000–05; 9% missing 2006–09). Hypertension was only available after 2003 (41% missing in 2004; 3% missing in 2008; 1% missing between 2006–08). Smoking was only available after 2004 (23% missing in 2005; 0.06% missing between 2006–08).
[b] Serum creatinine (n=58,599) was only available after 1998 (49% missing between 1999–2000; 4% missing between 2001–09). Cockcroft-Gault formula was used to obtain creatinine clearance estimates (n=21,295).
Source: Segev, Dorry L., M.D., et al. "Perioperative Mortality and Long-term Survival Following Live Kidney Donation." *Journal of the American Medical Association* 303, no. 10 (2010): 961.

received their kidney from a live donor 10 years ago (as of 2008) were still alive, compared to 60.9 percent of individuals who received their kidney from a deceased person.

See Table 5 for basic characteristics of deceased donors and see Table 6 for characteristics of live donors, such as the gender of the donor and relation of the donor to the transplant recipient. For example, from 1998 to 2007 full siblings represented the greatest percentage of living donors each year.

Unfortunately, there are insufficient numbers of kidneys (from both deceased and live donors) available to the many individuals who urgently need kidney transplantations; thus most people who need a kidney transplant must go on a waiting list, and many people die while waiting for a transplant.

***Expanded criteria donors***  Some donors fit into a category known as expanded criteria donors (ECD), which means that either the donor or the organ is not considered as healthy as with the regular donor. Expanded criteria donors for kidneys include individuals who are ages 60 years and older; those who are 50–59 years but who have had two or more of several medical crises, such as a history of hypertension, a stroke that caused their death, or the organ was donated after the

## TABLE 5: DECEASED DONOR CHARACTERISTICS, 1998 TO 2007, KIDNEY DONORS

| | 1998 | 1999 | 2000 | 2001 | 2002 | 2003 | 2004 | 2005 | 2006 | 2007 |
|---|---|---|---|---|---|---|---|---|---|---|
| Total | 5,339 | 5,386 | 5,489 | 5,528 | 5,638 | 5,753 | 6,325 | 6,700 | 7,181 | 7,245 |
| **Donor Age** | | | | | | | | | | |
| <1 Year | 32 | 45 | 42 | 47 | 38 | 29 | 33 | 36 | 58 | 68 |
| 1–5 Years | 208 | 174 | 171 | 185 | 171 | 155 | 176 | 175 | 203 | 175 |
| 6–11 Years | 183 | 178 | 181 | 202 | 164 | 128 | 164 | 121 | 135 | 146 |
| 12–17 Years | 543 | 488 | 513 | 471 | 481 | 481 | 492 | 467 | 490 | 456 |
| 18–34 Years | 1,469 | 1,398 | 1,437 | 1,486 | 1,608 | 1,586 | 1,728 | 1,861 | 1,941 | 2,018 |
| 35–49 Years | 1,394 | 1,483 | 1,492 | 1,492 | 1,494 | 1,552 | 1,692 | 1,784 | 1,932 | 1,905 |
| 50–64 Years | 1,116 | 1,197 | 1,267 | 1,267 | 1,291 | 1,427 | 1,570 | 1,721 | 1,844 | 1,903 |
| 65+ Years | 394 | 423 | 378 | 378 | 391 | 395 | 468 | 535 | 578 | 574 |
| **Donor Age (%)** | | | | | | | | | | |
| <1 Year | 0.6% | 0.8% | 0.8% | 0.9% | 0.7% | 0.5% | 0.5% | 0.5% | 0.8% | 0.9% |
| 1–5 Years | 3.9% | 3.2% | 3.1% | 3.3% | 3.0% | 2.7% | 2.8% | 2.6% | 2.8% | 2.4% |
| 6–11 Years | 3.4% | 3.3% | 3.3% | 3.7% | 2.9% | 2.2% | 2.6% | 1.8% | 1.9% | 2.0% |
| 12–17 Years | 10.2% | 9.1% | 9.3% | 8.5% | 8.5% | 8.4% | 7.8% | 7.0% | 6.8% | 6.3% |
| 18–34 Years | 27.5% | 26.0% | 26.2% | 26.9% | 28.5% | 27.6% | 27.3% | 27.8% | 27.0% | 27.9% |
| 35–49 Years | 26.1% | 27.5% | 26.9% | 27.0% | 26.5% | 27.0% | 26.8% | 26.6% | 26.9% | 26.3% |
| 50–64 Years | 20.9% | 22.2% | 23.4% | 22.9% | 22.9% | 24.8% | 24.8% | 25.7% | 25.7% | 26.3% |
| 65+ Years | 7.4% | 7.9% | 7.0% | 6.8% | 6.9% | 6.9% | 7.4% | 8.0% | 8.0% | 7.9% |
| **Donor Ethnicity/Race** | | | | | | | | | | |
| White | 4,074 | 4,077 | 4,170 | 4,092 | 4,116 | 4,081 | 4,455 | 4,630 | 4,919 | 4,922 |
| African American | 592 | 569 | 610 | 635 | 698 | 740 | 824 | 938 | 1,042 | 1,044 |
| Other/Multi-race | 9 | 21 | 16 | 17 | 38 | 34 | 49 | 66 | 47 | 70 |
| Asian | 110 | 136 | 132 | 143 | 120 | 144 | 153 | 141 | 177 | 176 |
| Hispanic/Latino | 519 | 565 | 559 | 637 | 662 | 738 | 844 | 925 | 996 | 1,033 |
| Unknown | 35 | 18 | 2 | 4 | 4 | 16 | – | – | – | – |
| **Donor Ethnicity/Race (%)** | | | | | | | | | | |
| White | 76.3% | 75.7% | 76.0% | 74.0% | 73.0% | 70.9% | 70.4% | 69.1% | 68.5% | 67.9% |
| African American | 11.1% | 10.6% | 11.1% | 11.5% | 12.4% | 12.9% | 13.0% | 14.0% | 14.5% | 14.4% |
| Other/Multi-race | 0.2% | 0.4% | 0.3% | 0.3% | 0.7% | 0.6% | 0.8% | 1.0% | 0.7% | 1.0% |
| Asian | 2.1% | 2.5% | 2.4% | 2.6% | 2.1% | 2.5% | 2.4% | 2.1% | 2.5% | 2.4% |
| Hispanic/Latino | 9.7% | 10.5% | 10.2% | 11.5% | 11.7% | 12.8% | 13.3% | 13.8% | 13.9% | 14.3% |
| Unknown | 0.7% | 0.3% | 0.0% | 0.1% | 0.1% | 0.3% | – | – | – | – |

U.S. Department of Health and Human Services. *2008 Annual Report of the U.S. Organ Procurement and Transplantation Network and the Scientific Registry of Transplant Recipients: Transplant Data 1998–2007.* Health Resources and Services Administration, Healthcare Systems Bureau, Division of Transplantation, Rockville, Md. October 2009, pp. 2–5.

The data and analyses reported in the 2008 Annual Report of the U.S. Organ Procurement and Transplantation Network and the Scientific Registry of Transplant Recipients have been supplied by UNOS and Arbor Research under contract with HHS/HRSA. The authors alone are responsible for reporting and interpreting these data; the views expressed herein are those of the authors and not necessarily those of the U.S. Government.

death of the individual. The life expectancy with an expanded criteria donor's kidney is lower than with a non-ECD donor or a live donor.

A patient might accept an ECD donor because the waiting list is long, and it may be believed that the patient will not survive long enough to

## TABLE 6: LIVING DONOR CHARACTERISTICS, 1998–2007, KIDNEY DONORS

| | 1998 | 1999 | 2000 | 2001 | 2002 | 2003 | 2004 | 2005 | 2006 | 2007 |
|---|---|---|---|---|---|---|---|---|---|---|
| Total | 4,422 | 4,724 | 5,494 | 6,038 | 6,240 | 6,473 | 6,647 | 6,570 | 6,435 | 6,036 |
| **Donor Gender** | | | | | | | | | | |
| Female | 2,558 | 2,743 | 3,130 | 3,546 | 3,641 | 3,830 | 3,843 | 3,886 | 3,807 | 3,502 |
| Male | 1,864 | 1,981 | 2,364 | 2,492 | 2,599 | 2,643 | 2,804 | 2,684 | 2,628 | 2,534 |
| **Donor Gender (%)** | | | | | | | | | | |
| Female | 57.8% | 58.1% | 57.0% | 58.7% | 58.3% | 59.2% | 57.8% | 59.1% | 59.2% | 58.0% |
| Male | 42.2% | 41.9% | 43.0% | 41.3% | 41.7% | 40.8% | 42.2% | 40.9% | 40.8% | 42.0% |
| **Donor Relation** | | | | | | | | | | |
| Parent | 795 | 790 | 736 | 861 | 824 | 797 | 763 | 784 | 657 | 651 |
| Offspring | 679 | 760 | 965 | 1,043 | 1,139 | 1,117 | 1,159 | 1,162 | 1,145 | 977 |
| Identical Twin | 11 | 7 | 12 | 12 | 14 | 14 | 9 | 19 | 21 | 15 |
| Full Sibling | 1,629 | 1,654 | 1,834 | 1,876 | 1,808 | 1,845 | 1,835 | 1,650 | 1,626 | 1,431 |
| Half Sibling | 47 | 77 | 71 | 91 | 67 | 83 | 66 | 82 | 64 | 63 |
| Other Relative | 296 | 348 | 411 | 468 | 493 | 478 | 510 | 506 | 491 | 488 |
| Spouse Unrelated | 547 | 577 | 688 | 715 | 720 | 728 | 784 | 790 | 780 | 737 |
| Other Unrelated | 362 | 476 | 774 | 930 | 1,116 | 1,328 | 1,435 | 1,496 | 1,570 | 1,416 |
| Unknown | 56 | 35 | 23 | 42 | 59 | 83 | 86 | 81 | 81 | 258 |
| **Donor Relation (%)** | | | | | | | | | | |
| Parent | 18.0% | 16.7% | 13.4% | 14.3% | 13.2% | 12.3% | 11.5% | 11.9% | 10.2% | 10.8% |
| Offspring | 15.4% | 16.1% | 17.6% | 17.3% | 18.3% | 17.3% | 17.4% | 17.7% | 17.8% | 16.2% |
| Identical Twin | 0.2% | 0.1% | 0.2% | 0.2% | 0.2% | 0.2% | 0.1% | 0.3% | 0.3% | 0.2% |
| Full Sibling | 36.8% | 35.0% | 33.4% | 31.1% | 29.0% | 28.5% | 27.6% | 25.1% | 25.1% | 23.7% |
| Half Sibling | 1.1% | 1.6% | 1.3% | 1.5% | 1.1% | 1.3% | 1.0% | 1.2% | 1.0% | 1.0% |
| Other Relative | 6.7% | 7.4% | 7.5% | 7.8% | 7.9% | 7.4% | 7.7% | 7.7% | 7.6% | 8.1% |
| Spouse Unrelated | 12.4% | 12.2% | 12.2% | 11.8% | 11.5% | 11.2% | 11.8% | 12.0% | 12.1% | 12.2% |
| Other unrelated | 8.2% | 10.1% | 14.1% | 15.4% | 17.9% | 20.5% | 21.6% | 22.8% | 24.4% | 23.5% |
| Unknown | 1.3% | 0.7% | 0.4% | 0.7% | 0.9% | 1.3% | 1.3% | 1.2% | 1.3% | 4.3% |

U.S. Department of Health and Human Services. *2008 Annual Report of the U.S. Organ Procurement and Transplantation Network and the Scientific Registry of Transplant Recipients: Transplant Data 1998–2007.* Health Resources and Services Administration, Healthcare Systems Bureau, Division of Transplantation, Rockville, Md. October 2009, pp. 2–32.

The data and analyses reported in the 2008 Annual Report of the U.S. Organ Procurement and Transplantation Network and the Scientific Registry of Transplant Recipients have been supplied by UNOS and Arbor Research under contract with HHS/HRSA. The authors alone are responsible for reporting and interpreting these data; the views expressed herein are those of the authors and not necessarily those of the U.S. Government.

receive a non-ECD donor; thus, an ECD donation may be beneficial, as it can improve both the quality and quantity of life, even though it is not quite as effective and is at a slightly higher risk than a non-ECD donor kidney. Lisa Vierira summarized the benefits and risks of expanded criteria donors:

The benefits of ECD transplantation include decreased waiting time for transplantation, decreased risk of the complications that can occur while the patient is receiving dialysis, and being able to stop dialysis if transplantation is successful. The risks include the chances of delayed graft function and decreased duration of graft survival. Delayed graft function is frequently encountered with transplants from deceased organ donors. Poor function of the transplanted organ can also occur from damage to any part of the organ during the transplantation process. If the kidney cannot function soon after transplantation, the risk of rejection increases and dialysis may become necessary. Dialysis may last from days to months, with no certainty that it will end.

In his article on expanded criteria donors, A. O. Ojo noted that some patients are statistically less likely to benefit from using an ECD. This includes individuals who are younger than age 40, those who are African American or Asian, and those whose median waiting time for an ECD is less than 1,350 days. In such individuals, the increased risk of complications associated with an ECD kidney may be greater than the risks associated with waiting only for a conventional criteria kidney.

In a study by Sheila M. Fraser and colleagues on the outcomes after expanded criteria donor grafts, based on 1,053 transplants with ECDs from 1995 to 2005, the researchers found that the five-year survival rate was comparable to survival with standard grafts. They also noted that donor hypertension and/or ischemic heart disease reduced graft survival in older patients but not in younger patients. The recipients themselves were older by an average of nine years compared to the standard kidney transplant recipients, and they had a higher rate of hypertension (14.5 percent) compared to the standard group (7.4 percent).

### Individuals Waiting for Kidneys

Many people wait for kidneys. In 2007, the largest percentage of people on this list were white/Caucasian (38 percent), followed by African Americans (34 percent). As seen in Table 7, in considering age alone, the greater percentage of those waiting for a kidney in 2007 are those ages 50–64 years, or 42 percent, followed by those ages 35–49 years (30 percent). In their article on kidney and pancreas transplantations among diabetics with end-stage renal disease (ESRD) over the period 1998–2007, K. P. McCullough and colleagues explain that although the total number of candidates on the kidney transplant waiting list increased from 40,825 in 1998 to 76,070 in 2007, in actuality, the number of active patients seeking kidney transplants increased by only 4,510 from 2002 to 2007 because many candidates on the list were in an inactive status.

Patients are placed into an inactive status if they previously have been approved for a kidney transplant, but then they have developed an infection or other complication which necessitates a delay in receiving a kidney transplant.

### State Differences for Diabetic Patients Receiving Transplants

There is a broad variation by state among the percentage of diabetics with ESRD for the percentage placed on the waiting list, the percent who receive their kidney transplant from living or deceased donors, and also the percent who receive simultaneous pancreas-kidney transplantation (SPK). These differences are depicted in Table 8. The range of patients with ESRD ages 50–75 years waitlisted for a kidney transplant or an SPK transplant was 5.6 percent to 24.1 percent, with a nationwide average of 14 percent. Among those receiving a kidney from a live donor, the range was even broader, from less than 1 percent to 10.1 percent and with an average of 2.3 percent. The range for those receiving a kidney from a deceased donor was 1.4 percent to 10.2 percent with an average of 3.9 percent nationwide. According to McCullough and colleagues, geographic differences continued even when adjustments were made for age, race, sex, insurance status, and other factors.

### Evaluation of the Recipient Candidate Prior to Approval of the Transplant

If the treating physician and the patient and the family agree that transplantation is an option for treatment, then such patients are referred to a kidney transplant center. The choice of which center to be referred to can include factors such as the geographical proximity to the patient, differences in insurance coverage for different transplant programs, and differences in reported outcomes from a kidney transplant at different centers. The transplant center then evaluates the patient in a multidisciplinary team approach. Each patient is evaluated by a transplant surgeon, a nephrologist, a social worker, and a transplant coordinator, as well as a dietitian.

**TABLE 7: KIDNEY WAITING LIST PATIENT CHARACTERISTICS AT END OF YEAR, ACTIVE WAITLIST PATIENTS, 1998 TO 2007**

| | 1998 | 1999 | 2000 | 2001 | 2002 | 2003 | 2004 | 2005 | 2006 | 2007 |
|---|---|---|---|---|---|---|---|---|---|---|
| Total | 34,496 | 36,948 | 39,956 | 42,219 | 44,263 | 45,479 | 45,294 | 46,120 | 47,060 | 48,773 |
| **Current Age** | | | | | | | | | | |
| <1 Year | 2 | 1 | 1 | None | None | 3 | 3 | 2 | 1 | 2 |
| 1–5 Years | 61 | 48 | 65 | 68 | 64 | 59 | 77 | 72 | 62 | 50 |
| 6–11 Years | 124 | 115 | 132 | 156 | 144 | 113 | 125 | 103 | 93 | 88 |
| 12–17 Years | 356 | 340 | 364 | 387 | 437 | 384 | 414 | 321 | 265 | 230 |
| 18–34 Years | 6,074 | 6,197 | 6,156 | 6,210 | 6,302 | 6,341 | 6,108 | 5,894 | 5,749 | 5,642 |
| 35–49 Years | 12,604 | 12,975 | 13,572 | 13,827 | 14,165 | 14,345 | 13,852 | 14,066 | 14,179 | 14,518 |
| 50–64 Years | 12,285 | 13,717 | 15,408 | 16,627 | 17,752 | 18,386 | 18,522 | 19,06 9 | 19,566 | 20,464 |
| 65+ Years | 2,990 | 3,555 | 4,258 | 4,944 | 5,399 | 5,848 | 6,193 | 6,593 | 7,145 | 7,779 |
| **Current Age (%)** | | | | | | | | | | |
| 1–5 Years | 0.2% | 0.1% | 0.2% | 0.2% | 0.1% | 0.1% | 0.2% | 0.2% | 0.1% | 0.1% |
| 6–11 Years | 0.4% | 0.3% | 0.3% | 0.4% | 0.3% | 0.2% | 0.3% | 0.2% | 0.2% | 0.2% |
| 12–17 Years | 1.0% | 0.9% | 0.9% | 0.9% | 1.0% | 0.8% | 0.9% | 0.7% | 0.6% | 0.5% |
| 18–34 Years | 17.6% | 16.8% | 15.4% | 14.7% | 14.2% | 13.9% | 13.5% | 12.8% | 12.2% | 11.6% |
| 35–49 Years | 36.5% | 35.1% | 34.0% | 32.9% | 32.0% | 31.5% | 30.6% | 30.5% | 30.1% | 29.8% |
| 50–64 Years | 35.6% | 37.1% | 38.6% | 39.4% | 40.1% | 40.4% | 40.9% | 41.3% | 41.6% | 42.0% |
| 65+ Years | 8.7% | 9.6% | 10.7% | 11.7% | 12.2% | 12.9% | 13.7% | 14.3% | 1 5.2% | 15.9% |
| **Ethnicity/Race** | | | | | | | | | | |
| White | 15,113 | 15,782 | 16,643 | 17,121 | 17,527 | 17,710 | 17,445 | 17,679 | 18,071 | 18,467 |
| African American | 12,493 | 13,485 | 14,563 | 15,343 | 15,987 | 16,340 | 15,876 | 15,914 | 16,003 | 16,632 |
| Other/Multi-race | 416 | 426 | 479 | 512 | 586 | 600 | 672 | 691 | 658 | 699 |
| Asian | 2,154 | 2,386 | 2,678 | 2,964 | 3,319 | 3,465 | 3,605 | 3,806 | 3,812 | 4,148 |
| Hispanic/Latino | 4,320 | 4,869 | 5,593 | 6,279 | 6,844 | 7,364 | 7,696 | 8,030 | 8,516 | 8,827 |
| **Ethnicity/Race (%)** | | | | | | | | | | |
| White | 43.8% | 42.7% | 41.7% | 40.6% | 39.6% | 38.9% | 38.5% | 38.3% | 38.4% | 37.9% |
| African American | 36.2% | 36.5% | 36.4% | 36.3% | 36.1% | 35.9% | 35.1% | 34.5% | 34.0% | 34.1% |
| Other/Multi-race | 1.2% | 1.2% | 1.2% | 1.2% | 1.3% | 1.3% | 1.5% | 1.5% | 1.4% | 1.4% |
| Asian | 6.2% | 6.5% | 6.7% | 7.0% | 7.5% | 7.6% | 8.0% | 8.3% | 8.1% | 8.5% |
| Hispanic/Latino | 12.5% | 13.2% | 14.0% | 14.9% | 15.5% | 16.2% | 17.0% | 17.4% | 18.1% | 18.1% |

Source: U.S. Department of Health and Human Services. *2008 Annual Report of the U.S. Organ Procurement and Transplantation Network and the Scientific Registry of Transplant Recipients: Transplant Data 1998–2007.* Health Resources and Services Administration, Healthcare Systems Bureau, Division of Transplantation, Rockville, Md. October 2009.

The data and analyses reported in the 2008 Annual Report of the U.S. Organ Procurement and Transplantation Network and the Scientific Registry of Transplant Recipients have been supplied by UNOS and Arbor Research under contract with HHS/HRSA. The authors alone are responsible for reporting and interpreting these data; the views expressed herein are those of the authors and not necessarily those of the U.S. Government.

The patient evaluation is then discussed in a multidisciplinary meeting, and a common consensus is developed as to the feasibility of the transplant candidate. If all agree that he or she is a suitable candidate, then diagnostic studies and tests are performed to evaluate the individual for any serious other illnesses. If those test results are favorable, and the person is considered a good candidate for kidney transplantation, then the individual is registered with the Organ Procurement and Transplantation Network (OPTN). This is an organization that maintains a centralized computer database on organ transplants. The United Network for

**TABLE 8: PERCENTAGE OF PATIENTS WITH DIABETES (BY AGE) PLACED ON THE KIDNEY WAITING LIST AND RECEIVING A TRANSPLANT, BY STATE, 1998–2007**

| State | Age < 50 Years | | | | | Age 50–75 Years | | | | |
|---|---|---|---|---|---|---|---|---|---|---|
| | Number | Waitlisted for KI or SPK (%) | Living donor transplants (%) | Deceased donor KI transplants (%) | Deceased donor SPK transplants (%) | Number | Waitlisted for KI or SPK (%) | Living donor transplants (%) | Deceased donor KI transplants (%) | Deceased donor SPK transplants (%) |
| AK | 66 | 40.9 | 13.6 | 1.5 | 12.1 | 241 | 14.5 | 3.3 | 5.4 | 0.4 |
| AL | 1,272 | 39.1 | 8.2 | 5.1 | 4.2 | 4,611 | 13.9 | 1.8 | 2.0 | 0.0 |
| AR | 635 | 26.5 | 6.9 | 10.1 | 4.6 | 2,211 | 7.0 | 1.8 | 3.6 | 0.2 |
| AZ | 1,345 | 33.4 | 7.8 | 5.9 | 6.3 | 5,448 | 14.0 | 3.1 | 3.5 | 0.2 |
| CA | 6,532 | 50.5 | 5.0 | 6.4 | 8.5 | 30,788 | 21.8 | 1.7 | 3.6 | 0.3 |
| CO | 626 | 47.3 | 11.5 | 8.3 | 11.5 | 2,358 | 19.6 | 3.3 | 4.7 | 0.1 |
| CT | 447 | 33.8 | 12.8 | 6.5 | 2.9 | 2,275 | 10.8 | 2.5 | 2.5 | 0.0 |
| DC | 252 | 30.2 | 5.6 | 4.8 | 5.2 | 1,065 | 15.4 | 2.0 | 3.2 | 0.4 |
| DE | 197 | 39.6 | 8.6 | 7.6 | 3.0 | 757 | 20.1 | 2.1 | 6.2 | 0.4 |
| FL | 2,972 | 28.9 | 3.4 | 7.1 | 10.1 | 13,876 | 10.2 | 1.2 | 4.3 | 0.3 |
| GA | 2,149 | 23.2 | 2.8 | 4.4 | 7.6 | 8,344 | 8.5 | 0.9 | 3.0 | 0.3 |
| HI | 401 | 31.4 | 2.7 | 6.5 | 4.0 | 1,986 | 15.4 | 1.4 | 2.7 | 0.0 |
| IA | 400 | 46.0 | 12.3 | 10.0 | 16.5 | 1,712 | 15.4 | 4.3 | 6.7 | 0.2 |
| ID | 192 | 34.9 | 13.5 | 10.9 | 9.9 | 546 | 13.7 | 3.8 | 6.8 | 0.2 |
| IL | 2,258 | 45.2 | 7.7 | 7.9 | 11.5 | 10,289 | 15.5 | 2.9 | 4.0 | 0.4 |
| IN | 1,185 | 37.6 | 7.6 | 8.4 | 14.1 | 5,048 | 10.2 | 2.0 | 3.9 | 0.5 |
| KS | 405 | 29.9 | 5.4 | 8.1 | 10.1 | 1,756 | 7.9 | 1.6 | 3.6 | 0.6 |
| KY | 875 | 28.3 | 4.0 | 6.3 | 11.1 | 3,489 | 8.4 | 1.3 | 3.9 | 0.5 |
| LA | 1,347 | 26.9 | 3.9 | 5.0 | 8.2 | 5,771 | 8.2 | 1.1 | 2.2 | 0.3 |
| MA | 738 | 48.5 | 21.4 | 10.8 | 3.9 | 3,647 | 19.7 | 3.6 | 6.2 | 0.2 |
| MD | 1,088 | 40.2 | 10.4 | 9.4 | 7.4 | 5,269 | 17.7 | 3.1 | 5.2 | 0.4 |
| ME | 135 | 41.5 | 16.3 | 7.4 | 8.9 | 755 | 11.1 | 3.0 | 4.8 | 0.0 |
| MI | 2,145 | 42.3 | 13.8 | 8.8 | 6.0 | 8,845 | 15.1 | 3.8 | 4.2 | 0.1 |
| MN | 683 | 51.2 | 36.0 | 9.4 | 7.5 | 2,377 | 24.0 | 10.1 | 7.5 | 0.9 |
| MO | 1,117 | 32.6 | 6.6 | 8.1 | 6.9 | 4,937 | 11.0 | 2.1 | 4.3 | 0.3 |
| MS | 836 | 31.2 | 3.1 | 7.7 | 4.7 | 3,146 | 8.7 | 1.0 | 1.7 | 0.0 |
| MT | 153 | 45.1 | 19.6 | 9.8 | 11.8 | 543 | 20.6 | 6.8 | 9.0 | 0.4 |
| NC | 2,070 | 28.9 | 4.6 | 5.0 | 7.6 | 8,246 | 10.4 | 1.6 | 2.7 | 0.3 |
| ND | 146 | 43.8 | 26.0 | 7.5 | 9.6 | 469 | 21.7 | 7.9 | 9.2 | 0.2 |
| NE | 284 | 36.6 | 10.6 | 8.8 | 13.7 | 1,205 | 12.6 | 3.5 | 5.1 | 0.2 |
| NH | 156 | 41.7 | 14.7 | 14.1 | 5.1 | 586 | 14.8 | 2.2 | 7.2 | 0.3 |
| NJ | 1,439 | 46.8 | 11.9 | 8.7 | 6.8 | 7,671 | 17.3 | 3.0 | 3.9 | 0.2 |
| NM | 527 | 31.5 | 7.4 | 8.3 | 3.6 | 2,133 | 11.3 | 2.2 | 3.4 | 0.0 |
| NV | 375 | 40.0 | 5.1 | 11.2 | 7.7 | 1,799 | 16.0 | 2.0 | 3.6 | 0.2 |
| NY | 3,176 | 41.0 | 10.3 | 8.6 | 4.3 | 16,098 | 16.5 | 2.6 | 3.7 | 0.2 |
| OH | 2,416 | 35.4 | 10.0 | 7.3 | 12.4 | 11,557 | 10.4 | 3.0 | 3.4 | 0.3 |
| OK | 880 | 25.1 | 3.6 | 7.4 | 5.2 | 3,157 | 10.0 | 1.2 | 4.4 | 0.2 |
| OR | 512 | 30.5 | 10.0 | 12.1 | 8.8 | 1,842 | 11.4 | 3.9 | 6.8 | 0.1 |

*(table continues)*

TABLE 8: *(continued)*

| State | Age < 50 Years | | | | | Age 50–75 Years | | | | |
|---|---|---|---|---|---|---|---|---|---|---|
| | Number | Waitlisted for KI or SPK (%) | Living donor transplants (%) | Deceased donor KI transplants (%) | Deceased donor SPK transplants (%) | Number | Waitlisted for KI or SPK (%) | Living donor transplants (%) | Deceased donor KI transplants (%) | Deceased donor SPK transplants (%) |
| PA | 2,238 | 50.8 | 8.8 | 10.5 | 12.6 | 11,131 | 17.3 | 1.9 | 6.5 | 0.4 |
| PR | 965 | 22.7 | 4.1 | 5.0 | 4.9 | 4,761 | 5.6 | 0.8 | 1.4 | 0.0 |
| RI | 146 | 56.8 | 24.7 | 18.5 | 4.1 | 643 | 11.7 | 4.2 | 4.5 | 0.0 |
| SC | 1,073 | 26.8 | 4.4 | 5.6 | 7.5 | 4,695 | 8.6 | 0.7 | 3.4 | 0.2 |
| SD | 164 | 50.6 | 18.9 | 15.2 | 9.1 | 660 | 24.1 | 4.4 | 10.2 | 0.6 |
| TN | 1,397 | 33.5 | 7.5 | 8.4 | 8.9 | 5,222 | 10.2 | 1.8 | 3.4 | 0.2 |
| TX | 6,127 | 31.9 | 4.4 | 7.8 | 4.4 | 23,951 | 12.6 | 1.5 | 3.6 | 0.1 |
| UT | 342 | 30.7 | 18.1 | 9.4 | 12.9 | 1,039 | 11.7 | 6.5 | 7.3 | 0.3 |
| VA | 1,541 | 40.6 | 9.2 | 6.1 | 7.1 | 6,565 | 14.9 | 3.3 | 3.1 | 0.1 |
| VT | 50 | 44.0 | 18.0 | 8.0 | 12.0 | 175 | 17.7 | 2.9 | 9.1 | 0.0 |
| WA | 852 | 38.7 | 9.0 | 8.0 | 12.8 | 3,357 | 14.0 | 3.1 | 5.2 | 0.3 |
| WI | 827 | 52.5 | 9.4 | 8.7 | 21.6 | 3,355 | 18.1 | 4.5 | 6.3 | 0.8 |
| WV | 405 | 34.8 | 9.1 | 13.1 | 6.7 | 1,859 | 9.1 | 1.8 | 3.4 | 0.1 |
| WY | 58 | 48.3 | 19.0 | 8.6 | 6.9 | 178 | 15.2 | 3.4 | 6.7 | 0.0 |
| ALL | 58,617 | 37.6 | 7.8 | 7.6 | 8.0 | 254,444 | 14.1 | 2.3 | 3.9 | 0.3 |

Source: McCullough, K. P., et al. "Kidney and Pancreas Transplantation in the United States, 1998–2007: Access for Patients with Diabetes and End-Stage Renal Disease." *American Journal of Transplantation* 9, Part 2 (2009): p. 903; Source: U.S. Department of Health and Human Services. *2008 Annual Report of the U.S. Organ Procurement and Transplantation Network and the Scientific Registry of Transplant Recipients: Transplant Data 1998–2007.* Health Resources and Services Administration, Healthcare Systems Bureau, Division of Transplantation, Rockville, Md. October 2009.

The data and analyses reported in the 2008 Annual Report of the U.S. Organ Procurement and Transplantation Network and the Scientific Registry of Transplant Recipients have been supplied by UNOS and Arbor Research under contract with HHS/HRSA. The authors alone are responsible for reporting and interpreting these data; the views expressed herein are those of the authors and not necessarily those of the U.S. Government.

Organ Sharing (UNOS), a private organization, administers the OPTN.

Many transplant centers have patient videos that describe in detail all the steps that are involved before the transplantation, during the procedure, and after the completion of the transplant. These informational sessions are very important for patient education, and patients should be asked to attend these sessions along with their next of kin or other family members and friends.

### Beginning the Process: The Search for a Donor

The process of kidney transplantation begins with a referral from a physician, and then a determination by a transplant program as to whether the person is a candidate for trans-

plantation. If he or she is determined to be a candidate, then the person is registered on the national organ transplant waiting list—unless a relative or other person has volunteered to be an organ donor. If a relative or friend has volunteered to be an organ donor and is also a suitable match, then the person needing the kidney does not need to be on the waiting list, but this plan is still reported to the United Network of Organ Sharing. It is important for potential donors to know that they too will be screened by the transplant program to ensure that they are in good health and that donating a kidney will not put them at significant health risk.

If a patient in need of a kidney transplant does not have any available living donors, and the person is registered on the transplant waiting list, then when an organ becomes available, the information is entered into a computer system. This system provides a ranked list of potential recipients, based on their blood type, organ size, and their genetic makeup with regard to the human leukocyte antigen (HLA) blood type.

When a kidney becomes available, the transplant program with patients on the waiting list is contacted, in a predetermined priority order, according to the priority of patients. The transplant team at a transplant center is given one hour to either accept or reject the organ that is offered. If they turn the organ down, then the center with the next patient on the list is contacted, and they are also given one hour to accept or reject the organ, and so on.

Patients needing a kidney may be registered with multiple transplant centers, but each center will usually require a separate evaluation, even though the patient is already registered at another center. Patients acquire additional parity points the longer that they are on the waiting list, but these parity points can only be applied for consideration for a transplant at a single center. Thus, being registered at multiple centers typically has a minimal impact on the time to acquire a kidney transplant for a patient on the waiting list.

### Patients with Diabetes Mellitus

Patients with diabetes mellitus are among the most likely to need a kidney transplant because diabetes mellitus is one of the most common causes of end-stage renal disease. According to Erika B. Rangel and colleagues in their 2009 article for *Diabetology & Metabolic Syndrome*, patients with diabetes are likely to have a better outcome with a kidney transplant than with dialysis, in terms of a higher survival rate. This is true despite the fact that diabetic patients are more likely to have cardiovascular events and infectious complications than others.

The authors also noted that among patients with Type 1 diabetes, a simultaneous pancreas-kidney transplant has correlated with a decreased preva-lence of heart attack (myocardial infarction), stroke, or amputation, compared to those patients with type 1 diabetes who have only a kidney transplant or dialysis. With a simultaneous pancreas-kidney transplant, there is the potential to cure the underlying diabetes mellitus.

### The Kidney Transplant Procedure

The kidney transplant is performed by a surgical team that has been extensively trained in transplant surgical techniques. A kidney transplant is a complex procedure, but simply put, it involves placing the new kidney in the abdomen in either the right or left lower quadrant, based upon a variety of surgical factors.

An incision is made from the pubic bone toward the flank and extends long enough to provide the surgical team with what they feel is sufficient space to insert the donor kidney. One very important aspect of the procedure is the anastomosis (connection) of the donor kidney blood vessels (the renal artery and the renal vein) to the recipient's artery and vein in the lower abdomen (the external iliac artery and vein).

Another important part of the procedure is the connection of the donor kidney ureter with the recipient's bladder. To help this ureteric anastomosis heal properly, a catheter is placed in the bladder so that the postoperative urine can be drained by the catheter. This catheter remains in place for up to several days before it is removed.

Sometimes a drain is left in and around the new kidney to facilitate fluid or blood drainage that can accumulate. Such drains are usually removed several days after the transplant procedure.

### Post Transplant Care

Following a successful surgery, the transplant recipient is intensively monitored for any postoperative complications. Immunosuppressive medicines to prevent the rejection of the transplanted kidney are begun at the time of the transplant procedure and then must be continued throughout the life of the recipient. Patients whose donated kidney starts functioning immediately may be discharged from the hospital on the third or fourth hospital day.

Almost always, the recipients of living donor kidneys demonstrate immediate graft function, which means that the linkup between the new kidney and the patient's body is working. About 10–30 percent of the recipients of deceased donor kidneys develop a problem with delayed graft function (DGF) and may need dialysis therapy until the graft "takes." However, even patients who develop DGF are frequently discharged from the hospital in the first week after surgery to either home or to an intermediate facility, and then they receive outpatient follow-up of their transplanted kidney. It may take four to 12 weeks for the DGF issue to resolve itself.

A small number of patients will develop an acute rejection of the transplanted kidney as a result of either preexisting or new antibodies. This type of acute rejection is diagnosed by the findings in the biopsy as well as by the detection of donor specific antibodies in the blood. Such patients may need intensive therapy with plasmapheresis (the exchange of patient plasma with albumin) as well as the use of intravenous immunoglobulin (IVIG) for two to four weeks.

### The Post-Transplant Course in the First Year

Patients with a stable graft function resume normal daily activities shortly after the transplant procedure. Because the risk of rejection is greatest immediately after the transplant, close observation and follow-up with a transplant nephrologist and regular monitoring of kidney function, often with blood tests once every week or even more often, are necessary. After the first three months, patients will have blood work performed less frequently, possibly monthly, including tests for the antirejection drug levels of their immunosuppressive drugs such as cyclosporine, tacrolimus, or sirolimus.

*Immunosuppressive medications taken by transplant patients*  The person who receives a kidney transplantation must take IMMUNOSUPPRESSIVE DRUGS to prevent the rejection of the kidney by the immune system of the recipient's body. The problem with this is that the individual who has received the kidney is now at increased risk from many different infections that the body would normally fight against naturally, as well as at an increased risk for the development of cancer. The only patients who do not require immunosuppressive therapy are those who received a kidney transplant from an identical twin. According to the American Society of Transplantation (AST), patients with kidney transplants may require several different types of medications, including two to three different drugs that keep the body from fighting the new kidney (immunosuppressants), protect the patient from infection, and control the side effects that transplant drugs can cause.

*Advice on immunosuppressants*  In their booklet, *Medicines for Keeping Your New Kidney Healthy*, the AST notes that the following advice is very important for patients with kidney transplants:

- Never stop taking your medication without calling your doctor first.
- Tell your doctor or nurse if you think you are having side effects from a medicine.
- Always have enough medicine on hand. Get your prescriptions filled before you run out. You must have the right amount of medicine every day.
- If you cannot pay for your medicine, tell your doctors right away. Transplant medicines cost a lot of money. Most health plans will cover the costs of medicine for a while. Also talk to the social worker at the transplant center.

### Grafts and Graft Survival

The graft survival refers to the continued functioning of the transplant kidney. The graft itself may fail, necessitating a new transplant. As with patient survival, graft survival is much lower with an expanded criteria donor; in his article on expanded criteria donors, Oho noted that the risk for graft failure is between one-half and two times higher than for a regular criteria kidney.

According to the USRDS, overall kidney graft failure rates have improved steadily, and the failure rate fell from 9.3 per patient year in 1991 to 6.6 in 2007. (The term *patient year* is a way to determine trends and includes the number of patients and the number of years they are in a study.) Of patients with a graft failure in 2007, the median time to a new transplant is 7.5 years, about the same as in 1991.

In their 2010 article on kidney transplant outcomes for the *Journal of Clinical Investigation*, authors Bernd Schröppel and Peter S. Heeger say that the half-life of a transplanted kidney from a deceased donor is about eight years. They also noted that less than a third of grafts from older donors will be still functional 10 years later.

### *Who Should Not Have a Kidney Transplant*

In some cases, a patient is *not* considered a good candidate for a kidney transplant. The following categories of patients are usually not considered suitable for receiving either a living or deceased donor kidney transplantation. These are by no means absolute barriers, and they are also subject to regional and local policies and procedures, as well as the experience of the transplant team.

- patients who have had a cancerous tumor within the past five years and are still under treatment
- patients with primary oxalosis, unless such patients are wait-listed for a combination of liver and kidney transplants
- patients with dementia or an inability to provide their own self-care
- those who have previously exhibited noncompliance to treatment
- patients with an ongoing drug addiction or drug abuse
- patients with psychiatric diseases that preclude adherence to treatment or who have an inability to comprehend the consent process
- patients with untreated infection: However, patients with HIV who have tight control on antiretroviral therapy can receive a deceased donor or living donor kidney transplant.

### *Dental Issues*

According to the National Institute of Dental and Craniofacial Research, there are also dental issues that are involved with transplanted organs; for example, all active dental problems should be dealt with *before* the transplantation and also before immunosuppressive medications must be taken. Other actions should be taken as well, including the extraction of nonrestorable teeth and the removal of orthodontic bands or the adjustment of prostheses for patients who may take cyclosporine after the transplant, because this medication can cause gingival hyperplasia.

Other medications may affect dental health; for example, tacrolimus can cause oral ulcerations and numbness and tingling around the mouth. Corticosteroids can cause an increased risk for infection and may also mask the early indications of an oral infection. Sirolimus can cause oral ulceration.

After the transplantation, patients should avoid dental care other than routine homecare (such as brushing one's teeth) unless they have an emergency. Once the transplant graft has stabilized, in about three to six months after surgery, patients can return to their dentists for regular treatment, albeit with precautions. Patients who need invasive dental procedures may need to be premedicated with ANTIBIOTICS if the patient's physician agrees. Patients may also be taking blood thinners, which could cause bleeding problems with dental treatment, and the patient's doctor may wish to adjust such medications several days before an invasive dental procedure will occur.

Dentists should screen post-transplant patients at every appointment, because malignancies can sometimes occur with patients who have had an organ transplant, such as Kaposi's sarcoma, lymphoma, and squamous cell carcinoma of the lip. These cancers may occur decades before they would occur in individuals not taking immunosuppressants.

See also CHRONIC KIDNEY DISEASE

Aradhye, Sheeram, et al. *Medicines for Keeping Your New Kidney Healthy.* Mount Laurel, N.J.: American Society of Transplantation, 2006.

Centers for Medicare & Medicaid Services. *You Can Live: Your Guide for Living with Kidney Failure.* Baltimore, Md.: Centers for Medicare & Medicaid Services, 2007.

Fraser, Sheila M., et al. "Acceptable Outcome After Kidney Transplantation Using 'Expanded Criteria Donor' Grafts." *Transplantation* 89, no. 1 (2010): 88–96.

Hunter Campbell, Kellie, M.D., et al. "Older Adults and Chronic Kidney Disease Decision Making by Primary Care Physicians: A Scholarly Review and Research Agenda." *Journal of General Internal Medicine* 23, no. 3 (2009): 329–336.

Ibrahim, Hassan N., M.D., et al. "Long-Term Consequences of Kidney Donation." *New England Journal of Medicine* 360, no. 5 (2009): 459–469.

Jagbir, Gill, et al. "Outcomes of Kidney Transplantation from Older Living Donors to Older Recipients." *American Journal of Kidney Diseases* 52, no 3. (2008): 541–552.

McCullough, K. P., et al. "Kidney and Pancreas Transplantation in the United States, 1998–2007: Access for Patients with Diabetes and End-Stage Renal Disease." *American Journal of Transplantation* 9, Part 2 (2009): 894–906.

National Institute of Dental and Craniofacial Research. *Dental Management of the Organ Transplant Patient.* National Institutes of Health, October 2009.

National Kidney and Urologic Diseases Information Clearinghouse. *Treatment Methods for Kidney Transplantation.* Bethesda, Md.: National Institutes for Health, 2006.

Navaneethan, Sankar D., Sarah Aloudat, and Sonal Singh. "A Systematic Review of Patient and Health System Characteristics Associated with Late Referral in Chronic Kidney Disease." *BMC Nephrology* 9, no. 3 (2008). Available online. URL: http://www.biomedcenetral.com/1471-2369/9/3. Accessed November 8, 2010.

Ojo, A. O. "Expanded Criteria Donors: Process and Outcomes." *Seminars in Dialysis* 18, no. 6 (2005): 463–468.

Peitzman, Steven J. *Dropsy, Dialysis, Transplant: A Short History of Failed Kidneys.* Baltimore, Md.: Johns Hopkins University Press, 2007.

Rangel, Erika B., et al. "Kidney Transplant in Diabetic Patients: Modalities, Indications and Results." *Diabetology & Metabolic Syndrome* 1, no. 2 (2009). Available online. URL: http://www.dmsjournal.com/content/1/1/2. Accessed February 5, 2010.

Schröppel, Bernd and Peter S. Heeger. "Gazing into a Crystal Ball to Predict Kidney Transplant Outcome." *Journal of Clinical Investigation* 120, no. 6 (2010): 1,803–1,806.

Segev, Dorry L., M.D., et al. "Perioperative Mortality and Long-term Survival following Live Kidney Donation." *Journal of the American Medical Association* 303, no. 10 (2010): 959–966.

Vieira, Lisa. "Expanded Criteria Donors Offer Hope for Patients Needing Kidney Transplant." *Journal of the American Association of Physician Assistants* 22, no. 3 (2009): 33–36.

**lithium and bipolar disorder** Lithium is a naturally occurring element that is sometimes prescribed as a medication used to treat individuals who have bipolar disorder, a serious psychiatric disorder that was formerly known as manic-depression and that sometimes presents with psychotic features. Lithium can be harmful and even toxic to the kidneys. Bipolar disorder causes an alternation between depression and mania, with some individuals spending a greater time in depression or mania than others. Individuals who rapidly change from a state of DEPRESSION to a state of mania and back are said to be rapid cyclers, and they are more difficult to treat than others with bipolar disorder. (Many physicians treat depression, but most people with bipolar disorder are treated by psychiatrists because specialized knowledge is needed to treat this severe psychiatric disorder.)

Individuals with bipolar disorder who are manic are ruled by their immediate impulses, and they can exhibit very extreme behavior, such as engaging in excessive gambling although they do not normally gamble and participating in uncharacteristic (for them, when not manic) sexual excesses. When depressed, the bipolar patient may become suicidal. Treatment for bipolar disorder can considerably improve the behavior of the bipolar patient toward normalcy, although bipolar disorder is a chronic disease. Individuals with bipolar disorder may suffer from other psychiatric disorders as well, further complicating their treatment.

Lithium at very high levels in the blood can lead to serious and potentially fatal effects. The neurologic effects include tremulous-ness, decreased alertness, coma, and seizures. Kidney-related effects include acute renal failure. Because the kidneys are the major means through which the body removes lithium, kidney failure can prevent recovery from lithium toxicity unless the kidney failure is treated. If untreated, it can lead to death. If kidney failure cannot be treated rapidly or if the lithium levels are very high, dialysis may be necessary to more rapidly remove the lithium.

Even in the absence of excessively high levels of lithium, lithium can have major side effects, such as a severe weight gain (as much as 50–100 pounds), and its use can also lead to serious kidney disease. The kidney effects include either chronic kidney disease or the excretion of very high volumes of urine. With lithium-induced nephrogenic diabetes insipidus, people may excrete six quarts of more of urine each day.

In a study of 24 patients with proven lithium toxicity by biopsy, reported by Glen S. Markowitz and colleagues in the *Journal of the American Society of Nephrology* in 2000, the researchers reported that 25 percent of the subjects with lithium-induced kidney damage had nephritic-range proteinuria and 87 percent had nephrogenic diabetes insipidus while 33.3 percent had hypertension.

The researchers also reported that a KIDNEY BIOPSY showed chronic tubulointerstitial nephropathy in all subjects, and about two-thirds (62.5 percent) had associated cortical and medullary tubular cysts, while a third had issues with dilation. Even with the discontinuation of lithium, seven of nine patients with high blood levels of lithium ultimately developed END-STAGE RENAL DISEASE (ESRD).

The researchers said, "In conclusion, lithium nephrotoxicity primarily targets distal and collecting tubules, with a higher incidence of proteinuria and associated glomerular pathology than recognized previously. Renal dysfunction is often irreversible despite lithium withdrawal, and early detection is essential to prevent progression to ESRD."

Bipolar disorder can be also treated with mood stabilizing medication such as valproate (Depakote and Depakene), which is not associated with the risks for kidney disease that has been linked to lithium. In addition, newer antipsychotic medications such as aripiprazole (Abilify) are also used to treat bipolar disorder, and they do not harm the kidneys as does lithium.

As a result, if lithium must be used, then physicians should carefully monitor the level of lithium in the patient's blood as well as the patient's kidney function. High lithium levels can cause potentially serious short-term neurologic disease and may lead to an increased risk of long-term kidney damage. In general, kidney disease should be an indication to discontinue lithium in order to minimize the risk of progressive chronic kidney disease. Unfortunately, even some individuals in whom lithium is discontinued will develop progressive worsening of their kidney disease.

See also CHRONIC KIDNEY DISEASE; MEDICATIONS THAT CAN HARM THE KIDNEYS.

Markowitz, Glen S., et al. "Lithium Nephrotoxicity: A Progressive Combined Glomerula and Tubulointerstitial Nephropathy." *Journal of the American Society of Nephrology* 11 (2000): 1,439–1,448.

**lithotripsy**    A commonly used procedure that is usually performed on an outpatient basis and is used to break up painful kidney stones into smaller particles with painless shock waves. The procedure is used to break up kidney stones in the kidney, ureters, or bladder. There are different forms of lithotripsy, including extracorporeal shock wave lithotripsy (ESWL), shock wave lithotripsy, laser lithotripsy, percutaneous lithotripsy, and endoscopic lithotripsy. The most commonly used form of lithotripsy is ESWL.

### Procedure

Patients are told to avoid food or fluids for several hours before having the procedure. The patient should inform the doctor about any medications that have been taken or that are normally taken. Patients scheduled for a lithotripsy may be told to stop taking warfarin (Coumadin), aspirin, ibuprofen, or any other drugs that affect blood clotting for several days before the procedure will occur. Lithotripsy should not be performed on a pregnant patient. Tests such as blood and urine tests, X-rays, and sometimes an electrocardiogram are performed before the procedure.

Before the procedure begins, the patient is often given a mild painkiller or sedative, since it can sometimes cause minor pain. X-rays or ultrasound help the doctor to determine where the kidney stones are located, and once identified, high-energy shock waves are sent through the body directly to the location of the kidney stones. The shock waves break up the stones so that they are easier to pass into the urine. The procedure often takes about an hour, and then the patient is in the recovery room for about two hours.

Most lithotripsy procedures are noninvasive, but sometimes the physician must use a laser to reach an obstructive kidney stone. The laser is inserted into an endoscope, and the endoscope is inserted into the urinary tract. Laser lithotripsy usually requires a general anesthesia.

With a percutaneous lithotripsy, the doctor accesses the stone from the back and into the kidney. This procedure is used if the patient has large kidney stones. Patients who have a percutaneous lithotripsy will stay overnight in the hospital.

### Risks and Complications

In general, lithotripsy works well for the patient. However, complications of the procedure may include the following:

- bleeding around the kidney, which rarely may require a blood transfusion
- pieces of stone left in the body which may require further treatment
- damage to the kidney tissue or nearby structures with ESWL
- blockage of urine flow from the kidney caused by pieces of stone

Infection is another risk and is also a complication of the procedure. Infection is generally indicated if the patient has excessive blood in the urine, severe pain, and an intense need to urinate frequently. Infection is treated with antibiotics.

### Outlook and Lifestyle Modifications

After the kidney stones are broken up and excreted, the symptoms will disappear and the patient will feel normal again. However, it is important to try to determine the cause of the kidney stones, and doctors may order a 24-hour urine collection so that any subsequent kidney stones can be collected and analyzed by a laboratory. Lithotripsy deals only with the kidney stones that are present at the time of the procedure. In the absence of effective long-term therapies directed at the etiology of the kidney stone, the risk of recurrence is very high.

See also KIDNEY STONES.

**lupus**  See LUPUS NEPHRITIS.

**lupus nephritis**  A serious kidney disorder that is a complication of systemic lupus erythematosus (SLE), which is an immune system disorder that affects up to an estimated 322,000 adults in the United States. Lupus nephritis is also known as lupus glomerular disease. In addition to harming the kidneys, SLE harms the joints, skin, blood cells, and the brain. According to Derek M. Fine, M.D., in his article for the *Journal of the American Medical Association* in 2005, as many as 60 percent of adults with systemic lupus erythematosus will develop lupus nephritis, and up to 50 percent of them will experience kidney disease early in the course of the disease.

Lupus nephritis is diagnosed when there is a buildup of antibodies in the kidneys that cause inflammation. This inflammation frequently leads to NEPHROTIC SYNDROME (an excessive level of excretion of protein), hematuria (blood cells in the urine), or both, and may quickly worsen to END-STAGE RENAL DISEASE (ESRD)/kidney failure, necessitating DIALYSIS or KIDNEY TRANSPLANTATION in order for the person to stay alive.

According to the National Institutes of Medicine, about three of 10,000 people in the United States are affected by lupus nephritis. Among children with SLE, about half of them will develop some form of kidney disease.

The causes of SLE are unknown, although it may be caused by an infection, by an inherited gene, by a virus, or by an environmental cause.

### Symptoms and Diagnostic Path

Key symptoms caused by lupus nephritis may include:

- hematuria (blood in the urine)
- PROTEINURIA (protein in the urine)
- a foamy appearance to the urine
- swelling in any body part
- darkened urine
- hypertension
- weight gain
- swelling of the eyes, legs, ankles, or fingers

Physicians may order urine and blood tests in order to diagnose lupus nephritis. They may also order testing to diagnose that the person has SLE, because less than half the patients with lupus nephritis were previously diagnosed with lupus. Lupus nephritis has many patterns of involvement of the kidney, and different patterns require different treatments. While the blood and urine testing can suggest which pattern is most likely, only a KIDNEY BIOPSY can tell for certain.

The patient may also have an abnormal GLOMERULAR FILTRATION RATE based on the creatinine measurement and the estimated glomerular filtration (eGFR) calculation. Other diagnostic tests that may be ordered to detect lupus nephritis include a urinalysis with microscopic examination, a urine protein measurement, an ANA titer, and the measurement of specific antibodies in the blood which are present frequently in patients with SLE and with lupus nephritis. (See URINE/URINALYSIS/URINE CULTURE.) In addition, the physical examination will often show high blood pressure and/or edema (fluid retention).

Individuals with lupus nephritis may have blood testing that shows a false positive test for syphilis, which means that the test is positive but they do not actually have syphilis. Anyone who is quite certain that he or she could not have syphilis should ask the doctor if they could possibly have lupus.

### Treatment Options and Outlook

Treatment of lupus nephritis is based upon the specific pattern of lupus nephritis in the individual. The World Health Organization categorizes lupus nephritis into classes I through V, ranging in severity from the least severe Class I to the most severe Class V. Some types of lupus nephritis, such as Classes I and II, generally do not require treatment. Class III may require treatment if the clinical symptoms, such as impaired estimated glomerular filtration rate (eGFR), the degree of proteinuria and the amount of edema are severe.

Class IV almost always requires very aggressive, and intense, therapy. Without treatment, ~50 percent of people with Class IV lupus nephritis will develop irreversible renal failure and require either dialysis or a kidney transplant within two years. Class V lupus nephritis often requires treatment, but typically not as aggressive therapy as Class IV. Treatment of lupus nephritis frequently involves very strong medications to suppress the immune system for the initial component of therapy. Once the disease has improved, less intense immunosuppressive medications can be substituted.

Many patients benefit from therapy for six to 12 months after all symptoms are maximally improved before discontinuing medications. Early discontinuation risks an increased likelihood of disease recurrence. If lupus nephritis recurs, then a repeat renal biopsy is often needed because approximately 20 percent of people who have a recurrence will develop a different pattern, which will require a different treatment regimen.

If the kidney disease progresses further to kidney failure, the patient will need dialysis or a kidney transplantation.

### Risk Factors and Preventive Measures

Because women have a greater risk for developing SLE than men, women also have a greater risk for developing lupus nephritis. SLE is most commonly diagnosed among females between ages 20 and 40 years. There are no known preventive measures for lupus nephritis.

Fine, Derek M., M.D. "Pharmacological Therapy of Lupus Nephritis." *Journal of the American Medical Association* 293, no. 24 (2005): 3,053–3,060.

Helmick, Charles G., et al. "Estimates of the Prevalence of Arthritis and Other Rheumatic Conditions in the United States. Part I." *Arthritis & Rheumatism* 58, no. 1 (January 2008): 15–25.

Houssiau, Frédéric A. "Management of Lupus Nephritis: An Update." *Journal of the American Society of Nephrology* 15 (2004): 2,694–2,704.

Waldman, M., and G. B. Appel. "Update on the Treatment of Lupus Nephritis," *Kidney International* 70, no. 8 (2006): 1,403–1,412.

**magnesium** The fourth most commonly appearing mineral in the human body, according to the Office of Dietary Supplements, and a mineral that is needed for more than 30 different biochemical reactions within the body; for example, magnesium is vital to the bones and is also important in the regulation of blood pressure, as well as in maintaining healthy nerve and muscle functioning. Only about 1 percent of the magnesium in the body is found in the blood but the body works hard to maintain a constant level of magnesium.

Magnesium is present in many foods, such as green vegetables, as well as nuts, seeds, peas, beans, and unrefined grains. Sometimes magnesium is also taken as a dietary supplement; for example, women who suffer from preeclampsia of pregnancy, a hypertensive condition that is unique to pregnancy, may obtain relief with the administration of magnesium, according to Catherine M. Champagne in her article on the role of magnesium in hypertension, cardiovascular disease, metabolic syndrome, and other conditions, published in 2008 in *Nutrition in Clinical Practice*.

Individuals suffering from dehydration may be deficient in magnesium as well as in other electrolytes, such as POTASSIUM and SODIUM, and thus may also suffer from an ELECTROLYTE imbalance. Research has also indicated that magnesium is important in the bone structure of the elderly, who may be deficient in this mineral because of an insufficient dietary intake of magnesium, impaired kidney absorption, or the use of DIURETICS.

Magnesium deficiencies are apparently linked with potassium deficiencies, and thus, if an individual is found deficient in one mineral, then he or she is likely also to be deficient in the other. Some early indications of a magnesium deficiency (hypomagnesemia) include the following:

- nausea and vomiting
- loss of appetite
- weakness
- fatigue

These manifestations are typically so mild that the diagnosis is made only by blood testing showing the low levels of magnesium. If the hypomagnesemia worsens further, the following signs and symptoms may occur:

- muscle contractions and cramps
- numbness and tingling
- seizures
- personality changes
- abnormal heart rhythms
- coronary spasms

Severe hypomagnesemia may cause HYPOCALCEMIA, or insufficient levels of calcium in the blood.

Males ages 31 years and older need the greatest amount of magnesium each day, or 420 mg per day. A close second is the category of males who are ages 14–18 years, who need 410 mg of magnesium per day, followed by pregnant women ages 14–18 years, who need 400 mg of magnesium per day. In contrast, small children ages 1–3 years need only 80 mg per day. (See Table 1.)

**TABLE 1: RECOMMENDED DIETARY ALLOWANCES FOR MAGNESIUM FOR CHILDREN AND ADULTS**

| Age (years) | Male (mg/day) | Female (mg/day) | Pregnancy (mg/day) | Lactation (mg/day) |
|---|---|---|---|---|
| 1–3 | 80 | 80 | n/a | n/a |
| 4–8 | 130 | 130 | n/a | n/a |
| 9–13 | 240 | 240 | n/a | n/a |
| 14–18 | 410 | 360 | 400 | 360 |
| 19–30 | 400 | 310 | 350 | 310 |
| 31+ | 420 | 320 | 360 | 320 |

Source: Office of Dietary Supplements. "Dietary Supplement Fact Sheet: Magnesium." National Institutes of Health. Available online. URL: http://ods.od.nih/gov/factsheets/Magnesium_pf.asp. Accessed December 30, 2009.

### Individuals Who May Need Extra Magnesium

Some categories of individuals need a greater amount of magnesium than others. For example, some medications deplete the body of magnesium, and thus, individuals taking these medications may need supplementation of their magnesium. Medications that may lead to a magnesium deficiency are diuretics, such as Lasix, Edecrin, Burmex, and hydrochlorothiazide. Some antibiotics, particularly Amphotericin and Gentamicin, can cause hypomagnesemia. Tetracyline, another antibiotic, may interact with magnesium and decrease the absorption of the tetracycline.

Patients with DIABETES MELLITUS are prone to hypomagnesemia, especially if their diabetes is not under good control. Individuals with alcoholism are a particularly high risk group for magnesium deficiencies, and as many as 60 percent of alcoholics may have hypomagnesemia, according to the Office of Dietary Supplements. This is likely related to poor nutrition; whether the excessive alcohol intake directly alters the body's handling of magnesium is another possible contributing factor. In addition, elderly individuals often have hypomagnesemia; this is often due to inadequate nutritional intake.

High blood levels of magnesium, hypermagnesemia, are substantially less frequently occurring. This can, however occur in patients with END-STAGE RENAL DISEASE who ingest large amounts of magnesium, which may occur with the use of magnesium-containing compounds to treat constipation or with the use of excessive amounts of magnesium-containing antacids in a patient with renal failure. The kidneys normally excrete excessive amounts of magnesium; patients with renal failure may be unable to do so.

See also CALCIUM; MEDICATIONS THAT CAN HARM THE KIDNEYS; PHOSPHORUS.

Champagne, Catherine M. "Magnesium in Hypertension, Cardiovascular Disease, Metabolic Syndrome, and Other Conditions: A Review." *Nutrition in Clinical Practice* 23, no. 2 (2008): 142–151.

Office of Dietary Supplements. "Dietary Supplement Fact Sheet: Magnesium." National Institutes of Health. Available online. URL: http://ods.od.nih/gov/factsheets/Magnesium_pf.asp. Accessed December 30, 2009.

**manic depression**   See LITHIUM AND BIPOLAR DISORDER.

**medications that can harm the kidneys**   Some medications that are commonly prescribed to treat many diseases and disorders, as well as some drugs that are infrequently prescribed, can be harmful to the kidneys, particularly if these medications are used on a regular basis. Also, some over-the-counter (OTC) drugs, or medications that are not prescribed and that can be readily purchased in pharmacies, supermarkets, and many other locations, may be harmful if used frequently, such as analgesics (painkillers), including OTC aspirin, NONSTEROIDAL ANTI-INFLAMMATORY DRUGS (NSAIDs), and other OTC medications. This overview covers these categories of medications, as well as broad subcategories of medications.

Just because a medication *may* be harmful to the kidneys does not mean that it inevitably *is* harmful. Many people take the medications that are described in this overview and never have a problem with them. Individuals with kidney disease (whether they know that they have kidney disease or not) are more likely to develop a problem, but even people with kidney disease may take many of these medications with no ill effect. It is best, however, for people with kidney disease to be carefully monitored on any medications that could be harmful to the kidneys.

Some medications are primarily processed or metabolized by the liver, while others are metabolized by the kidneys. Medications that are metabolized by the kidneys are more likely to be problematic in individuals with impaired kidney function, as with individuals with END-STAGE RENAL DISEASE. However, even if individuals have actively working kidneys with no CHRONIC KIDNEY DISEASE, some medications can be risky or harmful and should be used with caution, as is discussed in this overview.

Many medications are combined medications, including two or more different drugs, and some of these medications may include drugs that are harmful to the kidneys. For example, in a 2008 issue of the *Journal of the American Pharmacy Association,* J. Stroup and J. Stephens cited a case in which a man was receiving a combination therapy that included simvastatin (Zocor) and ezetimibe (Zetia). He was also prescribed simvastatin as a stand-alone medication, and the inadvertent high dosages of statins led to the development of RHABDOMYOLYSIS and kidney failure. Fortunately, the problem was identified and resolved with aggressive hydration (the administration of a high volume of fluids).

### Considering Potentially Nephrotoxic Medications

When doctors prescribe medications, whatever the disease or disorder that they are treating, they seek to avoid prescribing a medication that potentially might be harmful to a patient. One way they do this is by having a medical assistant or nurse review all current prescribed and OTC medications that patients take, as well as all herbal remedies and other supplements, even before a diagnosis of a new problem is made. Once the doctor diagnoses a disorder and prescribes a medication, there is another potential checkpoint for the patient: the pharmacist at the pharmacy. If the patient receives all prescribed medications from one pharmacy (which is advisable, whenever possible), then the pharmacist at this pharmacy will also use the information in their database to check whether a new medication could be potentially harmful to a patient.

Even these effective checks sometimes fail, for many reasons; for example, the doctor may not be aware that the patient has a kidney disease (or other disease), particularly when the illness is in the early stages. Also, even if the pharmacist is aware of an existing kidney disease that is being treated, he or she may be rushed and fail to perform the usual quick check. As a result, when patients know that they have kidney disease, they should always ask both their physician and their pharmacist if a newly-prescribed medication is safe for a person with kidney disease or with any other serious illnesses.

*Off-label prescriptions*  Some medications are prescribed on an off-label basis. This means that the physician prescribes a medication for a condition other than the one(s) for which it has specifically been approved by the Food and Drug Administration (FDA). For example, doctors may prescribe antidepressants for a temporary (or continued) period to treat not only depression but also such medical problems as migraine headaches or sleeplessness, even though there are specific migraine medications and sleep remedies that are FDA-approved for those problems.

This is a legal practice and is commonly done, although most physicians try medications that are FDA-approved for the condition first. They may resort to prescribing off-label uses of medications if they feel that such action is necessary to help the patient.

### Common Nephrotoxic Medications

Many medications can be harmful to the kidneys but this section covers some common categories of medications as well as some specific medications that are particularly known to be potentially harmful to the kidneys. A summary of many of these medications and their potentially toxic effects on the kidneys is also provided in Table 1.

*Analgesics*  Painkillers are commonly used by many people, particularly OTC analgesics such as aspirin or ibuprofen. Prescribed narcotics such as opioids are taken for extreme pain, such as with a patient with a severely strained muscle or very bad BACK PAIN. Both OTC analgesics and prescribed narcotics can lead to kidney damage, especially in those who are already at risk for kidney damage. For this reason, analgesics need to be carefully monitored among those with kidney disease.

According to M. Mazer and J. Perrone in their article on acetaminophen-induced nephrotoxicity for the *Journal of Medical Toxicology,* 1–2 percent of those who experience acetaminophen overdose will develop renal insufficiency. Renal failure may also follow after hepatoxicity (a toxic overdose to the liver).

As seen from Table 1, the overuse of analgesics can lead to the development of chronic interstitial nephritis.

*Antiarrhythmics*  Antiarrhythmic medications are prescribed for individuals who have, heart problems, particularly an unsteady or erratic heartbeat. These drugs are used to stabilize the heart rhythm. Some antiarrhythmics can be dangerous for patients with kidney disease, because they may accelerate the heartbeat too much, rather than achieving the desired opposite goal. If the doctor is considering prescribing an antiarrhythmic to a patient, whether the patient has been diagnosed with kidney disease or not, then the patient's MAGNESIUM and POTASSIUM blood levels should be checked first. If these levels are normal, then the physician can feel more confident with prescribing the antiarrhythmic.

Note that the antiarrhythmic medication disopyramide (Norpace) should be used only very cautiously with individuals who have impaired kidney function.

*Antibiotics*  ANTIBIOTICS are prescribed to treat bacterial infections, and there are many different types of antibiotics. Some can be potentially harmful to people who have poor kidney function, including such medications as nitrofurantoin (Macrodantin, Furandantin). Medications in the aminoglycoside class of antibiotics can lead to kidney damage. In addition, medications in the class of sulfonamides may lead to acute interstitial nephritis or a condition known as CRYSTAL NEPHROPATHY, in which the medication causes the creation and depositing of crystals in the urine that cannot be dissolved and that may obstruct the normal flow of urine.

Another issue is the frequency of the use of antibiotics. For people who suffer from numerous infections, physicians generally try to use antibiotics from different classes of medications so that a resistance to the antibiotic does not develop. Repeated courses of the same antibiotic may render that antibiotic less effectual or even incapable of killing the same type of bacteria. Sometimes individuals have repeated infections, even those whose doctors have used the common practice of "mixing up" the types of antibiotics to avoid the microbes having an opportunity to develop a resistance to the medication. Such individuals need to be evaluated for another underlying and previously unidentified immune system problem.

*Anticonvulsants*  Anticonvulsants, also known as antiseizure drugs, are medications that are used to treat individuals with seizure disorders, such as epilepsy. Some anticonvulsants are prescribed for other uses; for example, pregabalin (Lyrica) is approved by the Food and Drug Administration (FDA) to treat fibromyalgia. Anticonvulsants can interact with many different medications, and it is generally best for physicians to test the overall kidney function with laboratory tests before prescribing them, especially in elderly individuals. The anticonvulsant acetazolamide (Diamox) should be avoided in all patients with kidney disease.

Some antiseizure medications are associated with an increased risk for particular kidney diseases; for example, topiramate (Topamax) has been associated with an increased risk for the development of KIDNEY STONES.

*Antidepressants* Antidepressants are primarily used to treat depression, although some antidepressants have been employed for other uses; for example, duloxetine (Cymbalta) has been approved by the FDA to treat fibromyalgia. There are several major classes of antidepressants, including monoamine oxidase (MAO) inhibitors, tricyclics, selective serotonin reuptake inhibitors (SSRIs), serontonin norepinephrine inhibitors (SNRIs), and atypical antidepressants such as bupropion (Wellbutrin, Wellbutrin XL).

MAO inhibitors are not recommended for individuals with severe kidney disease. Individuals who do take an MAO inhibitor should avoid taking other antidepressants at the same time and they should also be very careful with any other medications that they take. In addition, a very strict dietary regimen is required with the use of MAO inhibitors because a possibly fatal elevated blood pressure may occur if individuals consume any foods containing a substance known as tyramine while on this medication. The problem is that many disparate foods contain tyramine (avocadoes, bananas, raisins, and salami are only a few of the many foods that have tyramine in them). Individuals must also avoid alcohol completely. For this reason, few physicians prescribe antidepressants that are in this class because it is so difficult for patients to adhere to the necessary dietary regimen.

Tricyclics are older antidepressants which are often sedating. They include such medications as amitriptyline (Elavil), clomipramine (Anafranil), desipramine (Norpramin, Pertofrane), doxepin (Sinequan), imipramine (Tofranil), nortriptyline (Pamelor), protriptyline (Vivactil), and trimipramine (Surmontil). Medications in this class are less commonly prescribed than SSRIs or SNRIs. Amtriptyline has been found to trigger rhabdomyolysis in some individuals.

SSRIs block the reuptake of serotonin, leading to the availability of more serotonin and thus alleviating depressive symptoms in many people. Examples of SSRIs include citalopram (Celexa), escitalopram (Lexapro), fluoxetine (Prozac), fluvoxamine (Luvox), paroxetine (Paxil), and sertraline (Zoloft). Some SSRIs are FDA-approved to treat other psychiatric disorders; for example, fluoxetine (Prozac) is also approved to treat panic disorder, obsessive-compulsive disorder (OCD), and bulimia nervosa. Fluoxetine has been known to trigger rhabdomyolysis in some individuals.

SNRIs act to inhibit the reuptake of serotonin and norepinephrine. Medications in this class include duloxetine (Cymbalta) and venlafaxine (Effexor).

*Antidiabetics* Antidiabetic medications generally refer to medications that are used by individuals with Type 2 diabetes. (All individuals with Type 1 diabetes must use insulin.) Among individuals with Type 2 diabetes, the most commonly prescribed medication is metformin (Glucophage, Glucophage XL), a medication in the biguanide class of antidiabetics, and the only biguanide approved by the FDA for use in the United States. Sometimes metformin is prescribed with other antidiabetic medications. One rare complication that may occur with the use of metformin in individuals with kidney disease is the development of lactic acidosis, a disorder resulting from a buildup of metformin, which can be fatal. This complication is more likely to occur with increasingly severe kidney disease; since kidney disease often escalates with age, older people taking metformin have a greater risk for this complication.

Alpha glucosidase inhibitors are antidiabetics that are not recommended for individuals with known kidney disease, because they may exacerbate the kidney disease.

*Antiemetics* Antiemetics are medications given to treat nausea and vomiting. Some antiemetics are not recommended for individuals with kidney disease; for example, droperidol (Inapsine), a dopamine antagonist, should be used cautiously in those with kidney dysfunction. Lorazepam (Valium), a drug which is used as an antiemetic as well as an antianxiety medication, should also be used cautiously among individuals with kidney disease.

*Antifungal drugs*  Some drugs that are used to treat fungus in the skin, nails, and other parts of the body should be carefully monitored because they may lead to kidney disease. One such medication is amphotericin B, and individuals who take this drug should have their kidney function monitored by the physician, because it may cause irreversible kidney disease and lead to kidney failure.

Among patients with existing kidney disease, the antifungal medication flucytosine (Ancobon) should be used only with caution and at lower than normal dosages.

*Antigout medications*  Some medications are given specifically to treat GOUT, a painful disease that often presents in the inflamed large toe. However, one gout medication, colchicine, has its own risks and should be used with caution in individuals with kidney disease. Chronic gout is often treated with allopurinol (Zyloprim) rather than colchicine; however, individuals who use allopurinol have an increased risk for acute interstitial nephritis.

*Antihistamines*  Antihistamines are medications prescribed for the treatment of allergies or severe colds; however, some antihistamines should be used with caution in patients with kidney disease and often should be used at a lower than normal dosage of the drug. They may be prescribed medications or OTC drugs.

Caution should be used with the following antihistamines: cetirizine (Zyrtec), desloratidine (Clarinex), and loratadine (Claritin), as well as fexofenadine (Allegra). Loratadine is available in a lower dosage as an over-the-counter medication also known as Claritin.

In addition, caution should be used with diphenhydramine (Benadryl) and doxylamine (Unisom), which may lead to the development of rhabdomyolysis.

*Antimigraine medications*  Some medications are prescribed to treat migraine headaches, which are extremely severe headaches that may be preceded by warning "auras," such as seeing lights flashing before the eyes or experiencing feelings of nausea. (Not all chronic migraineurs experience auras, and some patients with migraines experience auras on some occasions and not on others.)

Antimigraine medications are usually taken at the first sign of a migraine attack among those with chronic migraines. Medications that are known as triptans are often used to treat migraines, such as sumatriptan (Imitrex), almotriptan (Axert), rizatriptan (Maxalt), and zolmitriptan (Zomig). Other medications known as ergots are used to treat migraines, including dihydroergotamine (DHE-45, Migranal) and ergotamine tartrate (Ergomar). In general, almotriptan and rizatriptan should be used cautiously with migraine patients who also have kidney disease.

Sometimes medications in other classes of drugs are prescribed off-label to treat migraines, such as antidepressants or antiseizure medications. In such cases, any issues related to potential kidney damage caused by such drugs also apply to their off-label uses for treating migraines.

*Antipsychotics*  Antipsychotic medications are used to treat patients with psychotic disorders, such as schizophrenia, schizoaffective disorder, bipolar disorder, or depression with psychotic features. In general, antipsychotics should be prescribed with caution to individuals who also have kidney disease or disorders.

*Antiretrovirals*  Some antiretroviral medications used to treat individuals with hepatitis B can lead to kidney disease, such as adefovir (Hepsera), cidofovir (Vistide), or tenofovir (Viread). These medications have a risk of causing tubular cell toxicity.

*Calcineurin inhibitors*  Calcineurin inhibitors are medications that are used to suppress the immune system, and they are taken by individuals who receive kidney transplants or other organ transplants. They are also known as IMMUNOSUPPRESSIVE DRUGS. Sometimes their adverse effects may mimic the effect of a rejected organ. Some calcineurin inhibitors may cause chronic interstitial nephritis or thrombotic microangiopathy.

*Cardiovascular medications* Some medications used to prevent stroke or heart attack, sometimes known as antihypertensive medications, may lead to kidney disease; for example, medications in the angiotensin-converting enzyme inhibitor class (known as ACE inhibitors) and angiotensin receptor blockers (ARBs) may affect the dynamics of the kidney. Medications in the statin class may cause rhabdomyolysis. Other cardiovascular medications, such as clopidogreal (Plavix) and ticlopidine (Ticlid) may lead to thrombotic microangiopathy.

*Disease-modifying antirheumatic drugs (DMARDs)* DMARDs are medications that are used to treat rheumatoid arthritis and other serious diseases, and patients taking DMARDs need to be monitored carefully to ensure that their kidney function remains normal.

*Diuretics* Diuretics are medications used to move fluid out of the body and include such medications as thiazides or triamterene (Dyrenium). If overused, they may lead to an ELECTROLYTE imbalance. In addition, as seen in Table 1, the diuretic use of thiazide medications may lead to the development of acute interstitial nephritis, while the use of triamterene may lead to crystal nephropathy.

*Expectorants* Expectorants are prescribed or OTC medications that are used to treat cough and colds, including such medications as guaifenesin. However, over time, such medications may become harmful to the kidneys; for example, the heavy use of medications that are high in guaifenesin may induce the formation of kidney stones.

*Herbal remedies* There are far too many herbal remedies or supplements to describe in this entry; however, researchers do know that Chinese herbals with artistocholic acid can lead to acute interstitial nephritis. It should never be assumed that because herbal remedies, vitamin supplements or other "health" drugs are readily available, then they are automatically safe for everyone. This is not true, and some individuals have died from the use of some dietary supplements, particularly ephedra. As a result, it is important for all patients, with or without diagnosed kidney disease, to tell their physicians about every medication that they take.

*Laxatives* Laxatives are prescribed or OTC medications that are given to treat severe constipation. Many laxatives contain high dosages of SODIUM, and they should be used with care among patients with kidney disease. The excessive use of laxatives can lead to dehydration and electrolyte imbalances.

*Muscle relaxants* Muscle relaxants are drugs that are prescribed to treat people in severe pain from strain, arthritis, and other conditions that cause spasming and extreme muscle pain. They can be harmful to the kidneys over time.

*Nonsteroidal anti-inflammatory drugs (NSAIDs)* NSAIDs are one form of analgesic that needs its own category because medications in this class are used in a very prolific manner in the United States, and most families have OTC NSAIDs readily available in their medicine cabinets to treat everything from headache to back pain to the pain of minor injuries. However, the excessive use of NSAIDs can be harmful to the kidneys because this may lead to either chronic or acute interstitial nephritis, as well as glomerulonephritis.

*Proton pump inhibitors (PPIs)* Proton pump inhibitors are medications that are used to treat chronic gastroesophageal reflux disease, a disorder in which the acidic contents of the stomach move upwards into the esophagus. However, these medications can also be harmful to the kidneys, leading to acute interstitial nephritis.

*Psychiatric drugs* In addition to antidepressants and antipsychotics, there are other categories of medications prescribed for people with psychiatric problems, such as benzodiazepines (antianxiety drugs) and medications to treat alcohol dependence or drug dependence. Some medications can be harmful to the kidneys over time, and physicians should carefully note whether a medication may be harmful and the kidneys should be monitored.

Lithium, a medication that is used to treat bipolar disorder (formerly known as manic depression), can be harmful to the kidneys, causing

### TABLE 1: DRUGS ASSOCIATED WITH NEPHROTOXICITY

| Drug Class/Drug(s) | Pathophysiological Mechanism of Renal Injury |
|---|---|
| **Analgesics** | |
| Acetaminophen, aspirin | Chronic interstitial nephritis |
| Nonsteroidal anti-inflammatory drugs | Acute interstitial nephritis, altered intraglomerular hemodynamics, chronic interstitial nephritis, glomerulonephritis |
| **Antidepressants/mood stabilizers** | |
| Amitriptyline (Elavil*), doxepin (Zonalon), fluoxetine (Prozac) | Rhabdomyolysis |
| Lithium | Chronic interstitial nephritis, glomerulonephritis, rhabdomyolysis |
| **Antihistamines** | |
| Diphenhydramine (Benadryl), doxylamine (Unisom) | Rhabdomyolysis |
| **Antimicrobials** | |
| Acyclovir (Zovirax) | Acute interstitial nephritis, crystal nephropathy |
| Aminoglycosides | Tubular cell toxicity |
| Amphotericin B (Fungizone*); deoxycholic acid formulation more so than the lipid formulation) | Tubular cell toxicity |
| Beta lactams (penicillins, cephalosporins) | Acute interstitial nephritis, glomerulonephritis (ampicillin, penicillin) |
| Foscarnet (Foscavir) | Crystal nephropathy, tubular cell toxicity |
| Ganciclovir (Cytovene) | Crystal nephropathy |
| Pentamidine (Pentam) | Tubular cell toxicity |
| Quinolones | Acute interstitial nephritis, crystal nephropathy (ciprofloxacin [Cipro]) |
| Rifampin (Rifandin) | Acute interstitial nephritis |
| Sulfonamides | Acute interstitial nephritis, crystal nephropathy |
| Vancomycin (Vancodin) | Acute interstitial nephritis |
| **Antiretrovirals** | |
| Adefovir (Hepsera), cidofovir (Vistide), tenofovir (Viread) | Tubular cell toxicity |
| Indinavir (Crixivan) | Acute interstitial nephritis, crystal nephropathy |
| **Benzodiazepines** | Rhabdomyolysis |
| **Calcineurin inhibitors** | |
| Cyclosporine (Neoral) | Altered intraglomerular hemodynamics, chronic interstitial nephritis, thrombotic microangiopathy |
| Tacrolimus (Prograf) | Altered intraglomerular hemodynamics |
| **Cardiovascular agents** | |
| Angiotensin-converting enzyme inhibitors, angiotensin receptor blockers | Altered intraglomerular hemodynamics |
| Clopidogrel (Plavix), ticlopidine (Ticlid) | Thrombotic microangiopathy |
| Statins | Rhabdomyolysis |
| **Chemotherapeutics** | |
| Carmustine (Glidel), semustine (investigational) | Chronic interstitial nephritis |
| Cisplatin (Platinol) | Chronic interstitial nephritis, tubular cell toxicity |
| Interferon-alfa (Intron A) | Glomerulonephritis |
| Methotrexate | Crystal nephropathy |
| Mitomycin-C (Mutamycin) | Thrombotic microangiopathy |

| Drug Class/Drug(s) | Pathophysiological Mechanism of Renal Injury |
| --- | --- |
| **Contrast dye** | Tubular cell nephropathy |
| **Diuretics** | |
| Loops, thiazides | Acute interstitial nephritis |
| Triamterene (Dyrenium) | Crystal nephropathy |
| **Drugs of abuse** | |
| Cocaine, heroin, ketamine (Ketalar), methadone, methamphetamine | Rhabdomyolysis |
| **Herbals** | |
| Chinese herbals with aristocholic acid | Chronic interstitial nephritis |
| **Proton pump inhibitors** | |
| Lansoprazole (Prevacid), omeprazole (Prilosec), pantoprazole (Protonix) | Acute interstitial nephritis |
| **Others** | |
| Allopurinal (Zyloprim) | Acute interstitial nephritis |
| Gold therapy | Glomerulonephritis |
| Haloperidol (Haldol) | Rhabdomyolysis |
| Pamidronate (Aredia) | Glomerulonephritis |
| Phenytoin (Dilantin) | Acute interstitial nephritis |
| Quinine (Qualaquin) | Thrombotic microangiopathy |
| Ranitidine (Zantac) | Acute interstitial nephritis |
| Zoledronate (Zometa) | Tubular cell toxicity |

*Brand not available in the United States

Source: Naughton, Cynthia A. "Drug-induced Nephrotoxicity." *American Family Physician* 78, no. 6 (2008): p. 745. Reprinted with permission.

such disorders as chronic interstitial nephritis, glomerulonephritis, and rhabdomyolysis.

**Radiocontrast dye** Radiocontrast media is given to individuals receiving some imaging techniques in order to highlight potential problem areas. Among adults, from 1 to 20 percent have an adverse response to radiocontrast media, and the percentage of adverse responses is unknown in children. One serious adverse reaction to radiocontrast dye is the development of tubular cell nephropathy.

Once an adverse response occurs, that patient should avoid radiocontrast dyes in the future because the second reaction could be more amplified than the first reaction.

### Drugs of Abuse

Some individuals misuse or abuse both legal and illegal drugs, and such abuse can lead to serious kidney problems. For example, the abuse of drugs such as cocaine, ketamine (Ketalar), methadone, or methamphetamine can lead to rhabdomyolysis. Cocaine can be used legally by physicians to treat eye disorders, and ketamine is used as an anesthetic. Methadone is used to treat individuals with a heroin addiction, and some forms of amphetamine are used to treat attention deficit/hyperactivity disorder (ADHD).

### Special Populations of Individuals

Some individuals have a greater risk for harm to their kidneys from medication use than others, particularly those whose kidneys have already begun to fail, elderly people who often have an impaired ability to metabolize medications, hospital patients with impaired kidney function, and children, who are vulnerable to the nephrotoxic effects of medications and other chemicals. This section covers these four groups of people.

***Individuals whose kidneys have begun to fail***   When kidney failure has begun, it becomes increasingly difficult to identify medications that are safe for the individual to use. As a result, it is very important for the individual with worsening kidney disease to consult with a nephrologist about all medications that are used.

***Elderly individuals and medications that may harm their kidneys***   Many older individuals need to take lower dosages of medications because they metabolize the drug at a slower rate than younger individuals, whether the medication is metabolized by the liver or the kidneys. Higher dosage of medications, including dosages which would be safe for a healthy younger person, could be toxic to the older individual.

***Hospital patients and renal risk drugs***   One place where it would seem to be safe to conclude that patients with impaired kidney function would not receive renal risk drugs is the hospital environment. Yet such an assumption would be incorrect, based on research performed in Norway by Hege Salvesen Blix and colleagues and reported in *Nephrology Dialysis Transplantation* in 2006. In this study of 808 hospitalized patients, the researchers found that 36 percent had normal kidney function and the rest had some level of impairment based on their glomerular filtration rates, which were assessed by a multidisciplinary hospital team.

The researchers found that all but six patients with moderate to severe kidney disease received two or more renal risk drugs. The most commonly used medications were the following: antibacterials (antibiotics), antithrombotics, angiotensin-converting enzyme (ACE) inhibitors, opioids, and NSAIDs. Other drugs that were given were medications such as allopurinol and colchicines (antigout medications), statins such as simvastatin, and benzodiazepines such as diazepam (Valium), among others. The researchers also found that the patients with moderate to severe impaired renal function were prescribed more medications than those with mild renal impairment.

The researchers said, "The main reason for this was that the patients in the former group were older and had more accompanying comorbidities; for example, diabetes, hypertension and cardiac diseases, which evoke decline of renal function in addition to the genuine age-related decine. Thus, the pharmacotherapy of the elderly becomes more abundant and more complex, contributing to the high proportion of renal risk drugs being used in patients with non-adequate renal function. We did, however, find a lower ratio of renal risk drugs in the patients with the most severe RI [renal impairment], indicating somewhat heightened awareness directed towards that group."

The researchers also noted that the list of renal risk drugs is extensive and includes some medications that may benefit patients with some kidney disease, such as ACE inhibitors, which generally do not cause a problem. They also speculated that since ACE inhibitors are on the list of renal risk drugs, the assumption may be made that the renal risk drug list is overcautious. However, there is a risk for kidney disease with these medications, and thus kidney function should be monitored in patients taking these drugs.

In addition, they noted that dosages regarding combinations of renal risk drugs were not addressed in literature, although the researchers found that most patients received two or more renal risk medications. Thus, physicians had to decide for themselves how to judge risks and, if they decided the medications were needed, to determine the dosage themselves.

***Children and nephrotoxicity***   Sometimes renal risk drugs can cause nephrotoxicity in children, as described by Ludwig Patzer in *Pediatric Nephrology* in 2008. According to Patzer, nephrotoxic drugs represent about 16 percent of all causes of ACUTE KIDNEY INJURY in children and adolescents. Patzer said, "Nonsteroidal anti-inflammatory drugs (NSAIDs), antibiotics, amphotericin B, antiviral agents, angiotensin-converting enzyme (ACE) inhibitors, calcineurin inhibitors, radiocontrast media, and cytostatics are the most important drugs to indicate AKI as significant risk in children." Patzer says that these substances can lead to acute tubular necrosis, acute interstitial nephritis, and sometimes tubular obstruction.

Patzer says that some medications are known to cause acute kidney injury; for example ACE inhibitors, NSAIDs, diuretics, and some medications such as norepinephrine (and others) are known to cause prerenal failure. Medications known to cause acute tubular necrosis include such drugs as cephalosporins (commonly prescribed antibiotics), amphotericin B, rifampicin, foscarent, pentamidine, and vancomycin. In addition, NSAIDs, acetaminophen, contrast media (radiocontrast material that is used in some diagnostic tests) and other drugs can lead to acute tubular necrosis. (See Table 1.)

See also ANALGESIC NEPHROPATHY.

Blix, Hege Salvesen, et al. "Use of Renal Risk Drugs in Hospitalized Patients with Impaired Renal Function—An Underestimated Problem?" *Nephrology Dialysis Transplantation* 21 (2006): 3,164–3,171.

Cassell, Dana K., and Cynthia A. Sanoski. *The Encyclopedia of Pharmaceutical Drugs.* New York: Facts On File. In press for 2012.

Mazer, M., and J. Perrone. "Acetaminophen-Induced Nephrotoxicity: Pathophysiology, Clinical Manifestations, and Management." *Journal of Medical Toxicity* 4, no. 1 (2008): 2–6.

Naughton, Cynthia A. "Drug-Induced Nephrotoxicity." *American Family Physician* 78, no. 6 (2008): 743–750.

Patzer, Ludwig. "Nephrotoxicity as a Cause of Acute Kidney Injury in Children." *Pediatric Nephrology* 23 (2008): 2,159–2,173.

Stroup, J., and J. Stephens. "Combination Drug Products: An Indication for Medication Reconciliation and Pharmacist Counseling." *Journal of the American Pharmacy Association* 48, no. 4 (2008): 541–543.

Taber, S. S., and D. A. Pasko. "The Epidemiology of Drug-Induced Disorders: The Kidney." *Expert Opinions on Drug Safety* 7, no. 6 (2008): 679–690.

**medullary sponge kidneys (MSK)** Kidneys with a birth defect inside the tiny tubes (tubules) of the kidneys. With normal kidneys, the urine travels through these tubules, but with medullary sponge kidneys (MSK), tiny cysts form in terminal portions of the renal tubules and create a spongy appearance to the kidney. These cysts can lead to an increased risk of KIDNEY STONES, and a frequent recurrence of stones, if they do occur. The actual number of people with medullary sponge kidney disease is unknown, as it is usually not diagnosed unless it causes symptoms. As many as 20 percent of people with recurrent kidney stones, however, have medullary sponge kidney disease. MSK does not usually cause kidney failure or other serious kidney diseases except kidney stones.

### Symptoms and Diagnostic Path

A kidney stone or a urinary tract infection (CYSTITIS) is often the first indicator of MSK, and often does not occur until the person is 30–40 years old. Sometimes there are no symptoms or signs of the disorder, and it goes undiagnosed. Other signs and symptoms may include the following:

- BACK PAIN and pain in the lower abdomen or groin
- fever and chills
- urine that is cloudy, dark, or bloody
- pain or burning with urination
- excretion of large amounts of urine

If an individual has repeated kidney stones or urinary tract infections (UTIs), the doctor may suspect that they are caused by MSK. The diagnosis can be confirmed with an intravenous pyelogram (IVP), in which dye is injected into a vein and travels to the kidneys. The IVP will show the accumulation of the contrast dye in the dilated cysts. Because IVP is less commonly used in the 21st century than in past years, other tests may be necessary for diagnosis. An abdominal computerized tomography (CT) scan can detect calcium deposition in these dilated terminal cysts, but the findings are not diagnostic of medullary sponge kidney disease. The use of specialized testing, such as helical CT or CT urography, may enable a more accurate diagnosis.

### Treatment Options and Outlook

MSK cannot be cured but the symptoms can be treated. Individuals with frequent UTIs are treated with ANTIBIOTICS and may be given a low dose of antibiotic to prevent an infection from occurring. Kidney stones are treated with LITHOTRIPSY, a procedure that is used to break the kidney stones up. Some stones may be prevented in the future by the individual increasing the intake of fluid. The patient with recurrent kidney stones should have a routine evaluation to determine whether there are abnormal amounts of specific solutes in the urine, and if present, they should be treated.

### Risk Factors and Preventive Measures

There are no known risk factors or preventive measures for MSK. If symptoms develop, then they should be treated.

## membranoproliferative glomerulonephritis

**(MPGN)**   A rare autoimmune kidney disease that primarily affects children and young adults. MPGN causes an inflammation of the kidneys, scarring the glomeruli (the tiny filtration units within the kidneys), and resulting in blood in the urine (hematuria). MPGN may lead to CHRONIC KIDNEY DISEASE and to the development of END-STAGE RENAL DISEASE (kidney failure). This disorder may be triggered by an infection with HEPATITIS C or the human immunodeficiency virus (HIV).

There are two forms of MPGN, including membranoproliferative GN Type I and membranoproliferative GN Type II. Type I is much more common.

### Symptoms and Diagnostic Path

Urinary symptoms are common with MPGN, including hematuria, cloudy urine, dark urine, and a decrease in the overall urinary volume. Some individuals with MPGN experience decreased mental concentration or decreased alertness. Edema (swelling) is another common symptom and can occur anywhere in the body. The person often has high blood pressure as well.

Individuals who may have MPGN are tested with a urinalysis, a test of urine protein levels (PROTEINURIA), and also tests for the levels of blood urea nitrogen (BUN) and creatinine. Confirmation of the diagnosis requires a KIDNEY BIOPSY, as many other forms of glomerulonephritis can cause similar symptoms.

### Treatment Options and Outlook

The physician treats the symptoms of MPGN and tries to slow them from worsening. Patients may be prescribed ANTIHYPERTENSIVE DRUGS as well as DIURETICS and steroids. DIETARY CHANGES may be recommended, such as limiting the consumption of SODIUM and fluids. Treating the underlying disease is the most effective therapy. This is particularly true for the person with hepatitis C that is causing their membranoproliferative GN. In these patients, effective treatment of the hepatitis C infection can result in stabilization and sometimes improvement and even resolution of the kidney disease.

Many people with MPGN develop chronic kidney failure and in about half the cases, the kidneys fail within 10 years.

### Risk Factors and Preventive Measures

Most people affected by MPGN are males and females younger than age 30. Effective therapy of hepatitis C infection can prevent the development of hepatitis C-associated membranoproliferative glomerulonephritis.

See also GLOMERULONEPHRITIS; URINE/URINALYSIS/URINE CULTURE.

## membranous nephropathy   A disorder that

causes harmful deposits and a thickening on the glomerular membrane, which is the part of the kidneys that filters waste and extra fluid from the blood; as a result, membranous nephropathy impairs this ability. The disorder can be a primary membranous disease, in which the underlying cause is not known. It can also be a secondary membranous disease that develops in patients with other types of systemic diseases. Membranous nephropathy is a common cause of NEPHROTIC SYNDROME in adults.

### Symptoms and Diagnostic Path

Sometimes there are no symptoms of membranous nephropathy. When symptoms occur, the following symptoms may indicate its presence:

- edema in any part of the body
- weight gain
- poor appetite
- a foamy appearance of the urine

The physician will evaluate the patient's symptoms and usually order a urinalysis, which may show blood in the urine (hematuria) or protein in the urine (PROTEINURIA). Blood levels of albumin may be low, while blood lipid levels may be elevated. A KIDNEY BIOPSY is necessary to confirm the presence of membranous nephropathy, as many other conditions can cause similar symptoms.

### Treatment Options and Outlook

The treatment goal is to resolve the symptoms and delay the progression of the disease. General supportive care is needed, including control of blood pressure and edema and control of the lipid abnormalities that often accompany heavy proteinuria. Decreasing salt consumption may help the patient to decrease edema. Some patients may need vitamin D supplements if nephrotic syndrome is a chronic problem that does not respond to therapy.

Patients with membranous nephropathy are at risk for blood clots in the legs and lungs, and they may be prescribed blood thinner medications to prevent clots. In addition to the treatment of edema, hyperlipidemia, and hypertension, the inhibition of the renin-angiotensin system is necessary to help to reduce the degree of proteinuria. In some cases, ANGIOTENSIN-CONVERTING ENZYME INHIBITOR medications combined with ANGIOTENSIN II RECEPTOR BLOCKERS (ARBs) will reduce proteinuria further. Therapy with IMMUNOSUPPRESSIVE DRUGS can be used in patients with primary membranous disease and persistent proteinuria (more than 3.0 g/24 hours).

The outlook varies, and 30 to 50 percent of patients with membranous nephropathy may develop irreversible kidney damage within two to 20 years. Of those patients, an estimated 20 percent will develop END-STAGE RENAL DISEASE (kidney failure), according to the National Institutes of Health. Progressive disease that eventually leads to end-stage renal disease can develop in 14 percent of patients after five years, 35 percent at 10 years, and 41 percent at 15 years. Patients with nonselective proteinuria may develop thrombotic complications. However, patients with membranous disease are at the highest risk for such complications. MPGN has the highest reported incidences of renal vein thrombosis, pulmonary embolism, and deep vein thrombosis.

On a positive note, spontaneous remissions occur in one-third of patients and may occur after a long period with nephrotic syndrome. Another one-third of patients continue to have relapsing nephrotic syndrome but they usually maintain normal renal function. The final one-third of patients may develop renal failure, and they will need DIALYSIS therapy or KIDNEY TRANSPLANTATION. Occasionally patients may die from the complications of nephrotic syndrome.

### Risk Factors and Preventive Measures

Risk factors that may lead to a bad prognosis include male gender, older age, the concomitant presence of HYPERTENSION, greater degrees of proteinura, and the persistence of proteinuria that does not resolve spontaneously or with therapy. The use of blood thinner medication to decrease the risk of blood clots is controversial, but it has been recommended for patients with severe or prolonged proteinuria in the absence of risk factors for bleeding.·

Researchers have found that some diseases can cause membranous nephropathy; for example, the presence of some autoimmune diseases such as systemic lupus erythematosus (SLE), rheumatoid arthritis, and ankylosing spondylitis may increase the risk for membranous nephropathy. Infectious diseases, such as hepatitis B, HEPATITIS C, syphilis, leprosy, and recurrent malaria also can cause membranous nephropathy.

In patients older than 60 years, 5–10 percent of the cases of membranous nephropathy can be due to an underlying malignancy. Such malignancies include solid organ tumors, such as colon cancer, lung cancer, or lymphomas. Treating the cancer can cause the membranous nephropathy to resolve. Some drugs can cause membranous type disease, such as the use of gold, captopril, penicillanine, and rarely, the use of NONSTEROIDAL ANTI-INFLAMMATORY DRUGS (NSAIDs).

Membranous nephropathy may be diagnosed in individuals of any age but it most commonly occurs in those older than 40 years. The disease may manifest with the onset of allergic reactions, a viral infection, or with recent immunizations.

See also LUPUS NEPHRITIS; URINE/URINALYSIS/URINE CULTURE.

**minimal change disease (MCD)** A kidney disorder that results in the loss of proteins into the urine. A protein leak in itself does not mean that the disease is minimal change disease (MCD) because there are many causes of urinary protein losses. Because different causes require different treatments, a person with high levels of urinary protein losses may need to be evaluated with a KIDNEY BIOPSY. Most of the time minimal change disease (MCD) is associated with a protein leak in combination with generalized swelling. This disease is termed "minimal change disease" because the changes to the kidney are so minimal that they cannot be seen with a light microscope and require a specialized electron microscope to visualize.

Minimal change disease is the most common cause of NEPHROTIC SYNDROME (NS) in children and adolescents (70–90 percent). It is so common in children that children with nephrotic syndrome are often treated for this condition without a kidney biopsy. Children who do not respond well to treatment may then undergo a kidney biopsy in order to define the exact cause of their protein leak. In adults, MCD is a cause of NS in less than 15 percent of people with nephrotic syndrome, and requires a renal biopsy.

According to Abeera Mansur, M.D., and colleagues, MCD may be caused by medications, especially NONSTEROIDAL ANTI-INFLAMMATORY DRUGS (NSAIDs), as well as interferon, some ANTIBIOTICS, such as ampicillin/penicillin, and other medications. In addition, infections with infectious mononucleosis or the human immunodeficiency virus (HIV) may cause a secondary MCD. Some tumors, most commonly Hodgkin's lymphoma, may lead to MCD. MCD that has an identifiable cause is termed secondary MCD.

### Symptoms and Diagnostic Path

Patients with MCD typically have the symptoms of nephrotic syndrome, and high (greater than 3.5 gm per day) levels of urinary protein losses, edema, high cholesterol levels, and low albumin levels in their blood. Occasionally, MCD may result in hematuria (blood in the urine), although the presence of hematuria should lead to an aggressive search for the underlying cause, most commonly, systemic lupus erythematosus. MCD may rarely lead to blood clots in the renal veins (renal vein thrombosis), which can lead to flank pain and acute renal failure. In the absence of renal vein thrombosis, kidney failure is rarely seen with MCD.

Other symptoms may include poor appetite, weight gain caused by fluid retention, and foamy urine.

Blood and urine tests show abnormalities, including proteinuria, low blood levels of albumin, and high cholesterol. A kidney biopsy of tissue examined under an electron microscope will reveal signs of minimal change disease.

### Treatment Options and Outlook

Almost all children with MCD are treated with glucocorticoid steroids, and almost all will respond with a dramatic decrease in the urinary protein loss and with improvement in their edema and cholesterol and albumin levels. After stopping the steroids, approximately one in three will have rare (less than twice a year) recurrences, and about one in three will have frequent (twice a year or more often) recurrences. Children who do not respond to steroids or have frequent recurrences may need a kidney biopsy to confirm the diagnosis and evaluate the possibility of a different cause. Most children with MCD develop a complete remission after six to eight weeks of steroid therapy. However, most adults with MCD need more than six months of steroid therapy before achieving a remission.

Children with MCD who do not respond to steroids may have FOCAL SEGMENTAL GLOMERULOSCLEROSIS (FSGS) instead of MCD. This disorder can be identified with a kidney biopsy. It is important to recognize that patients with FSGS may not have identifiable changes of FSGS on a renal biopsy and may be mistakenly identified as having MCD. In the case of a person not responding well to therapy for MCD, one or more kidney biopsies may be necessary to consider, and even reconsider, the possibility of FSGS.

Relapses occur in many children after the first remission, and an early relapse is predictive for future relapses. Relapses are less common in adults but are more resistant to subsequent therapy.

### Risk Factors and Preventive Measures

MCD is about twice as common in boys as in girls. Among adults, the frequency is the same among men and women.

There are no known preventive measures to minimal change disease.

See also CHILDREN AND KIDNEY DISEASE.

Mansur, Abeera, M.D., Florin Georgescu, M.D., and Susie Lew, M.D. "Minimal-Change Disease." eMedicine Nephrology. June 11, 2007. Available online. URL: http://emedicine.medscape.com/article/243348-overview. Accessed September 14, 2009.

**multiple myeloma**   See MYELOMA KIDNEY.

**myeloma kidney**   Kidney disease that is caused by multiple myeloma, a bone marrow cancer that is caused by the excessive growth of the plasma cells. According to the National Cancer Institute (NCI), this disease affects about 16,000 people in the United States and is more common among the elderly. Because the disease causes an excessive production of CALCIUM (HYPERCALCEMIA) or myeloma protein, it can damage the kidneys, leading to weakness and lethargy. The disease also causes high levels of protein in the blood and urine (PROTEINURIA) and ANEMIA. DIALYSIS may be needed if the kidneys fail, or alternatively, a KIDNEY TRANSPLANTATION may be given.

The cause of multiple myeloma is unknown. Patients with multiple myeloma are more susceptible to dehydration-induced acute renal failure. It is important to differentiate this condition from myeloma kidney, as dehydration-induced acute renal failure can be treated with intravenous fluids and hydration.

### Symptoms and Diagnostic Path

According to the NCI, common symptoms of multiple myeloma are the following:

- bone pain in the back and ribs
- broken bones, usually in the spine
- weakness and fatigue
- extreme thirst
- frequent infections and fevers
- weight loss
- nausea or constipation
- frequent urination

A bone marrow biopsy and various blood tests can help to diagnose multiple myeloma; for example, a complete blood count (CBC) is needed to check for anemia, along with chemistry panels that assess kidney function, such as tests for creatinine and blood urea nitrogen (BUN) levels. It is also important to test for calcium levels and CHOLESTEROL levels. The urine can be tested for abnormal myeloma protein, testing for Bence Jones protein over 24 hours. The bones can be tested for bone damage with X-rays or computerized tomography (CT) scans. The presence of abnormal immunoglobulin proteins, which results from the plasma cell cancer, can be detected either in the blood or the urine. Testing for these abnormal proteins in both the urine and the blood is important because some patients may have the abnormal proteins only in the blood or only in the urine.

### Treatment Options and Outlook

Multiple myeloma and myeloma kidney cannot usually be cured (although a bone marrow transplant could mean a cure and some medications provide remission of the symptoms), so the goal is often to stabilize the disease. Medications are given to reduce the high levels of calcium, and plasmapheresis, a process that removes proteins from the blood, is given to thin the blood when necessary.

Older medications that may be used are thalidomide combined with dexamethasone or melphalan/prednisone. (Thalidomide is known for having caused birth defects many years ago;

it can be effective in treating some diseases in nonpregnant women.) Newer medications that may bring remission are VAD (Vincristine/Adriamycin/dexamethasone) and Velcade alone or combined with Melphalan and prednisone. These medications have benefits and side effects. Consultation with an experienced oncologist is important in the treatment of multiple myeloma. (For more information, go to the International Myeloma Foundation Web site at www.myeloma.org.)

Some people are treated with a stem cell transplant from a family member or other donor. Stem cells can also be removed from the patient, treated, frozen, and stored. Then they are thawed and returned to the patient.

### Risk Factors and Preventive Measures

The onset of multiple myeloma usually occurs in individuals ages 60 years and older. It is more common in men and in African Americans. According to the NCI, Asians have the least risk for this disorder. Only patients suffering from multiple myeloma can develop myeloma kidney.

See also BLADDER CANCER; KIDNEY CANCER.

Durie, Brian G. M., M.D. *Multiple Myeloma: Cancer of the Bone Marrow. Patient Handbook.* North Hollywood, Calif.: International Myeloma Foundation, 2009.
National Cancer Institute. What You Need to Know about Multiple Myeloma. National Institutes of Health, September 2008.

**nephritic syndrome** A condition that is defined by the presence of HYPERTENSION, microscopic hematuria (blood in the urine), and red blood cell casts in the urine. Nephritic syndrome is a GLOMERULAR DISEASE, as is nephrotic syndrome.

### Symptoms and Diagnostic Path

Many patients with nephritic syndrome experience high blood pressure. If renal function is impaired, they may develop peripheral edema. Some causes of nephritic syndrome are associated with the effects in tissues other than the kidneys. This may include skin rashes; sinus disease; lung disease and bleeding into the lung; fever, particularly at nighttime while the patient is sleeping and leading to otherwise unexplained sweating at nighttime; unexplained weight loss, and unexplained malaise and fatigue.

Laboratory tests help the doctor with diagnosis. The level of proteinuria is generally modest with nephritic syndrome, and is less than 2 g/day in adults. In contrast, NEPHROTIC SYNDROME is a condition of higher levels of proteinuria than with nephritic syndrome, or greater than 3.5 g/day in adults and greater than 40 mg/kg in children, and in which hematuria is either absent or minimal. In addition, the person with nephrotic syndrome also has edema (excess fluid and swelling) and low levels of serum albumin, as well as elevated levels of blood CHOLESTEROL. Nephritic syndrome is often associated with clinically important kidney disease and may require investigation into the etiology, which may even require a KIDNEY BIOPSY.

### Treatment Options and Outlook

The identification of nephritic syndrome indicates the presence of substantial amounts of ongoing inflammation in the kidney, particularly in the glomeruli, the filtering unit of the kidney. If nephritic syndrome is not treated, it can progress to irreversible damage to the kidney in many cases and lead to irreversible renal failure. There are multiple causes of nephritic syndrome, ranging from slowly progressive, as commonly is found with IgA NEPHROPATHY, to rapidly progressive, as may occur with lupus nephritis, Wegener's granulomatosis, and anti-GBM disease. Appropriate treatment can prevent many of the complications of nephritic syndrome and can even result in reversal of existing disease. The appropriate treatment regimens differ substantially with different causes of nephritic syndrome. An accurate diagnosis depends upon laboratory studies. In many cases, a renal biopsy is important in order to guide therapy.

The outlook for nephritic syndrome depends on how early it is diagnosed and the specific cause of an individual patient's nephritic syndrome. In general, the earlier that the syndrome is diagnosed and the less irreversible kidney damage has occurred, the better the likelihood for restoration of normal renal function and avoidance of or minimization of irreversible damage and avoidance of need for dialysis or a renal transplant. Also, the more rapidly nephritic syndrome has developed, the greater the chance for speedy improvement, and vice versa.

### Risk Factors and Preventive Measures

Individuals with serious kidney disease are at risk for nephritic syndrome. There are no known preventive measures.

**nephritis, interstitial**    See INTERSTITIAL NEPHRITIS.

**nephrogenic diabetes insipidus**    See DIABETES INSIPIDUS.

**nephrolithiasis**    See KIDNEY STONES.

**nephrologists**    Physicians who specialize in the treatment of kidney disease and its related disorders. Because nephrologists have an active knowledge of and interest in kidney disease, it is best that patients with kidney disease are treated by these specialists. In fact, one study that was published in *Archives of Internal Medicine* in 2008 showed that those patients who were diagnosed with a moderate to severe kidney disease that was also combined with DIABETES MELLITUS actually had a *lower* risk of death when their treatment team included a nephrologist. Yet disturbingly, the study also showed that many patients who had a serious kidney disease that had occurred prior to their beginning DIALYSIS were not treated by a nephrologist.

According to data released in 2009 by the United States Renal Data System (USRDS), an organization that tracks data on individuals with END-STAGE RENAL DISEASE (ESRD) and who receive dialysis or KIDNEY TRANSPLANTATION, only 27 percent of new dialysis patients have received more than 12 months of pre-ESRD care from a nephrologist.

To locate a nephrologist, individuals should ask their primary care physician for a recommendation. Their health insurance company may also have a list of nephrologists in the area. Verify that the nephrologist is board-certified in nephrology by not only asking the staff if the doctor is board-certified but also by checking with the American Board of Internal Medicine at http://www.abim.org/services/physver.aspx.

See also CHRONIC KIDNEY DISEASE.

eHow. "How to Find a Nephrologist." Available online. URL: http://www.ehow.com/how_2071732_find-nephrologist.html. Accessed November 5, 2010.

Tseng, Chin-Lin, et al. "Survival Benefit of Nephrologic Care in Patients with Diabetes Mellitus and Chronic Kidney Disease." *Archives of Internal Medicine* 168, no. 1 (January 14, 2008): 55–62.

United States Renal Data System. *USRDS 2009 Annual Data Report: Atlas of Chronic Kidney Disease and End-Stage Renal Disease in the United States.* Bethesda, Md.: National Institutes of Health, National Institute of Diabetes and Digestive and Kidney Diseases, 2009.

**nephropathies of systemic lupus nephritis**    See LUPUS NEPHRITIS.

**nephropathy, analgesic**    See ANALGESIC NEPHROPATHY.

**nephropathy, crystal**    See CRYSTAL NEPHROPATHY.

**nephropathy, diabetic**    See DIABETIC NEPHROPATHY.

**nephropathy, IgA**    See IGA NEPHROPATHY.

**nephropathy, membranous**    See MEMBRANOUS NEPHROPATHY.

**nephropathy, reflux**    See REFLUX NEPHROPATHY.

**nephrotic syndrome**    A set of symptoms that indicates that a person's kidneys are losing excessive amounts of protein, and therefore is an indication of relatively severe kidney disease. These symptoms include losing more than 3.5 g per day of protein in the URINE, a high blood CHOLESTEROL level, a low level of the protein albumin in the blood, and the presence of peripheral edema. Nephrotic syndrome is also known as nephrosis. The most common cause of nephrotic syndrome among children is MINIMAL CHANGE DISEASE. In adults, nephrotic syndrome may result from many different causes, such as genetic disorders, autoimmune disorders, the use of some medications, and diseases such as AMYLOIDOSIS, cancer, DIABETES MELLITUS, and systemic lupus erythematosus (SLE). (See LUPUS NEPHRITIS.) In adults, the most likely cause of nephrotic syndrome not associated with any of the diagnoses listed above differs depending on the individual's race. For example, FOCAL SEGMENTAL GLOMERULOSCLEROSIS (FSGS) is the most common cause of nephrotic syndrome in African-American adults, while membranous glomerulonephritis is the most common cause in Caucasian adults.

### Symptoms and Diagnostic Path

The most common symptom related to nephrotic syndrome is peripheral edema. In children, it particularly involves the tissues around the eyes, and is most prominent in the morning. Peripheral edema may even lead to fluid accumulation in the abdominal cavity, known as ascites. In adults, peripheral edema typically involves the ankles and feet. The large amounts of proteinuria that are present can lead to a frothing appearance of the urine in the toilet. The low serum albumin and high cholesterol levels may be identified by appropriate blood testing. Some other common symptoms of nephrotic syndrome include

- abdominal swelling
- facial swelling
- unintentional weight gain caused by fluid retention
- poor appetite

Nephrotic syndrome is often initially suspected because the urinalysis shows substantial amounts of proteinuria. The diagnosis should then be confirmed by either a 24-hour urine collection for protein quantification that shows greater than 3.5 g per day proteinuria or by a random urine protein to creatinine ratio showing a ratio greater than 3.5 g protein per gram creatinine.

A blood test for diabetes may be ordered to rule out diabetes mellitus and tests for hepatitis B and C may be indicated as well. In selected cases, serologic testing for systemic lupus erythematosus (SLE) and for other autoimmune diseases may be helpful.

The physician may order imaging of the kidneys with ultrasound. In many cases, a KIDNEY BIOPSY is necessary to determine the specific cause of the nephrotic syndrome.

### Treatment Options and Outlook

Treatment depends on the disease or disorder that is diagnosed. An accurate diagnosis is necessary in order to guide therapy. Medications may be prescribed for swelling and edema, such as DIURETICS. ANGIOTENSIN-CONVERTING ENZYME INHIBITOR (ACEI) medications are often prescribed irrespective of the specific cause of the nephrotic syndrome because of their generalized effectiveness in decreasing proteinuria. If the patient is hypertensive, then the high blood pressure must be treated. In addition, individuals with nephrotic syndrome are restricted with regard to both their water and salt consumption. Corticosteroids may also be needed.

### Risk Factors and Preventive Measures

Nephrotic syndrome generally occurs among young children with kidney disease. In adults, avoidance and/or treatment of conditions that can cause the renal diseases that cause nephrotic syndrome is key to avoiding this complication. This includes aggressive control of blood pressure and blood glucose in patients with diabetes mellitus, weight loss in the obese patient, immunization to prevent hepatitis B infections, and avoidance of risk factors for hepatitis C infection.

**nephrotoxicity of medications** See CHILDREN AND KIDNEY DISEASE; MEDICATIONS THAT CAN HARM THE KIDNEYS.

**nonsteroidal anti-inflammatory drugs (NSAIDs)** Prescribed or over-the-counter (OTC) medications that are taken to relieve inflammatory pain, such as the pain that is caused by rheumatoid arthritis, various other forms of arthritis, BACK PAIN, or menstrual cramps; however, NSAIDs can also cause damage to the kidneys over time, up to and including kidney failure. They can also impair the effectiveness of ANTIHYPERTENSIVE DRUGS and DIURETICS, leading to worsening of HYPERTENSION and ineffective therapy for peripheral edema and/or pulmonary edema. In addition, individuals taking NSAIDs may develop bleeding and ulcers in the stomach and intestine.

A specialized class of nonsteroidal anti-inflammatory drugs, termed cyclooxygenase-two (Cox-two) inhibitors, are used frequently because they are associated with a lesser risk of gastro-intestinal irritation and bleeding. However, they appear to have similar effects as conventional nonsteroidals on the kidneys and on responsiveness to diuretics.

NSAIDs are among the most widely used drugs in the United States, both among prescribed and OTC medications. The use of these types of painkillers can sometimes result in different types of kidney diseases, including

- acute kidney injury, also known as acute renal failure
- NEPHROTIC SYNDROME
- INTERSTITIAL NEPHRITIS
- development of KIDNEY CANCER

Typically, the development of nephrotic syndrome and interstitial nephritis occur in parallel. This occurrence is frequently an unpredictable side effect and resolves with discontinuation of the medication. ACUTE KIDNEY INJURY may occur in patients with congestive heart failure, volume depletion, or acute or chronic liver disease who are treated with nonsteroidal anti-inflammatory drugs. Typically, this will also resolve with discontinuation of the medication.

Individuals taking NSAIDs who experience the following symptoms should contact their physicians right away:

- shortness of breath or trouble breathing
- chest pain

- weakness in one part or one side of the body
- slurred speech
- swelling of the face or throat

According to the Food and Drug Administration (FDA), an NSAID medication should be stopped immediately and the health care provider called if any of the following symptoms occur:

- nausea
- feeling more tired or weaker than usual
- itching

| TABLE 1: NSAID MEDICATIONS THAT NEED A PRESCRIPTION | |
|---|---|
| **Generic Name** | **Trade Name** |
| Celecoxib | Celebrex |
| Diclonfenac | Cataflam, Voltaren, Arthrotec (combined with misoprostol) |
| Diflunisal | Dolobid |
| Etodolac | Lodine, Lodine XL |
| Fenoprofen | Nalfon, Nalfon 200 |
| Flurbiprofen | Ansaid |
| Ibuprofen | Motrin, Tab-Profen, Vicoprofen * (combined with hydrocodone), Combunox (combined with oxycodone) |
| Indomethacin | Indocin, Indocin SR, Indo-Lemmon, Indomethagan |
| Ketoprofen | Oruvail |
| Ketolorac | Toradol |
| Mefenamic acid | Ponstel |
| Meloxicam | Mobic |
| Nabumetone | Relafen |
| Naproxen | Naprosyn, Anaprox, Anaprox DS, EC-Naprosyn, Naprelan, NapraPAC (copackaged with lansoprazole) |
| Oxaprozin | Daypro |
| Piroxicam | Feldene |
| Sulindac | Clinoril |
| Tolmetin | Tolectin, Tolectin DS, Tolectin 600 |

*Vicoprofen contains the narcotic analgesic, hydrocodone, in conjunction with the same dose of ibuprofen as in over-the-counter (OTC) NSAIDs, and is usually used for less than 10 days to treat pain. The OTC NSAID label warns that long-term continuous use may increase the risk of heart attack or stroke.

Source: Food and Drug Administration. Available online. URL: http://www.fda.gov/downloads/Drugs/DrugSafety/ucm088646.pdf. Undated. Accessed February 9, 2010.

- skin or eyes that look yellow (jaundiced)
- stomach pain
- flu-like symptoms
- vomiting blood
- blood in the bowel movement or a bowel movement that is black and sticky like tar
- skin rash or blisters with fever
- unusual weight gain
- swelling of the arms, legs, hands, and feet

Many NSAIDS are over-the-counter drugs but some require a prescription, as noted in the table.

See also ANALGESIC NEPHROPATHY; LITHIUM AND BIPOLAR DISORDER; MEDICATIONS THAT CAN HARM THE KIDNEYS.

Food and Drug Administration. Available online. URL: http://www.fda.gov/downloads/Drugs/Drug Safety/ucm088646.pdf. Undated. Accessed February 9, 2010.

**obesity** Excessive weight, as defined by the body mass index (BMI) of the individual. Obesity is a risk factor for kidney disease and kidney failure. Obesity is linked to HYPERTENSION and DIABETES MELLITUS, and both hypertension and diabetes are directly correlated with the development of CHRONIC KIDNEY DISEASE (CKD) as well as with kidney failure. In occasional individuals, obesity can lead to a specific type of kidney disease, such as FOCAL SEGMENTAL GLOMERULO-SCLEROSIS (FSGS), which can lead to NEPHROTIC SYNDROME, decreased kidney function and even kidney failure.

About 27 percent of all adults in the United States are obese, according to the Centers for Disease Control and Prevention, and rates are higher among some groups, such as blacks and Hispanics and women with less than a high school education. (See Table 1.)

Body mass index (BMI) is a measure that compares the height and weight of an individual, using mathematical calculations, to determine whether people are underweight, of normal weight, overweight, obese, or morbidly obese. A BMI of 25 to 29.9 means that a person is overweight. A BMI of 30.0 or greater means that a person is obese. A morbidly obese person has a BMI of greater than 40 and is more than 100 pounds overweight.

Morbid obesity increases the risk for many types of illnesses, such as diabetes and hypertension as well as kidney disease and kidney failure. According to Ion D. Bucaloiu, M.D., and colleagues in their 2010 article for *Critical Care Clinics* on acute kidney injury in the critically ill, morbidly obese individuals may represent

**TABLE 1: SELF-REPORTED PREVALENCE OF OBESITY AMONG ADULTS, BY SEX AND SELECTED CHARACTERISTICS. BEHAVIORAL RISK FACTOR SURVEILLANCE SYSTEM, UNITED STATES, 2009.**

| | Overall (N=405,102) | Men (n=158,455) | Women (n=246,647) |
|---|---|---|---|
| **Characteristic** | % | % | % |
| Total | 26.7 | 27.4 | 26.0 |
| **Age group (years)** | | | |
| 18–29 | 20.3 | 20.1 | 20.6 |
| 30–39 | 27.8 | 29.4 | 26.2 |
| 40–49 | 29.4 | 31.0 | 27.8 |
| 50–59 | 31.1 | 31.9 | 30.3 |
| 60–69 | 30.9 | 30.4 | 31.3 |
| ≥70 | 20.5 | 19.8 | 21.0 |
| **Race/Ethnicity** | | | |
| White, non-Hispanic | 25.2 | 27.1 | 23.3 |
| Black, non-Hispanic | 36.8 | 30.9 | 41.9 |
| Hispanic | 30.7 | 30.6 | 30.8 |
| Other race | 16.7 | 16.9 | 16.5 |
| **Educational level** | | | |
| Less than high school graduate | 32.9 | 29.6 | 36.4 |
| High school graduate | 29.5 | 29.5 | 29.5 |
| Some college | 29.1 | 30.6 | 27.9 |
| College graduate | 20.8 | 22.9 | 18.6 |
| **Census region** | | | |
| Northeast | 24.3 | 25.2 | 23.4 |
| Midwest | 28.2 | 29.2 | 27.2 |
| South | 28.4 | 28.8 | 28.1 |
| West | 24.4 | 25.1 | 23.7 |

Source: Adapted from Centers for Disease Control and Prevention. "Vital Signs: State-Specific Obesity Prevalence among Adults— United States, 2009." *Morbidity and Mortality Weekly Report*, Early Release. Available online. URL: http://www.cdc.gov/mmwr/preview/mmwrhtml/mm59e0803a1.htm?s_cid=mm59e0803a1_e% 0D%0A. Accessed November 9, 2010.

7 percent of patients in intensive care units. They also noted that morbid obesity is a risk factor by itself for kidney disease, citing obesity-related glomerulopathy, a disorder that may increase the risk for acute kidney injury (AKI) among the morbidly obese. Some reasons for the AKI among the morbidly obese may be the physician's lack of awareness of the kidney damage, which may then lead to the prescribing of nephrotoxic medications such as nonsteroidal anti-inflammatory drugs (NSAIDs). In addition, because of the lack of awareness of existing kidney damage, the patient is at risk for kidney disease caused by the use of contrast material in imaging tests. One treatment for obesity is bariatric surgery, which is major surgery that alters the stomach capacity to process food; however, there are risks to the kidneys with this treatment. For example, according to Bucaloiu and colleagues, some risks for AKI after gastric bypass are such factors as a BMI greater than 50, preoperative chronic kidney disease, the presence of diabetes and hypertension, and an operative time of greater than 210 minutes. The authors also noted that morbidly obese patients who undergo gastric bypass have an elevated risk for needing intensive care subsequent to their surgery, and postoperative AKI may occur at a higher level in the morbidly obese.

See also DIABETIC NEPHROPATHY; END-STAGE RENAL DISEASE.

Bucaloiu, Ion D., M.D. "Acute Kidney Injury in the Critically Ill, Morbidly Obese Patient: Diagnostic and Therapeutic Challenges in a Unique Patient Population." *Critical Care Clinics* 26 (2010): 607–624.

**one kidney** See SOLITARY KIDNEY.

**oxalate stone disease** See HYPEROXALURIA; KIDNEY STONES.

**papillary necrosis**  See RENAL PAPILLARY NECROSIS.

**pediatric end-stage renal disease**  See CHILDREN AND KIDNEY DISEASE.

**pediatric kidney disease**  See CHILDREN AND KIDNEY DISEASE.

**peritoneal dialysis**  One of the two primary methods that are used to treat individuals with END-STAGE RENAL DISEASE (ESRD), also known as kidney failure. (The other method is HEMODIALYSIS.) Peritoneal dialysis is used less commonly than hemodialysis. According to the United States Renal Data System (USRDS), in 2007, 25,752 individuals received peritoneal dialysis. Dialysis is a process that cleans out impurities from the bloodstream when the kidneys can no longer perform this function. Peritoneal dialysis uses the internal lining of the abdomen as a filter to clean the blood. There are three types of peritoneal dialysis, including continuous ambulatory peritoneal dialysis (CAPD), continuous cycle-assisted peritoneal dialysis (CCPD), and a combination of CAPD and CCPD.

### Procedure

With peritoneal dialysis, a special catheter fills the inside of the abdomen with dialysis solution. The solution itself draws waste and extra fluid from within the abdominal cavity, and all of these fluids are drained out with the dialysis solution, which is thrown away. It takes about 40 minutes to fill and drain the abdomen, and this procedure needs to occur at least four times each day in most individuals. With CAPD, the individual can walk around while the process occurs and no machine is required. The other processes require a machine called a cycler to fill up and drain out the abdomen; this is often performed at night while the person sleeps.

Whatever form of peritoneal dialysis is used, the individual must have a soft catheter inserted into the abdomen so that the solution can travel through it. It takes several weeks for scar tissue to build up so that the catheter will be held in place and the fluids do not leak out of the abdomen around the catheter.

Nocturnal intermittent peritoneal dialysis (NIPD) is another form of peritoneal dialysis, but the dialyzing occurs only at night. This procedure may be used for those who still have some kidney function but not enough to handle all their needs.

### Risks and Complications

The most common complication that a person using peritoneal dialysis will develop is intraabdominal infection, termed peritonitis. This may present with cloudy dialysis fluid, a low-grade fever, and abdominal pain. Antibiotics are needed to treat the peritonitis. In rare cases, the catheter may have to be removed. If a fungus is causing the infection, then antifungal agents are needed and the catheter will generally have to be removed.

ANEMIA is another common problem among patients who receive dialysis. In addition, many dialysis patients have what was once called renal osteodystrophy and is now referred to as CHRONIC KIDNEY DISEASE–MINERAL BONE DISORDER (CKD-MBD). This is a disorder that causes bone to become weak, and it can cause rickets in children who receive dialysis. Another problem for many people receiving dialysis is extreme itching, also known as pruritus. This problem is generally greater before or directly after a dialysis treatment. It may also be related to excess levels of parathyroid hormone, or HYPERPARATHYROIDISM. Antihistamines may help as may treatments with ultraviolet light or phosphate binder medications.

Many people on dialysis suffer from SLEEP PROBLEMS, such as insomnia or sleep apnea syndrome. These disorders may lead to a day-night reversal, in which the individual is awake all night and sleeps or is sleepy for most of the day. Sleep apnea may stem from the failed kidney. Nasal continuous positive airway pressure may help some individuals. "Restless legs" syndrome is another problem for many people with dialysis, who cannot settle down and instead feel like they must kick their legs. This syndrome may be caused by nerve damage. Individuals with restless legs syndrome should avoid consuming food or beverages with caffeine before they go to bed and should also avoid tobacco and alcohol. Benzodiazepines, such as diazepam (Valium) or clonazepam (Klonopin), may provide some relief.

### Outlook and Lifestyle Modifications

Peritoneal dialysis (PD) is far less efficient than are working kidneys, and thus the individual on PD needs to be very careful with his or her diet. A dietitian can provide an individualized program for what foods to eat and what to avoid.

### Questions to Ask Prior to Peritoneal Dialysis

According to the National Institute of Diabetes and Digestive and Kidney Diseases, patients considering peritoneal dialysis should ask their health care team the following questions:

- Is peritoneal dialysis the best treatment choice for me? Why? If yes, which type is best?

- How long will it take me to learn how to do peritoneal dialysis?
- What does peritoneal dialysis feel like?
- How will peritoneal dialysis affect my blood pressure?
- How will I know if I have peritonitis? How is it treated?
- As a peritoneal dialysis patient, will I be able to continue working?
- How much should I exercise?
- Where do I store supplies?
- How often do I see my doctor?
- Who will be on my health care team? How can these people help me?
- Whom do I contact with problems?
- With whom can I talk about finances, sexuality, or family concerns?
- How/where can I talk with other people who have faced this decision?

See also CHRONIC KIDNEY DISEASE; DIALYSIS.

**phosphate** See PHOSPHORUS.

**phosphorus** A substance that is important to health and referred to as phosphate when combined with oxygen. Phosphorus builds up and maintains the bones and is also important in the metabolism of energy. Low levels of phosphate are unusual. Excessively high levels of phosphate lead to low levels of CALCIUM in the blood (HYPOCALCEMIA). High levels of phosphate in the blood (HYPERPHOSPHATEMIA) are linked to the presence of CHRONIC KIDNEY DISEASE, and children with kidney failure may have growth failure because of high levels of blood phosphorus that interfere with the formation of healthy bone and growth. The abnormal metabolism of phosphorus is also linked to CHRONIC KIDNEY DISEASE–MINERAL BONE DISORDER. Chronically elevated phosphorus levels lead to an increased risk for atherosclerosis and CARDIOVASCULAR DISEASE.

Phosphorus is present in many foods, such as meat, whole-grain bread, cereals, egg yolk, poultry, and fish. Phosphorus is particularly high in some foods, and individuals with already high levels of phosphorus are advised to limit their consumption of milk, cheese, cocoa, peas, nuts, peanut butter, and dried beans. In addition, medications that increase the binding of phosphorus may be recommended to rid the body of excessive phosphorus, such as over-the-counter (OTC) drugs like calcium carbonate or prescribed drugs such as sevelamer bicarbonate (Renvelal) or lanthanum carbonate (Fosrenol).

See also CALCIUM; MAGNESIUM; POTASSIUM; SODIUM.

**polycystic kidney disease (PKD)** A genetic disorder that is characterized by numerous fluid-filled cysts that are found in both kidneys. These cysts eventually cause the kidneys to become enlarged and to destroy the functioning kidney tissue. According to the National Institute of Diabetes and Digestive and Kidney Diseases, about 600,000 people in the United States have PKD, and it is the fourth leading cause of kidney failure.

Polycystic kidney disease leads to CHRONIC KIDNEY DISEASE, and in about half the cases of individuals with this disease, it leads to kidney failure (END-STAGE RENAL DISEASE [ESRD]). Once the kidneys fail, the individual with PKD must have either DIALYSIS or KIDNEY TRANSPLANTATION in order to survive. The majority of cases are inherited as an autosomal dominant PKD, while rarely, the disease is inherited as an autosomal recessive form of PKD. In about 10 percent of the cases of PKD, a spontaneous genetic mutation caused the disease. A cyst-filled kidney is common in individuals with this disease, and often the kidney is markedly enlarged up to the size of a professional-sized football; the normal size of a kidney is approximately the size of an adult male's fist.

In most cases of autosomal dominant PKD, symptoms develop between ages 30 and 40 years. With autosomal recessive PKD, symptoms begin in early infancy and may lead to death in infancy or childhood.

Individuals with PKD are more likely to develop KIDNEY STONES than others. In addition, they are also more likely to have brain aneurysms, as well as cysts in their testes, liver, or pancreas, and also diverticula of the colon. If a patient with autosomal dominant polycystic kidney disease has a family history of cerebral vessel aneurysm or intracranial hemorrhage, the patient may have as much as a 10 percent chance of also having an intracranial aneurysm. In the absence of such a family history, the risk is substantially lower.

### Symptoms and Diagnostic Path

Many people with autosomal dominant PKD have no symptoms. If symptoms are present, they may include the following:

- blood in the urine (hematuria)
- abdominal pain
- infections
- urinary tract infections
- abnormal heart valves
- high blood pressure
- kidney stones
- brain aneurysms
- diverticulosis (small pouches that bulge out from the colon)
- liver and pancreatic cysts

Ultrasound is often used to diagnose PKD, although computerized tomography (CT) scans or magnetic resonance imaging (MRI) scans may also help diagnose this disease.

With autosomal recessive PKD (ARPKD), symptoms may include high blood pressure, frequent urination and urinary tract infections. The liver is often also involved. Some infants may need dialysis during the first week of birth.

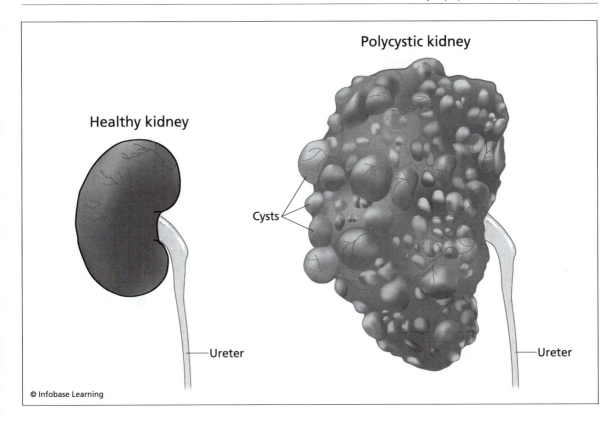

Polycystic kidney

Healthy kidney

Cysts

Ureter

Ureter

© Infobase Learning

Children with autosomal recessive PKD are usually small in size because of decreased kidney function. Growth problems are common among children with this disease.

### Treatment Options and Outlook

With autosomal dominant PKD, the physician treats the symptoms, such as pain, INFECTIONS, HYPERTENSION, and ESRD. Cysts which are painful and/or bleeding may be drained. In most cases of PKD, there are too many cysts to make their removal practical.

Patients with autosomal dominant polycystic kidney disease are at very high risk of having spontaneous bleeding into the cysts. This can be very painful and often requires the use of narcotic analgesics for adequate pain control. Infections of the cysts are also common. Only certain antibiotics can be used because of the difficulty of the antibiotic gaining entry into the cyst fluid.

Very rarely, the kidneys become so enlarged that they almost completely fill the abdomen, making space available for the intestinal tract very limited and thereby limiting adequate oral nutrition.

Women in particular with this genetic disorder can develop substantial enlargement of their liver due to innumerable liver cysts. Rarely, this may cause a doubling or more of the size of the liver, which can also lead to recurrent liver infections or difficulty obtaining adequate nutrition because of limited available abdominal space. In contrast to the kidney disease that is associated with autosomal dominant polycystic kidney disease, liver cysts do not cause abnormalities in liver function.

In some cases, the removal of one or both kidneys may be indicated (nephrectomy); if both kidneys are removed, this will cause the patient to have kidney failure and need dialysis or kidney transplantation.

With autosomal recessive PKD, medications are given to control hypertension, and ANTIBIOTICS are administered to control urinary tract infections. Sometimes growth hormones are also administered to children with this form of PKD. If the child develops a serious liver disease in addition to kidney failure, caused by scarring of the liver, then he or she may need a combined liver and kidney transplantation.

### Risk Factors and Preventive Measures

If one parent has PKD, then a child has a 50 percent risk of also developing the disorder. There are no known preventive measures for PKD as of this writing. As of this writing, several medications are undergoing clinical trials to determine whether they slow the progression of chronic kidney disease associated with autosomal dominant polycystic kidney disease. These studies are hoped to identify new treatments which can be used in the future to treat this very common disease.

See also CHILDREN AND KIDNEY DISEASE.

**poststreptococcal glomerulonephritis (PSGN)** Inflammation and damage to the kidneys that is caused by a streptococcus infection, usually a Group A streptococcus (GAS) infection but occasionally by infection with *Streptococcus zooepidemicus*. According to the National Institute of Diabetes and Digestive and Kidney Diseases (NIDDK), the streptococcus bacteria do not attack the kidneys directly but an infection can cause the immune system to produce an excessive level of antibodies. These antibodies circulate in the blood and are eventually deposited in the glomeruli of the kidneys, damaging them. Rarely, impetigo, a skin infection, can cause poststreptococcal glomerulonephritis (PSGN).

According to Bernardo Rodriguez-Iturbe and James M. Musser, PSGN is among the oldest known kidney diseases in history. Although streptococcus is commonly present in the United States, it is readily identified and eradicated with antibiotics. Even if untreated, few individuals in the United States and Canada develop PSGN, and epidemics are virtually unknown. However, this infection continues to affect an estimated 9.5–28.5 individuals per 100,000 people every year among those who reside in developing countries as well as among indigenous populations within developing countries, such as the Aborigines in Australia. Rodriguez-Iturbe and Musser report that in India, 73 percent of the cases of acute glomerulonephritis that occur among the elderly are caused by PSGN.

Sometimes epidemic outbreaks of streptococcus cause glomerulonephritis, as with an outbreak in Brazil in 1997–98, according to Ricardo Sesso and Sergio Wyton L. Pinto. In the group of 135 mostly adult subjects at the beginning of their study, three patients died and five patients required DIALYSIS. In this study, the microbe that was responsible for the epidemic was *Streptococcus zooepidemicus*. This microbe is more commonly found in adults.

In a follow-up study of 56 subjects about five years later, Sesso and Pinto found that 57 percent of the subjects had either reduced creatinine clearance or increased microalbuminuria. The researchers found that the patients at greatest risk for reduced renal function were older than 54 years.

### Symptoms and Diagnostic Path

PSGN can cause sudden symptoms of a reduced urinary output (oliguria), blood in the urine (hematuria), and body swelling (edema). Tests of the urine will show large amounts of protein (proteinuria) and high levels of creatinine and urea, indicating kidney damage. HYPERTENSION is another common symptom. An ASO titer or streptozyme assay will commonly be elevated following streptococcal pharyngitis, and can suggest the diagnosis of the streptococcal glomerulonephritis. Because other conditions, most commonly IGA NEPHROPATHY, can also cause hematuria and proteinuria following an upper respiratory tract infection, and because the treatment of poststreptococcal glomerulonephritis differs from that of IgA nephropathy and other types of glomerulonephritis, a renal biopsy is necessary in order to guide appropriate therapy.

### Treatment Options and Outlook

Individuals with streptococcal pharyngitis or with streptococcal skin infections should be treated with antibiotics early on to avoid the progression of the disease to PSGN. If there is an epidemic outbreak level of streptococcus, Rodriguez-Iturbe and Musser recommend treatment in individuals with or without symptoms as a protective measure. They also report that the prognosis is usually excellent in children and most adults, but note that it is worse in elderly people and/or groups with other risk factors of CHRONIC KIDNEY DISEASE.

There is no specific therapy for PSGN once the glomerulonephritis has developed. Although it is not clear how effective they are, many nephrologists treat patients who have aggressive forms of poststreptococcal glomerulonephritis with aggressive IMMUNOSUPPRESSIVE DRUGS.

Otherwise, management of the patient with the streptococcal glomerulonephritis focuses on treating the clinical effects, particularly those related to volume overload. These include hypertension and, less commonly, pulmonary edema. If present, treatment should include sodium and water restriction and may require the use of loop diuretics. In rare occasions, severe high blood pressure may lead to neurologic abnormalities. These patients will likely require hospitalization and emergency therapy to reduce their blood pressure.

Renal function in patients with PSGN can be reduced, and may be reduced sufficiently that some patients will require dialysis during the acute episode. The management of acute kidney injury in children is discussed separately.

In addition, adults who have other conditions such as DIABETES MELLITUS, malnutrition, alcoholism, or other chronic illnesses have a risk for a poor prognosis from PSGN, and death may occur in up to 25 percent of these individuals. Individuals at risk for kidney failure are also those with persistent proteinuria. In an Australian Aboriginal population with PSGN, kidney failure is common and is often linked to low birth weight of infants and diabetes.

### Risk Factors and Preventive Measures

Children and adults in developing countries have a greater risk for PSGN than children and adults in developed countries. PSGN most commonly affects boys ages 3–7 years according to the NIDDK, although individuals of any age may be affected. Better rates of sanitation and cleanliness could help prevent such infections. Early identification and treatment of existing infections could prevent the progression to PSGN.

See also CHILDREN WITH KIDNEY DISEASE; GLOMERULONEPHRITIS.

Rodriguez-Iturbe, Bernardo, and James M. Musser. "The Current State of Poststreptococcal Glomerulonephritis." *Journal of the American Society of Nephrology* 19 (2008): 1,855–1,864.

Sesso, Ricardo, and Sergio Wyton L. Pinto. "Five-Year Follow-up of Patients with Epidemic Glomerulonephritis due to *Streptococcus zooepidemicus*." *Nephrology Dialysis Transplantation* 20 (2005): 1,808–1,812.

Steer, Andrew C., Margaret H. Danchin, and Jonathan R. Carapetis. "Group A Streptococcal Infections in Children." *Journal of Paediatrics and Child Health* 43 (2007): 203–213.

**potassium** An important mineral that is essential to normal electrolyte functioning and which directly affects the blood pressure. HYPERKALEMIA refers to high blood levels of potassium which may be caused by diseases or medications, while HYPOKALEMIA refers to insufficient blood levels of potassium, which may be caused by DIURETIC medications, diarrhea, or vomiting.

Hyperkalemia is often caused by decreased kidney function in combination with medications that decrease the kidney's ability to excrete potassium. It may also occur with acute kidney failure, DIABETES MELLITUS, LUPUS NEPHRITIS, rejection of a KIDNEY TRANSPLANTATION, or obstructive uropathy.

ALDOSTERONE, a hormone, regulates the removal of potassium and SODIUM by the kidneys. An insufficient amount of aldosterone may lead to hyperkalemia, as among patients with Addison's disease.

Many medications increase the risk for hyperkalemia. These include NONSTEROIDAL ANTI-INFLAMMATORY DRUGS (NSAIDs) and COX-2 inhibitors, BETA BLOCKERS, ANGIOTENSIN-CONVERTING ENZYME INHIBITORS (ACEIs), and ANGIOTENSIN II RECEPTOR BLOCKERS (ARBs) as well as potassium-sparing diuretics. In addition, mineralocorticoid receptor blockers, such as sprionolactone and eplerenone, frequently lead to hyperkalemia. Digoxin, a cardiac medication sometimes used for either congestive heart failure or atrial fibrillation, can cause hyperkalemia. Finally, certain ANTIBIOTICS, such as trimethoprim (a component of Bactrim and Septra) and pentamidine, function as potassium-sparing diuretics and can lead to hyperkalemia, particularly when used in high doses.

When laboratory tests are ordered during routine checkups, most physicians order a measure of the potassium level; thus high or low levels are discovered and a further investigation is made by the physician to determine the cause and then make a treatment plan. Patients receiving any of the medications discussed above, particularly those who are taking more than one of these medications or who have CHRONIC KIDNEY DISEASE (CKD) may need regular monitoring of their blood potassium level.

An individual's diet may affect his or her level of potassium as well as health. For example, a diet that is low in potassium but is high in sodium can lead to elevated blood pressure, and can further lead to hypokalemia. This is because high sodium intake increases renal potassium excretion, which can lead to worsening of hypokalemia. Moreover, animal studies have shown that the lower the potassium intake, the greater an effect that sodium chloride intake has on blood pressure. Increasing potassium intake can decrease blood pressure, and may decrease the risk of strokes.

According to Horacio Adrogué and Nicolaos E. Madias in their 2007 article for the New England Journal of Medicine, increasing the potassium levels can reduce the need for taking ANTIHYPERTENSIVE DRUGS to either fewer drugs or no drugs.

Many different foods contain high amounts of potassium, such as tomatoes, bananas, and many other fruits and vegetables, as well as chocolate, nuts and seeds, and nutritional supplements. Such foods may need to be limited among individuals with chronic kidney disease or who are on DIALYSIS because their kidney disease limits the body's ability to excrete the potassium.

According to the United States Renal Data System, with higher levels of the five stages of chronic kidney disease also comes an increased risk for an abnormal potassium level. For example, according to the United States Renal Data System in their 2009 report and based on 1999–2006 data, 8.3 percent of individuals without CKD had abnormal potassium levels. At Stages 4–5 of the five stages of CKD, 47.5 percent had abnormal potassium levels.

Severe hyperkalemia can be life-threatening due to effects on the heart. An electrocardiogram (ECG) may need to be performed to assess the cardiac effects. If heart disease is present, the patient may need emergency intravenous medications to block the effects on the heart, followed by either specific medications or by emergency HEMODIALYSIS to remove the excess potassium from the body.

Hypokalemia has several important adverse effects. These include the development of or worsening of hypertension, an increased risk of sudden death from a heart attack (myocardial infarction), muscle weakness, RHABDOMYOLYSIS, cardiac arrhythmias, and progressive renal failure. Treatment may require oral medications, of if the hypokalemia is severe or the person is unable to take oral medications, then intravenous potassium is administered.

See also CALCIUM; ELECTROLYTES AND ELECTROLYTE IMBALANCES; HYPERTENSION; MAGNESIUM; MEDICATIONS THAT CAN HARM THE KIDNEYS; SODIUM.

Adrogué, Horacio, M.D., and Nicolaos E. Madias, M.D. "Sodium and Potassium in the Pathogenesis of Hypertension." *New England Journal of Medicine* 356, no. 19 (May 10, 2007): 1,966–1,978.

**prediabetes** A condition defined by a glucose level that is close to but not high enough to be diagnosed as DIABETES MELLITUS. It indicates one's heightened risk for developing diabetes and other diseases. Specifically, prediabetes is measured by a blood test and a fasting plasma glucose level of greater than 100 but less than 126 mg/dl. Individuals with prediabetes are at an increased risk of developing Type 2 diabetes. There are usually no symptoms of prediabetes, although individuals with this condition are often overweight or obese and have a family history of diabetes. In a study by L. S. Geiss and colleagues published in 2010, the researchers found that based on their analysis of 1,402 subjects, nearly 30 percent of adults in the United States had prediabetes in 2005–06, but only 7 percent were aware that they had this condition. Of those with prediabetes who took actions to change their behavior to avoid the development of diabetes (such as exercising and losing weight), most were previously advised by their doctors that they had prediabetes, were female, and were either overweight or obese.

Some researchers have concluded that prediabetes is a risk factor for CHRONIC KIDNEY DISEASE (CKD). Using data from more than 8,000 subjects over the period 1999–2006 from the National Health and Nutrition Examination Survey (NHANES), a study by Laura C. Plantinga and colleagues found that the overall prevalence of CKD was 17.1 percent among those with prediabetes, compared to 11.8 percent among those without diabetes. (The prevalence of CKD was 39.6 percent among those with diagnosed diabetes and 41.7 percent among those with undiagnosed diabetes.)

Among those with prediabetes and CKD, risks were higher among individuals ages 60 years and older, non-Hispanic blacks, people with a body mass index (BMI) equal to or greater than 30, and those with self-reported HYPERTENSION. As can be seen from the table, individuals with prediabetes who were ages 60 and older had more than three times the risk for having CKD compared to those who were ages 20–59 years. Also note that the sections in parentheses in the second and third columns of the table indicate the range of percentages. (This ratio was even greater for those without diabetes, although the percentages of having CKD were lower.) Females with prediabetes had a greater risk for CKD than males with prediabetes. In addition, 29.5 percent of those with self-reported hypertension had prediabetes, compared to 10.7 percent of those with prediabetes and no hypertension. (See the table.)

People with diagnosed diabetes generally are informed by their physicians that they are at risk for kidney disease and their kidney function is also regularly tested with tests such as the estimated GLOMERULAR FILTRATION RATE (eGFR). However, those with undiagnosed diabetes or prediabetes usually are not aware of their risks for kidney disease. It is clear that it is important for more people to be screened for diabetes and prediabetes and also to be screened for chronic kidney disease at the same time, before symptoms become present and when actions can be taken to prevent the development of diabetes and the escalation of the risk for CKD. Such an intervention could alleviate a significant level of kidney disease and kidney failure in the United States.

See also DIABETIC NEPHROPATHY.

**TABLE 1: ADJUSTED PREVALENCE OF CKD, BY MDRD STUDY EQUATION ESTIMATE OF GFR, AMONG THOSE WITH PREDIABETES VERSUS NO DIABETES, BY SELECTED CHARACTERISTICS, NHANES 1999 THROUGH 2006**

| Characteristic | % with Stages 1 through 4 CKD (95% CI) | | |
| | Prediabetes | No Diabetes | $p^a$ |
| --- | --- | --- | --- |
| **Overall** | 17.1 (15.9 to 18.5) | 11.8 (10.5 to 13.3) | <0.001 |
| **Age (years)** | | | |
| 20 to 59 | 11.7 (10.6 to 12.9) | 6.3 (5.4 to 7.4) | 0.001 |
| ≥60 | 36.9 (34.3 to 39.5) | 31.5 (28.4 to 34.8) | 0.164 |
| **Gender** | | | |
| Male | 14.3 (12.9 to 15.8) | 8.1 (6.9 to 9.6) | 0.172 |
| Female | 18.6 (17.0 to 20.4) | 13.3 (11.5 to 15.4) | 0.001 |
| **Race/ethnicity[b]** | | | |
| Non-Hispanic white | 15.8 (14.4 to 17.2) | 10.7 (9.3 to 12.3) | 0.005 |
| Non-Hispanic black | 20.4 (18.3 to 22.7) | 12.9 (10.9 to 15.3) | 0.036 |
| Mexican-American | 14.5 (12.7 to 16.6) | 7.6 (6.0 to 9.5) | 0.035 |
| **BMI (kg/m²)** | | | |
| <30 | 14.6 (13.1 to 16.3) | 9.7 (8.5 to 11.2) | 0.017 |
| ≥30 | 17.9 (15.8 to 20.2) | 11.5 (9.6 to 13.8) | 0.008 |
| **Self-reported hypertension** | | | |
| Yes | 29.5 (27.1 to 31.9) | 21.6 (18.7 to 24.8) | 0.011 |
| No | 10.7 (9.3 to 12.4) | 7.1 (6.0 to 8.3) | 0.121 |

CKD defined by MDRD Study equation-calculated eGFR <60 ml/min per 1.73 m² or single micro/macroalbuminuria measurement; prediabetes, FPG ≥100 and <126 mg/dl and no self-report of diabetes; no diabetes, FPG <100 mg/dl and no self-report of diabetes. BMI, body mass index; CI, confidence interval.

[a] Prevalence estimates adjusted for age, gender, and race/ethnicity only. Models that produced prevalence estimates included individuals in all four categories of diabetes status; models that produced P values included only those with prediabetes or no diabetes.

[b] Prevalence for other race/ethnicity not shown because of small sample sizes, but individuals in category are included in all analyses.

American Society of Nephrology. Clinical Journal by Laura C. Plantinga et al. Copyright 2010 by American Society of Nephrology. Reproduced with permission of American Society of Nephrology in the format Tradebook via Copyright Clearance Center.

Source: Plantinga, Laura C., et al. "Prevalence of Chronic Kidney Disease in U.S. Adults with Undiagnosed Diabetes or Prediabetes." *Clinical Journal of the American Society of Nephrology* 5 (2010): p. 679.

Geiss, L. S. "Diabetes Risk Reduction Behaviors among U.S. Adults with Prediabetes." *American Journal of Preventive Medicine* 38, no. 4 (2010): 403–409.

Plantinga, Laura C., et al. "Prevalence of Chronic Kidney Disease in U.S. Adults with Undiagnosed Diabetes or Prediabetes." *Clinical Journal of the American Society of Nephrology* 5 (2010): 673–682.

**proteinuria** Protein in the urine, which is usually a sign of kidney disease. (Exercise and fever can also sometimes temporarily increase the protein levels in the urine.) When detected early enough, the underlying abnormality causing the proteinuria may be treated to prevent progression of the kidney dysfunction or insufficiency; however, when there are large amounts of proteinuria, there is generally an increased risk of developing irreversible kidney failure. In addition, proteinuria can be used as an indicator of cardiovascular risk. Recent evidence shows that the greater the amount of proteinuria, the greater the risk of cardiovascular-related death.

Albumin is one form of a protein that can be found in the urine, and when this protein is identified, the condition is known as albuminuria. When the relative levels of albumin in the urine are low (between 30 and 300 mg/gm creatinine) but above normal, this is termed microalbuminuria. If the levels are higher, or greater than 300 mg/gm creatinine, the condition is called macroalbuminuria. This indicates the presence of serious kidney disease.

Proteinuria is often caused by DIABETES MELLITUS, HYPERTENSION, GLOMERULONEPHRITIS, or other illnesses (or the patient may have two or more illnesses, such as having both hypertension and diabetes simultaneously). An estimated 20–40 percent of Type 2 diabetes patients will develop DIABETIC NEPHROPATHY, as defined by persistent proteinuria, hypertension, and a decline in their kidney function.

In rare cases, proteinuria and/or albuminuria are benign conditions that do not indicate kidney disease or an increased cardiovascular risk. Some individuals have a condition known as orthostatic proteinuria, in which they have proteinuria only when standing and not while lying down. This condition has no associated long-term risk. Other individuals will have proteinuria in response to physical exertion. If they have no proteinuria when not exercising, then this too, is a benign condition and is not associated with long-term risk. Finally, a urinary tract infection can cause proteinuria that is present only during the infection.

When a person has either Type 1 or Type 2 diabetes, even the presence of microalbuminuria is an indication of an early kidney malfunction, and in the absence of specific therapy, the person is at increased risk for worsening kidney function. Extensive evidence indicates that treatment with an ANGIOTENSIN-CONVERTING ENZYME INHIBITOR (ACEI) medication or with an ANGIOTENSIN II RECEPTOR BLOCKER (ARB) can be protective to the kidneys.

### Symptoms and Diagnostic Path

There are no specific symptoms that are experienced by those with low-grade proteinuria, and consequently, the only way to tell if the problem exists is to test the urine. One such test is done with a urinary dipstick to test for albumin. If the urine dipstick is negative, then the patient at risk for proteinuria (such as a patient with diabetes or hypertension) should have a yearly spot urine test for microalbumin by radioimmunoassay. This is a very sensitive test that detects tiny amounts of protein.

With large amounts of proteinuria, a person may develop a condition known as NEPHROTIC SYNDROME. This condition involves proteinuria of more than 3.5 mg/d, development of peripheral edema, low serum albumin (hypoalbuminemia), and elevated cholesterol levels (hypercholesterolemia). Nephrotic syndrome is indicative of significant glomerular and kidney damage.

Another test for proteinuria is a 24-hour urine collection, in which urinary protein excretion is measured over the course of one day by having the patient collect all urine passed over a 24-hour period. At the same time frame, an estimate of kidney function (known as the creatinine clearance) is also measured. In general, the 24-hour test is used on adults and adolescents rather than on children, because it is usually more difficult to collect the child's urine for such a long time frame.

Because of the inconvenience of a 24-hour urine collection, it is also possible to assess the protein excretion rate from measuring the ratio of protein to creatinine in the urine. While this test may not yield an absolute measure of protein excretion, it does enable serial measurements of protein excretion rates that can be used to assess the patient's response to therapy.

If protein is found in the urine, then blood tests are usually ordered. The doctor will generally order a test for creatinine and urea nitrogen levels, because creatinine and urea nitrogen are normally removed from the blood by the kidneys. High levels of creatinine and urea nitrogen in the blood are an indication that the kidneys are not functioning normally.

### Treatment Options and Outlook

After diagnosing proteinuria, the medical goal usually is to determine and treat the underlying cause. For example, if the primary problem is hypertension, then the goal is to reduce the blood pressure to as close to normal levels as possible. The person with diabetes should work to improve his or her glucose level to as close to normal as possible. Certain medications, such as ACEIs and ARBs, predictably decrease protein excretion and may decrease the risk of progressive loss of kidney function and the associated cardiovascular risk.

The greater the amount of protein in the urine, the more important it is to bring blood pressure levels under control. For example, if the proteinuria exceeds 1 g per 24 hours, the National Heart, Lung, and Blood Institute recommends that the blood pressure be maintained below 125/75 mm Hg. Note: 125/75 is considered a normal and not hypertensive blood pressure level; however, when the person has proteinuria that is caused by diabetes, then attaining an even lower blood pressure will work to improve the prognosis for the individual.

If proteinuria is identified in the microalbuminuria phase and is treated, then the outlook is very good. If the proteinuria has advanced further and the person is treated early in the overt proteinuria phase, the outcome depends upon the amount of proteinuria, the level of effective blood pressure control, and also other factors that contribute to inflammation and atherosclerosis (such as SMOKING, lipid levels, and so forth).

Nephrotic syndrome indicates the presence of a severe glomerular disease and also indicates that the risk of progressive loss of kidney function, possibly leading to end-stage renal disease, is substantial. There are many causes of nephrotic syndrome, and the treatments differ with different causes. A KIDNEY BIOPSY may be necessary to determine the specific cause and to guide therapeutic decisions.

### Risk Factors and Preventive Measures

Some groups of people are more likely than others to have proteinuria, including:

- people with diabetes (including both Type 1 and Type 2 diabetes)
- people with hypertension
- African Americans
- American Indians
- Hispanic Americans
- Pacific Islander Americans
- elderly individuals
- obese individuals
- those with a family history of kidney disease

It is difficult to prevent proteinuria without knowing that it is present, but once it is identified, it is very important to identify and treat the underlying cause of the proteinuria.

See also CHRONIC KIDNEY DISEASE; END-STAGE RENAL DISEASE.

**purpura, Henoch-Schönlein** See HENOCH-SCHÖNLEIN PURPURA.

**pyelonephritis** An infection of the kidneys, which is sometimes caused by an untreated bladder infection (CYSTITIS) that has ascended into the kidneys. Other causes include KIDNEY STONES and a weak immune system caused by taking IMMUNOSUPPRESSIVE DRUGS to prevent the rejection of a transplanted kidney or other transplanted organ. Few people die of a kidney infection; according to the National Center for Health Statistics in their 2009 report, only 673 people died because of a kidney infection in the United States in 2006. However, kidney infections can be extremely painful, and they can also lead to other serious diseases and complications.

Some people have recurrent bouts of pyelonephritis and cystitis. In some cases, this may indicate another underlying disease which should be identified and treated. For example, in their article on recurrent pyelonephritis for the *Cleveland Journal of Medicine* in 2009, Hung-Yi Chu, M.D., and colleagues reported that frequent infections of the kidney may be an indicator of MEDULLARY SPONGE KIDNEY, a serious disorder. The authors say that up to 20 percent of patients with urolithiasis (kidney stones) have medullary sponge kidneys and also that more than 70 percent of patients with medullary sponge kidneys develop kidney stones. The presence of medullary sponge kidney also causes recurrent kidney infections.

Sometimes the use of a catheter to drain urine from the bladder or the examination of the bladder with a cystoscope can lead to a kidney infection. A prostate enlargement may also cause a kidney infection. Sexual activity, particularly in women, can lead to cystitis, which, if untreated, can lead to pyelonephritis.

### Symptoms and Diagnostic Path

The most common symptoms of pyelonephritis are fever, flank pain, dysuria (pain when urinating), frequent urination (the need to urinate often, generally with small volumes), and urinary urgency (the need to urinate quickly, without an ability to delay urinating). Other symptoms may include:

- blood in the urine (hematuria)
- cloudy or abnormal urine color
- foul or strong urine odor
- nausea and vomiting
- chills and shaking

A physical examination and a history may indicate a kidney infection to the physician. Laboratory testing of the urine can show evidence of infection. For example, dipstick testing can show the presence of nitrite and leukocyte esterase, which indicate infection. Microscopic examination of the urine can show white blood cells (leukocyturia) and bacteria (bacteruria). A URINE culture can identify the specific bacteria causing the infection and can be used to show which antibiotics will be effective against that bacteria.

### Treatment Options and Outlook

Kidney infections are treated with common antibiotics, such as amoxicillin, or sulfa drugs, such as sulfimethoaxole/trimethoprim. Recurrent or complicated infections may be treated with a medication in the fluoroquinolone class, such as levofloxacin (Floxin). Often the results of a urine culture and sensitivity analysis can be used to choose the best antibiotic. Pain medications may also be required, either over-the-counter (OTC) or prescribed medications.

It is important for patients to take all the medication unless directed otherwise by the doctor. Often patients feel well in a few days, and they may mistakenly assume that they are cured and stop taking the medication. But if all of the bacteria are not eliminated, they can proliferate after the antibiotics are stopped prematurely, and this may result in a rapid recurrence of the infection.

After the completion of medication therapy, pregnant women and individuals with diabetes should have a repeat urine culture to ensure there are no bacteria present in the urine.

### Risk Factors and Preventive Measures

Individuals with vesicoureteric reflux (backing up of the urine) have an increased risk for kidney infections, as do those with kidney stones or RENAL PAPILLARY NECROSIS.

Individuals with a past history of kidney infections have an increased risk for the development of more infections. To prevent further kidney infections, individuals should empty the bladder completely when they need to urinate (even if it may be inconvenient).

Other suggestions to avoid kidney infections include the following:

- After women use the toilet, wipe from front to back to avoid introducing bacteria into the urethra.
- Urinate after sexual intercourse to help get rid of any bacteria that were introduced during sexual activity.
- Drink a lot of fluids, at least 64 ounces per day. This will encourage frequent urination and help flush bacteria out of the bladder.

Individuals with recurrent infections may also benefit from drinking cranberry juice, which can help prevent some bacteria from attaching to the bladder wall and causing an infection.

Chu, Hung-Yi, M.D., Ming-Tso Yan, M.D., and Shih-Hua Lin, M.D. "The Clinical Picture: Recurrent Pyelonephritis as a Sign of 'Sponge Kidney.'" *Cleveland Clinic Journal of Medicine* 76, no. 8 (2009): 479–480.

Heron, Melonie, et al. "Deaths: Final Data for 2006." *National Vital Statistics Report* 57, no. 14 (April 17, 2009): 43.

McGregor, Jessica C., George P. Allen, and David T. Bearden. "Levofloxacin in the Treatment of Complicated Urinary Tract Infections and Acute Pyelonephritis." *Therapeutics and Clinical Risk Management* 4, no. 5 (2008): 843–853.

**racial differences** See KIDNEYS AND KIDNEY DISEASE.

**reflux nephropathy** A condition that damages the kidney because of a backward flow of the urine up into the kidney. Reflux nephropathy is also referred to as vesicoureteric reflux and ureteral reflux. Reflux nephropathy occurs when the one-way valves in the ureters (the tubes that extend into the bladder) fail for some reason, thus allowing the urine to back up. If the backed-up urine is infected, this can cause a kidney infection as well (PYELONEPHRITIS). Since the bladder pressure is usually higher than the pressure in the kidneys, reflux nephropathy can cause damage and scarring to the kidneys. The exact relationship between ureteral reflux and kidney disease is controversial among experts as of 2010. Experts disagree whether ureteral reflux causes kidney damage by itself, the kidney damage results from subsequent bacterial infections, or the reflux is just a marker of abnormal kidney development, which causes kidney damage.

Other causes for reflux nephropathy besides a bladder infection may include the following diagnoses:

- bladder stones
- abnormal ureters
- a bladder outlet obstruction
- a neurogenic bladder

### Symptoms and Diagnostic Path
There may be no symptoms. When there are symptoms of reflux nephropathy, they may resemble the symptoms of a urinary tract infection, and they may include

- repeated urinary tract infections in a female
- even one urinary tract infection in a male
- back pain or abdominal pain
- blood in the urine (hematuria)
- stinging or burning with urination
- a feeling that the bladder does not empty completely

Vesicoureteral reflux is the most common urologic disease in children, and is present in 30–45 percent of children with a urinary tract infection. In addition, the person may have an elevated blood pressure.

The patient is diagnosed based on symptoms as well as the results of tests such as a renal ultrasound, an abdominal computerized tomography (CT) scan, or a retrogradepyelogram that shows evidence of urinary reflux. In some cases, a radionuclide cystogram is used to detect the reflux. Rarely, an intravenous pyelogram (IVP) is also used, although this test is used much less frequently in modern times than in the past.

### Treatment Options and Outlook
If the reflux is uncomplicated, then antibiotics and the prompt treatment of urinary tract infections may prevent progressive loss of kidney function. A yearly ultrasound of the kidneys may also be helpful. In the case of more severe reflux nephropathy, a reconstructive repair of the ureters may be needed. Because reflux leads to an increased risk for urinary tract infections,

and these infections lead to substantial morbidity (disease) and may also lead to a worsening of the kidney disease, long-term prophylactic (preventive) antibiotics are generally prescribed for children with vesicoureteral reflux.

Kidney damage from reflux nephropathy may be permanent, although the other kidney can usually take over the entire function. If both kidneys are involved, however, the patient may worsen and develop END-STAGE RENAL DISEASE (ESRD).

### Risk Factors and Preventive Measures

Repeated bouts of CYSTITIS may lead to reflux nephropathy. Other risk factors are abnormalities within the urinary tract, as well as a family or personal history of reflux.

**renal artery stenosis (RAS)** A disorder in which one or both of the arteries that carry blood to the kidneys is significantly narrowed. This disorder can cause elevated blood pressure and can also impede the overall kidney function. Renal artery stenosis (RAS) is usually caused by atherosclerosis, or a hardening of the arteries of the kidneys. (Other arteries may also be affected by atherosclerosis.) Atherosclerosis is a buildup of a plaque-like material that makes it difficult for blood to travel through the arteries, similar to the plaque that builds up in the arteries of the heart, leading to myocardial infarction (heart attack), or in arteries going to the brain, which can cause strokes.

### Symptoms and Diagnostic Path

Individuals with RAS may have no symptoms but high blood pressure is frequently a sign, and the hypertension may not be as responsive as anticipated to antihypertensive medications. If a person suddenly develops hypertension with no family history of high blood pressure and is either relatively young or if at more than 50–60 years old a person develops high blood pressure after having normal blood pressure throughout a long life, the physician may suspect RAS. RAS can also cause patients to have rapidly worsening shortness of breath due to fluid accumulation in the lungs, sometimes termed flash pulmonary edema, and it sometimes can cause rapidly worsening renal failure. Still, the majority of people with RAS have no signs or symptoms that can be clearly attributed to their RAS.

RAS that develops in relatively young people, such as less than about 30 years old, may be due to a condition termed fibromuscular dysplasia (FMD). In FMD, fibrous bands develop inside the renal arteries, leading to RAS. FMD typically occurs in young women, but may also occur in young men, causes fairly severe hypertension, and may affect either one or both kidneys. Sometimes, FMD can also involve arteries other than the renal arteries, including the carotid arteries that supply the brain.

Multiple tests can be used to diagnose RAS. A renal ultrasound is a noninvasive test that uses sound waves to create an image of the kidneys. A specialized version of an ultrasound test, termed a Doppler ultrasound, uses Doppler-based analysis of the ultrasound waves to determine whether there is likely to be a blockage of the renal artery. Sometimes a computerized tomography angiogram (CTA) scan or magnetic resonance angiogram (MRA) is used to diagnose RAS. These procedures are noninvasive, but their usefulness is partially limited because the contrast agents which may be used to image the blood vessels have risks to their use which increase as renal function decreases. The primary usefulness of these noninvasive tests is that they provide a high degree of, but not perfect, accuracy in diagnosing renal artery stenosis, without having an invasive procedure performed.

The definitive test to diagnosis RAS is a renal angiogram. An angiogram is an invasive test in which a tiny catheter is inserted into large arteries and threaded all the way to the arteries of the kidney. Special radiocontrast agents are then injected into the renal arteries, which enables direct visualization of the renal arteries. In this way, it is similar to a cardiac catheterization, with the exception that the kidney's arteries, not the heart's arteries, are being evaluated.

## Treatment Options and Outlook

The goal with treating RAS is to lower blood pressure and relieve the blockage or obstruction within the arteries of the kidney. This is achieved in part with antihypertensive medications, and often a combination of medications is required. In addition, cholesterol-lowering medications may be prescribed to prevent any further plaque buildup, and a blood thinner medication is given to help the blood pass through the arteries more freely.

In selected patients, direct procedures to reverse the RAS may be helpful. The most common procedure uses angioplasty, a procedure in which a tiny deflated balloon is inserted into the renal artery at the site of the stenosis; this is performed as a part of a renal angiogram described above. The balloon is inflated after insertion so that it can squash the plaque against the arterial wall, relieving the obstruction. A stent is often needed to hold the artery open. Another procedure that may be used is bypass surgery, in which a surgeon makes a new connection of the kidney to the aorta, using a vein or a synthetic tube. Sometimes an endarterectomy is the chosen procedure, in which the surgeon cleans out the plaque from the affected artery, leaving it clean and free-flowing. Surgical procedures are being used less often due to the greatly increased time required to recover after surgery, typically measured in weeks, as compared to the time to recover after angioplasty, where patients can return to near normal activities as early as the next day.

The choice of which patients with RAS should undergo invasive intervention, with either angioplasty or, rarely, surgery, is difficult. Recent evidence suggests that most patients with RAS do not benefit from these interventions and should instead focus their treatment on controlling their blood pressure, blood glucose, and cholesterol and optimizing other cardiovascular risk factors. However, patients with flash pulmonary edema, or those with reversible acute renal failure in response to the use of an ACEI or ARB medication, and who have recently worsening and difficult to control hypertension, or the onset of hypertension at a young age, typically less than 30 years old, are likely to benefit. In particular, the hypertension in patients with FMD is typically greatly improved with angioplasty, and these patients should routinely receive this therapy.

## Risk Factors and Preventive Measures

Individuals who have atherosclerosis in other arteries have an increased risk for developing RAS. Approximately 20 percent of patients with a history of a stroke, myocardial infarction, or claudication (a condition in which atherosclerosis limits blood flow to the legs and causes leg pain with exercise) will also have renal artery stenosis. Because cigarette smoking, hypertension, hyperlipidemia, and a family history of cardiovascular disease are risk factors for atherosclerosis, they are also risk factors for RAS. Men ages 50–70 have the highest risk for RAS but the disorder may also occur in younger individuals and females of any age.

See also HYPERTENSION.

**renal cell carcinoma**   See KIDNEY CANCER.

**renal disease, end-stage**   See END-STAGE RENAL DISEASE.

**renal dysplasia**   A condition in which the internal structures of the kidneys fail to develop normally. Usually this problem occurs in only one kidney; if it occurs with both kidneys, the fetus may not survive the pregnancy. A child born with renal dysplasia in both kidneys often has decreased renal function at birth and is at increased risk of developing end-stage renal disease. If the problem occurs in only one kidney, the child can usually grow and develop normally. A pregnant woman's abuse of cocaine or other illegal drugs can lead to the development of kidney dysplasia in the fetus. Some prescription medications may also cause renal dysplasia if taken during pregnancy, specifically ANGIO-TENSIN-CONVERTING ENZYME (ACE) INHIBITORS or ANGIOTENSIN II RECEPTOR BLOCKERS (ARBs).

In some cases, renal dysplasia occurs as a result of a genetic trait that is passed on to the child.

### Symptoms and Diagnostic Path

Renal dysplasia may cause an enlargement of the affected kidneys, although if only one kidney is affected, there are often no signs or symptoms. Renal dysplasia is diagnosed with a fetal ultrasound (sonogram) that is administered during pregnancy. However, the condition sometimes is not detected during pregnancy.

### Treatment Options and Outlook

If the renal dysplasia is limited to one kidney, usually no treatment is needed and only periodic follow-ups are indicated. If the dysplasia occurs in both kidneys, usually DIALYSIS is needed. When one kidney is affected, this kidney may shrink and become invisible on an X-ray or an ultrasound by the time the child is five years old.

### Risk Factors and Preventive Measures

If the parents of the child have renal dysplasia, they may pass on this trait to the child. Often the parents do not realize that they are genetic carriers of the trait because they have not experienced kidney problems.

The only preventive measure is to avoid illegal drugs during pregnancy and also to avoid medications that could harm the fetus, particularly ACE inhibitors and ARBs.

**renal osteodystrophy**   See CHRONIC KIDNEY DISEASE–MINERAL BONE DISORDER (CKD-MBD).

**renal papillary necrosis**   A kidney disorder in which all or part of the renal papillae die. The renal papillae refer to the area where the opening of the collecting ducts enter the kidneys.

(*Necrosis* means tissue death.) Renal papillary necrosis is most commonly associated with ANALGESIC NEPHROPATHY or with SICKLE CELL DISEASE, but other conditions may cause this disorder, including the following:

- diabetic nephropathy
- kidney infection (PYELONEPHRITIS)
- KIDNEY TRANSPLANTATION rejection
- sickle cell anemia (particularly in children)
- urinary tract obstruction

### Symptoms and Diagnostic Path

Symptoms that may occur with renal papillary necrosis include the following:

- blood in the urine (hematuria)
- cloudy urine
- back or flank pain
- tissue found in the urine
- incontinence
- increased urinary urgency or frequency
- painful urination
- chills
- passing large amounts of urine
- frequent urination at night (nocturia)

The physician may find that the area over the affected kidney is very tender to the touch. The doctor may also note that the patient has had a history of recurrent urinary tract infections (CYSTITIS). An imaging test such as a renal ultrasound or computerized tomography (CT) scan may show an obstruction or may show tissue present in the renal pelvis or ureter. A urinalysis may show dead tissue in the urine.

### Treatment Options and Outlook

There is no specific treatment for this disorder, instead, the underlying cause is sought and treated. If analgesic nephropathy is the cause, the condition may improve over time with avoidance of analgesics.

### Risk Factors and Preventive Measures

Individuals at risk for renal papillary necrosis include those who rely heavily on painkillers, as well as those with some autoimmune diseases.

**renal risk drugs**  See MEDICATIONS THAT CAN HARM THE KIDNEYS.

**renal tubular acidosis (RTA)**  A disease that is caused by a kidney defect that impairs the excretion of acids, and which causes an excess of acid in the blood. Renal tubular acidosis can lead to weakened bones, abnormal bone growth in children, the failure to thrive (to grow normally and be healthy) in children, KIDNEY STONES, and recurrent, sometimes severe HYPOKALEMIA. In children, renal tubular acidosis can also cause poor growth. Pediatric neurologist Donald Lewis has hypothesized that Tiny Tim, a character in the popular Christmas story *A Christmas Carol* by Charles Dickens, may have had renal tubular acidosis because of his small stature, malformed limbs, and other symptoms. However, when Ebenezer Scrooge was willing to pay for treatment (probably sodium bicarbonate), the child improved dramatically.

### Symptoms and Diagnostic Path

The symptoms of proximal renal tubular acidosis may include

- confusion
- dehydration
- fatigue
- muscle pain
- weakness

In addition, the patient may also have

- blood in the urine (hematuria)
- decreased urinary output
- increased heart rate or irregular heart rhythm

- back pain or pain in the bones or flank
- muscle cramps

Blood chemistries may show electrolyte abnormalities and metabolic acidosis. A check of blood pH levels may show a systemic metabolic acidosis. Quantitative analysis of the urine may show abnormal amounts of urinary phosphate, glucose, proteins, and amino acids in selected patients with proximal RTA. This combination of urinary abnormalities with proximal RTA is termed the Fanconi syndrome. The urine pH may be helpful in differentiating different types of RTA. In the untreated patient, urine pH is typically 6 or less in patients with proximal Type II RTA or hyperkalemia Type IV RTA, whereas in a patient with Type I, or distal RTA, urine pH is typically 7 or greater.

Renal tubular acidosis is diagnosed when blood testing shows an excessive amount of acid in the blood associated with low levels of bicarbonate in the blood; there is no other systemic disease which can explain this occurrence. Frequently the serum POTASSIUM levels are also abnormal. In proximal and distal RTA, the serum potassium level is low, whereas in Type IV or hyperkalemic RTA, the serum potassium level is elevated.

Distal RTA, also known as Type I RTA, may be an inherited disorder or a symptom of a systemic disease, such as lupus or SJOGREN'S SYNDROME. Other diseases that are associated with distal RTA are sickle cell disease and HYPERPARATHYROIDISM. In addition, ANALGESIC NEPHROPATHY has been associated with distal RTA, as has rejection of a transplanted kidney. Distal RTA is typically associated with hypokalemia, severe metabolic acidosis, and recurrent kidney stones. Without sufficient potassium in the bloodstream, the individual can develop heart arrhythmias, paralysis, and death. Children with classic distal RTA experience growth retardation, and adults with the disease have bone and kidney disease.

With proximal renal tubular acidosis, also known as Type II RTA, the most common causes are cystinosis and the use of some drugs (such as the chemotherapy agent, ifosfamide; the carbonic anhydrase inhibitor, acetazolamide; and outdated tetracycline). Proximal renal tubular acidosis is typically associated with hypokalemia and moderate metabolic acidosis.

Hyperkalemic RTA, also known as Type IV RTA, occurs when serum potassium levels rise, and the effects of serum potassium on renal acid excretion lead to decreased acid excretion by the kidneys, the subsequent retention of acids, and the development of metabolic acidosis. In some cases, the primary cause of hyperkalemic RTA is a low level of ALDOSTERONE; those cases are typically associated with normal levels of renal function.

Some medications may cause Type IV hyperkalemic RTA, such as DIURETICS, including spironolactone or eplerenone, as well as some blood pressure drugs such as ANGIOTENSIN-CONVERTING (ACE) INHIBITORS and ANGIOTENSIN II RECEPTOR BLOCKERS (ARBs). Some ANTIBIOTICS may cause this disease, such as trimethoprim or pentamidine (used to treat pneumonia). Heparin, an anticlotting drug, may also cause this disorder. Some IMMUNOSUPPRESSIVE DRUGS, such as antirejection drugs used with patients with a KIDNEY TRANSPLANTATION or other organ transplant, may cause hyperkalemic RTA, as may NONSTEROIDAL ANTI-INFLAMMATORY DRUGS (NSAIDs). In each of these cases, the effect of these medications is to inhibit renal potassium excretion, leading to hyperkalemia and the subsequent development of Type IV renal tubular acidosis.

Some diseases may also cause hyperkalemic RTA, such as Addison's disease, DIABETIC NEPHROPATHY, SICKLE CELL DISEASE, and AMYLOIDOSIS. The removal or one or both adrenal glands or the rejection of a kidney transplantation may cause Type IV RTA.

### Treatment Options and Outlook

The primary base therapies are to identify the underlying cause of renal tubular acidosis and to correct it, when possible. Renal obstruction should be evaluated with renal ultrasound and corrected if present. The patient who has had a kidney transplantation may require a KIDNEY BIOPSY in order to exclude rejection of the organ. Serologic testing for autoimmune diseases is frequently performed so that such conditions can be diagnosed and treated.

If an underlying cause cannot be identified and treated, then the primary goal of treatment is to reduce the level of acidity in the blood. Alkaline medications such as potassium citrate and sodium bicarbonate may decrease the acidity sufficiently; the relative amount of each of these must be balanced in order to appropriately correct the hypokalemia.

Patients with distal Type I RTA generally require only modest amounts of sodium bicarbonate and potassium citrate to correct both the metabolic acidosis and the hypokalemia. However, when the person is first diagnosed, it is important to treat the hypokalemia aggressively, as treatment with sodium bicarbonate can worsen the hypokalemia and increase the risk of hypokalemia-associated cardiac arrhythmias.

Patients with proximal Type II RTA generally require very large amounts of potassium citrate in sodium bicarbonate. This is because as the acidosis is corrected, the renal losses of bicarbonate worsen. Very aggressive therapy with large doses is necessary in order to overcome the ongoing renal losses. This is particularly important in children with proximal RTA, because correction of the acidosis can completely normalize the failure to thrive symptoms and the bone growth defects associated with proximal RTA.

With hyperkalemic RTA, treatment should be directed at dealing with the hyperkalemia. Typically, dietary potassium restriction and addition of diuretics is necessary. In the patient with chronic kidney disease and Type IV RTA, use of mineralocorticoids should be avoided, if possible, because this class of medication can worsen the progression of chronic kidney disease. The patient will need alkaline agents but will also need medication to lower the potassium level in the blood.

### Risk Factors and Preventive Measures

Individuals with certain diseases, such as sickle cell disease and amyloidosis, have an increased risk for RTA, and physicians should monitor the individual's electrolyte levels carefully. There are no known preventive measures, and if the individual develops any form of RTA, the disorder should be treated.

John, R., and A. M. Herzenberg. "Renal Toxicity of Therapeutic Drugs." *Journal of Clinical Pathology* 62 (2009): 505–515.

**rhabdomyolysis**   The breakdown of muscle fibers and the release of their contents into the bloodstream, which is a process that can damage the kidneys, sometimes severely and to the point of the development of acute tubular necrosis or to kidney failure. There are many possible causes of rhabdomyolysis, including severe trauma to the muscles, the abuse of cocaine or amphetamines, alcoholism, abnormally low blood levels of phosphate, seizures, extreme physical activity, heat exhaustion and/or heat stroke, and genetic disorders. The prolonged interruption of the blood supply to the muscles, as may occur if a building collapses or heavy equipment falls on a person's legs, can also cause rhabdomyolysis.

### Symptoms and Diagnostic Path

The symptoms and signs of rhabdomyolysis include the following:

- urine that is an abnormal color, such as red or the color of a cola soft drink
- muscle stiffness and/or weakness
- muscle tenderness

Rhabdomyolysis is diagnosed based on its signs and symptoms, physical examination, and the results of tests. Blood testing will reveal high levels of proteins that are usually found in the muscle cells, such as CPK. The urine will reveal the presence of myoglobin, which is normally found in muscle cells and not in urine. A urinalysis may test positive for hemoglobin but a microscopic examination of the urine does not show red blood cells; in this case, the hemoglobin test is positive because of the myoglobin in the urine which cross-reacts with the testing for hemoglobin.

Patients with rhabdomyolysis may have a variety of other laboratory abnormalities that are detected by testing. The patient's blood level of potassium may be very high (HYPERKALEMIA) because of the release of potassium from the damaged muscle cells. The potassium level may also be low because low potassium levels can increase the person's susceptibility to rhabdomyolysis. The phosphate level may be either high or low for similar reasons. The blood calcium level is often mildly low because the calcium in the blood can chemically attach to the damaged muscle cells.

### Treatment Options and Outlook

Treatment involves the administration of massive amounts of fluids to prevent kidney damage by flushing out the myoglobin. This fluid should be administered intravenously. Once kidney damage has developed, the benefit of fluid administration decreases, and patients may become at risk for pulmonary edema if excessive amounts of fluid continue to be administered. Increasing the pH of the urine helps to minimize the renal toxicity from rhabdomyolysis. This can be performed either by adding sodium bicarbonate to the intravenous fluids or with the use of medications, such as acetazolamide, that directly increase urine pH. Some patients will need to receive DIALYSIS. Patients may also be given diuretics to flush fluids and the myoglobin out of the system.

Hypocalcemia, if present, should generally not be treated unless the patient has tetany (a symptom of dangerously severe hypocalcemia) or definitive clinical side effects from the hypocalcemia. Calcium is deposited in the damaged muscle during the early phase of rhabdomyolysis, and during the later phases, calcium can be released from the muscles and result in life-threatening HYPERCALCEMIA. Minimizing calcium administration during the early phase can minimize this late-phase complication.

The outlook of rhabdomyolysis is largely dependent on if and how severely the kidneys are damaged. Individuals with mild cases of rhabdomyolysis may recover within a few days or weeks. If a patient develops kidney failure to the extent that he or she needs dialysis, then the time to recovery is much more variable. Most people will recover renal function, but some will not and will need continued dialysis or a KIDNEY TRANSPLANTATION.

### Risk Factors and Preventive Measures

Individuals who abuse or are dependent on drugs or alcohol are at risk for rhabdomyolysis, as are those who are treated inappropriately with medications that harm the kidneys. There are no known preventive measures, and individuals who develop rhabdomyolysis need immediate treatment and careful monitoring.

See also MEDICATIONS THAT CAN HARM THE KIDNEYS.

**scleroderma/scleroderma renal crisis** Scleroderma is a systemic autoimmune disorder and
a connective tissue disease that causes multiple
problems, including kidney disease. It may also
be caused by genetic and environmental factors,
although this is unclear. A scleroderma renal crisis causes ACUTE KIDNEY INJURY (kidney failure).
Silvio Belland Randone and colleagues stated
that many bacterial and viral agents have been
proposed as possible triggers to scleroderma,
such as Epstein-Barr virus, Cytomegalovirus,
and Parvovirus B19, but as of this writing, the
cause remains unknown.

About 2.3 to 22.8 new cases per million of
individuals with systemic sclerosis are diagnosed
each year worldwide, based on an analysis of
studies by Hélène Chifflot, M.D., and colleagues.
When considering everyone with scleroderma
(prevalence), there are about 50 to 300 cases
per 1 million persons worldwide, although Chifflot said the prevalence was higher in the United
States (276 persons per million) and in Australia
(233 per million), as compared to the prevalence
of this disorder in many other countries.

According to Armando Gabrielli and colleagues, there are two forms of scleroderma,
limited cutaneous scleroderma and diffuse cutaneous scleroderma. Limited cutaneous scleroderma affects only the arms, hands, and face.
In contrast, diffuse scleroderma, also known as
systemic sclerosis, affects a much broader area of
the skin and also can harm the internal organs.
It is the diffuse scleroderma that can lead to a
scleroderma renal crisis. The internal organs
most likely to be affected by diffuse scleroderma
are the kidneys, heart, lungs, and esophagus.

### Symptoms and Diagnostic Path

Scleroderma causes chronic inflammations of
the skin. This may appear as ulcerations and
thickening in the fingers. Many patients may
experience Raynaud's phenomenon, which is a
condition of abnormal circulation in the hands
that is severely exacerbated by cold or by stress,
causing the fingers to radically change color; for
example, a white person's fingers may change
to a bluish purple or red color. Acid reflux is
another common symptom among those with
scleroderma.

In the case of a scleroderma renal crisis, the
patient with no previous hypertension may
develop severe high blood pressure and the
rapid loss of kidney function. The average time
from the onset of scleroderma to a scleroderma
renal crisis is about 7.5 months, but it can vary
widely in different patients, according to Chifflot and colleagues. Aggressive treatment of the
scleroderma renal crisis is critical for preventing
permanent, irreversible kidney disease that can
lead to END-STAGE RENAL DISEASE.

According to Monique Hinchcliff, M.D., and
John Varga, M.D., a scleroderma renal crisis
develops in up to 10 percent of patients with
systemic sclerosis. Factors that increase the risk
are the use of high doses of corticosteroids (such
as more than 15 mg of prednisone per day),
older age, pregnancy, and new-onset anemia.
Patients with a scleroderma renal crisis also have
PROTEINURIA.

Diagnosis of scleroderma is made with laboratory testing as well as with testing of pulmonary
(lung) function, Doppler echocardiograpy, and a
high-resolution computerized tomography (CT)

scan of the chest. A KIDNEY BIOPSY can provide a definitive diagnosis of scleroderma affecting the kidneys.

### Treatment Options and Outlook

Prior to the usage of ANGIOTENSIN-CONVERTING ENZYME INHIBITORS (ACEIs), the death rate was high among patients with scleroderma renal crisis, but it has fallen considerably since then. In the analysis by Penn et al., DIALYSIS was not needed in 36 percent of the cases and was needed temporarily, up to three years, among 23 percent. Forty-one percent required permanent dialysis. Treatment with ACE inhibitors is known to be the most important component of treating the scleroderma renal crisis. If ACE inhibitors are not sufficient at lowering the blood pressure to normal, then other medications should be added. Because of the role of the renin-angiotensin system in the scleroderma renal crisis, medications that stimulate the renin-angiotensin system, such as DIURETICS, should be avoided if possible.

### Risk Factors and Preventive Measures

Women have at least a three times greater risk for the development of scleroderma than men. Individuals of African origin also have an elevated risk for scleroderma. Toxic exposure to some materials, such as silica and solvents, is also a risk factor.

See also LUPUS NEPHRITIS; SICKLE CELL DISEASE/ SICKLE CELL NEPHROPATHY.

Bellando Randone, Silvia, Serena Guiducci, and Marco Matucci Cerinic. "Systemic Sclerosis and Infections." *Autoimmunity Reviews* 8, no. 1 (2008): 36–40.

Chifflot, Hélène, et al. "Incidence and Prevalence of Systemic Sclerosis: A Systematic Literature Review." *Seminars in Arthritis and Rheumatism* 37 (2008): 223–235.

Gabrielli, Armando, M.D., Enrico V. Avvedimento, M.D., and Thomas Krieg, M.D. "Scleroderma." *New England Journal of Medicine* 360, no. 19 (May 7, 2009): 1,989–2,003.

Hinchcliff, Monique, M.D., and John Varga, M.D. "Systemic Sclerosis/Scleroderma: A Treatable Multisystem Disease." *American Family Physician* 78, no. 8 (2008): 961–968.

Penn, H., et al. "Scleroderma Renal Crisis: Patient Characteristics and Long-Term Outcomes." *Q J Med* 200, no. 8 (2007): 485–494. Available online. URL: http://qjmed.oxfordjournals.org/content/100/8/485.long. Accessed March 9, 2010.

## sickle cell disease/sickle cell nephropathy

Sickle cell disease is a genetic blood disorder that primarily affects African Americans and individuals of Mediterranean descent. When it causes kidney disease, this is referred to as sickle cell nephropathy. Sickle cell disease is also known as sickle cell anemia or hemoglobin SS disease (Hb SS). An estimated 100,000 people in the United States have sickle cell disease, which decreases an individual's life span by an estimated 25 to 30 years.

The disease is present at birth but symptoms may not occur until the child is four months old or older. Sickle cell disease causes two primary types of health crises: a hemolytic crisis (when damaged red blood cells break down), and vaso-occlusive crisis. Vaso-occlusion results in severely painful episodes and serious organ complications. These crises may occur every few years or many times a year and frequently require hospitalization as well as pain control.

### Symptoms and Diagnostic Path

The primary symptoms of sickle cell disease include the following:

- abdominal pain
- bone pain
- breathlessness
- delayed growth and delayed puberty
- fatigue
- fever
- jaundice
- paleness
- rapid heart rate

- susceptibility to infections
- lower leg ulcers (in adolescents and adults)

Other symptoms and signs that may occur are painful erection (in 10–40 percent of men with sickle cell disease), poor vision or blindness, and strokes.

To diagnose sickle cell disease, patients are tested with a complete blood count (CBC) as well as a sickle cell test and a hemoglobin electrophoresis. If sickle cell disease is diagnosed, then family members are also tested for the disease. The patient with sickle cell disease often will have an elevated level of bilirubin and a decreased serum hemoglobin level.

Sickle cell nephropathy indicates the presence of direct effects of sickle cell disease on the kidney. This typically involves PROTEINURIA and can lead to a decreased glomerular filtration rate. The proteinuria can be modest or may be very severe: 20 gm per day or more. Patients with proteinuria and hypertension are at particular risk of developing CHRONIC KIDNEY DISEASE and even END-STAGE RENAL DISEASE.

Sickle cell disease can also cause acute renal failure and ACUTE KIDNEY INJURY (AKI). The most common event is RENAL PAPILLARY NECROSIS. Papillary necrosis commonly presents as painless gross hematuria (blood in the urine that can be seen without testing and that is seen solely by looking at the urine). It may be complicated by urinary tract infection or obstruction. Another manifestation is acute segmental or total renal infarcts, and these may present with such symptoms as nausea, vomiting, flank or abdominal pain, fever, and presumably renin-mediated hypertension.

Patients with sickle cell disease frequently have difficulty concentrating their urine and as a result, excrete large amounts of urine. This can lead them to be more susceptible to volume depletion, which may precipitate the painful crises that are a hallmark of vaso-occlusive crises.

Sickle cell disease also leads to a markedly increased risk of a specific type of kidney cancer, renal medullary carcinoma. This is a highly·aggressive malignancy that is found almost exclusively in young patients with sickle cell trait or sickle cell disease. It generally occurs in relatively young patients, less than 20 years of age, and it is more frequent in males than females. It often presents with weight loss, gross hematuria, a urinary tract infection, flank pain, and an abdominal mass. Because renal medullary carcinoma is often metastatic (spread beyond the kidneys) when it is diagnosed, either surgery or chemotherapy is often ineffective.

### Treatment Options and Outlook

Patients with sickle cell disease need regular monitoring. Most are given folic acid to help them produce red blood cells. ANTIBIOTICS are given to prevent bacterial infections, which are particularly common among children with sickle cell disease. Physicians work to limit the symptoms and to treat any symptoms that do appear.

A bone marrow transplant can cure sickle cell disease but it is very difficult to find a compatible donor. Also, there are risks with bone marrow transplantation, such as infection or the rejection of the donated marrow.

According to Sophie Lanzkron, M.D., in her 2008 article in the Annals of Internal Medicine, an analysis of existing studies has revealed that hydroxyurea is an effective treatment for adults with sickle cell disease, although possible adverse effects are unknown based on an insufficient number of studies. (Hydroxyurea does not work in all people.) This drug has been used to treat sickle cell disease since 1998. Other drugs that are used to treat sickle cell disease may lead to leg ulcers, which does not appear to be a problem with hydroxyurea.

Most people with sickle cell disease live until their forties or fifties before they die of organ failure and/or infection.

### Risk Factors and Preventive Measures

African Americans and individuals of Mediterranean descent have the greatest risk for developing sickle cell disease. An estimated one in 12 African Americans carries the sickle cell trait.

The disease can present only if both parents carry the sickle cell trait. As a result, individuals who carry the sickle cell trait should receive genetic counseling if they hope to have children.

Immediate treatment for any infections that occur can improve the prognosis of the disease, as can treatment with immunizations for pneumococcus, influenza, and hepatitis B. Individuals with sickle cell disease should avoid smoking, because the disease carries risk to the lungs even without smoking, while smoking would exacerbate the risk further.

See also DIABETES INSIPIDUS.

Lanzkron, Sophie, M.D., et al. "Systematic Review: Hydroxyurea for the Treatment of Adults with Sickle Cell Disease." *Annals of Internal Medicine* 148 (2008): 939–955.

Ojo, A. O., R. L. Schmouder, Govaerts, T. C., and A. B. Leichtman. "Renal Transplantation in End-Stage Sickle Cell Nephropathy." *Transplantation* 67 (1999): 291–295.

Platt, Orah S., M.D. "Hydroxyurea for the Treatment of Sickle Cell Anemia." *New England Journal of Medicine 358,* no. 13 (2008): 1,362–1,369.

Thompson, Joanne, et al. "Albuminuria and Renal Function in Homozygous Sickle Cell Disease: Observations from a Cohort Study." *Archives of Internal Medicine* 167 (2007): 701–708.

**Sjögren's syndrome**   An autoimmune disease that affects up to 3.1 million adults in the United States, which may be present either alone or in association with other autoimmune diseases, such as RHEUMATOID ARTHRITIS or systemic lupus erythematosus (SLE). (Sjögren's is pronounced "SHOW-grins.") Patients with Sjögren's syndrome are at risk for the development of kidney disease, and they may develop INTERSTITIAL NEPHRITIS, although kidney failure does not commonly occur. It may also lead to distal renal tubular acidosis, the excretion of large amounts of relatively dilute urine, or, less commonly, to proximal renal tubular acidosis (RTA) Fanconi syndrome. Sjögren's syndrome may also affect other organs in addition to the kidneys, such as the lungs, liver, thyroid, skin, pancreas, and brain. Some people experience only mild symptoms of Sjögren's syndrome, while others suffer severe and debilitating consequences of this disorder.

The syndrome was first identified by Henrik Sjögren in the early part of the 20th century when he identified symptoms in patients with chronic arthritis as well as with severely dry eyes and dry mouth.

***Symptoms and Diagnostic Path***

Sjögren's syndrome most commonly affects the tear glands of the eyes and the salivary glands, causing dry eyes and a dry mouth. Primary Sjögren's syndrome occurs in individuals who have no other arthritic disorders, while secondary Sjögren's occurs among individuals who do have other autoimmune forms of arthritis, primarily either rheumatoid arthritis or systemic lupus erythematosus.

The most common renal manifestations of Sjögren's syndrome include hyposthenuria (the inability to concentrate the urine, resulting in the excretion of relatively large amounts of dilute urine). Less commonly, it may lead to proximal RTA with Fanconi syndrome. These manifestations, if they occur, tend to occur early in the course of the disease. (They do not present at all in many patients.) Glomerulonephritis is a relatively uncommon complication of Sjögren's syndrome, and when it occurs, it typically appears late in the course of the disease. Glomerulonephritis causes hypertension, mild proteinuria, and microscopic hematuria (blood in the urine).

Because of the severity of the eye and salivary gland dryness, there is an increased risk for infections; for example, severe dry mouth may lead to dental decay and gum disease as well as thrush, an oral yeast infection. Individuals with severely dry eyes may develop eye infections.

Other symptoms that may occur include

- chronic dry cough
- hoarseness

- numbness and tingling
- severe fatigue
- skin rashes
- joint and muscle pain
- difficulty swallowing
- loss of the sense of taste

An eye examination can help the physician determine the presence of Sjögren's syndrome. Blood tests for rheumatoid factor also indicate the possibility of this disorder. Biopsies of the salivary glands are sometimes used to determine the diagnosis.

The ophthalmologist may use a slit lamp to examine the eyes, which will show dryness and its severity as well as any inflammation of the exterior eye. The Schirmer test measures how well the tear glands are working. With this test, thin paper strips are placed on the lower eyelids to measure the level of wetness after five minutes.

A mouth examination by the primary care physician will determine if there are severe signs of dryness as well as swelling of the salivary glands. A lip biopsy can confirm the presence of Sjögren's syndrome.

The physician may also order a chest X-ray because Sjögren's syndrome sometimes leads to lung inflammation. Blood chemistries, such as a basic or a complete metabolic panel, in conjunction with a urinalysis will provide information on kidney function and evaluate for distal renal tubular acidosis.

It often takes years before patients with Sjögren's syndrome are diagnosed, often because the disorder has symptoms in common with both rheumatoid arthritis and lupus.

### Treatment Options and Outlook

Treatment is directed at the symptoms. Artificial tears can be used to treat dry eyes, and anti-inflammatory eyedrops, such as cyclosporine (Restasis) can be used to reduce eye inflammation. Dry mouth is treated with water, chewing gum, or saliva substitutes. Some patients take medications that stimulate saliva production, such as cevimuline (Evoxac) or pilocarpine (Salagen).

Patients should also receive regular dental care, since individuals with Sjögren's syndrome are at high risk for dental decay.

Patients who experience joint pain and rash may be treated with an antimalarial drug, hydroxychloroquine (Plaquinel). Patients with kidney diseases may need to take corticosteroids such as prednisone or IMMUNOSUPPRESSIVE DRUGS such as methotrexate (Rheumatrex) or cyclophosphamide (Cytoxan). Joint or muscle pain can be treated with NONSTEROIDAL ANTI-INFLAMMATORY DRUGS (NSAIDs).

Glomerulonephritis may respond to immunosuppressive drugs, typically involving intravenous cyclophosphamide and oral corticosteroids. However, renal interstitial disease and either distal or proximal RTA typically do not respond to immunosuppressants; treatment of distal or proximal RTA is directed at replacing the alkali losses, typically with citrate-containing compounds.

***Recommendations for oral hygiene*** The National Institute of Arthritis and Musculoskeletal and Skin Diseases (NIAMS) recommends the following tips for those with Sjögren's syndrome:

- Visit a dentist at least twice a year to have teeth cleaned and examined.
- Rinse the mouth with water several times a day. Avoid mouthwash with alcohol because alcohol is drying.
- Use toothpaste with fluoride, and brush after each meal and at bedtime. Nonfoaming toothpaste is less drying.
- Floss the teeth daily.
- Avoid sugar between meals.
- See a dentist immediately if there is continuous mouth burning or other oral symptoms.
- Ask the dentist if he or she recommends fluoride supplements or a protective varnish on the enamel of the teeth.

*Risk Factors and Preventive Measures*

Most individuals with Sjögren's syndrome develop symptoms in middle age, between ages 45 and 55 years; however, symptoms can occur at any age. It is rare in childhood. Women have about 10 times the risk of developing this syndrome as males. The factors that precipitate the development of Sjögren's syndrome are incompletely understood as of this writing in 2011.

The disorder cannot be prevented but actions can be taken to protect the eyes. According to NIAMS, the following general tips on eye care should be followed:

- Do not use artificial tears that are irritating. If one brand or prescription irritates the eyes, another brand should be tried. Eye drops without preservatives may limit the development of irration over time and may be needed for long-term use.

- Practice blinking. Individuals tend to blink less when they are reading or using the computer. Blink five to six times per minute.

- Protect the eyes from drafts, breezes, and wind.

- Place humidifiers in rooms where the individual with Sjögren's syndrome spends most of the time, such as the bedroom, or install a humidifier in the heating and air conditioning unit.

- Do not smoke, and be sure to avoid smoky rooms.

- If eye makeup is used, then apply mascara only to the tips of the lashes so it will not get into the eyes. If eye liner or eye shadow is used, it should not be placed on the skin under the lashes. In addition, facial creams should not be used on the lower lid skin if the individual wakes up with eye irritation.

- Ask the doctor if any other medications could be contributing to dryness. If so, ask how this dryness could be reduced. Medications that may increase dryness of the mouth and/or eyes include antihistamines, decongestants, diuretics, some antidiarrhea drugs, some antipsychotic medications, tranquilizers, some blood pressure medications, and some antidepressants.

See also LUPUS NEPHRITIS, URINE/URINALYSIS/URINE CULTURE.

Dale, Erin E., and Nicholas G. Popovich. "Sjögren's Syndrome." *U.S. Pharmacist* 32, no. 3 (2007): 72–81.
Fulop, Milford, M.D., and Meggan Mackay, M.D. "Renal Tubular Acidosis, Sjögren Syndrome, and Bone Disease." *Archives of Internal Medicine* 164 (2004): 905–909.
Helmick, Charles G., et al. "Estimates of the Prevalence of Arthritis and Other Rheumatic Conditions in the United States. Part I." *Arthritis & Rheumatism* 58, no. 1 (January 2008): 15–25.
Kassan, Stuart S., M.D., and Haralampois M. Moutsopoulos, M.D. "Clinical Manifestations and Early Diagnosis of Sjögren Syndrome." *Archives of Internal Medicine* 164 (2004): 1,275–1,284.
National Institute of Arthritis and Musculoskeletal and Skin Diseases (NIAMS). *Questions and Answers about Sjögren's Syndrome.* Bethesda, Md.: National Institutes of Health, December 2006.

**sleep problems** Sleep difficulties encompass trouble getting to sleep, trouble staying asleep, frequent awakenings, waking too early in the morning, and feeling unrested after sleeping. Some individuals with kidney disease experience significant sleep difficulties, especially patients who have recently started DIALYSIS. Some may experience day-night reversal, in which the individual is awake all night and sleeps during the day. Both adults and children receiving dialysis experience sleep difficulties.

Sleep difficulties are very common among patients receiving dialysis, according to a study by Nancy G. Kutner and colleagues. In this study of about 240 patients receiving dialysis, the researchers found that nearly 60 percent of the subjects reported significant sleep difficulties. They noted that those patients with sleep difficulties were also the most likely to report a depressed mood and physical pain. In addition, the subjects with sleep difficulties were more likely to be taking a benzodiazepine medication. In contrast, those who reported fewer problems with sleep were predicted by having less body pain and a higher level of education. Sometimes ANTIHYPERTENSIVE DRUGS and other drugs can impede sleep and sleep quality.

The researchers also noted that sleep loss can affect an individual's cognition and behavioral performance. Some studies have shown that sleep fragmentation is predictive for cognitive impairments regardless of the total amount of sleep that was received by the individual. That means that many breaks in sleep, even if the total sleep amount would otherwise be considered sufficient, are problematic. This may be due to the individual not attaining deep sleep patterns. Some individuals with kidney disease may have difficulty with sleep due to other specific disorders, such as restless legs syndrome or obstructive sleep apnea. The researchers said, "Increased understanding of links among sleep difficulty, management of sleep difficulty, and cognitive function could benefit multiple dimensions of dialysis patients' quality of life and daily function."

To treat sleep disorders, medications such as nonbenzodiazepines may be used, including such drugs as zaleplon (Sonata), zolpidem (Ambien), or eszopiclone (Lunesta). In addition, the patient may be given daytime sleep restriction; for example, naps during the day are restricted so that the individual is more likely to be able to sleep all night long. Patients may also keep sleep diaries to help themselves and physicians determine if there are any patterns or likely causes of their sleep difficulties, so that they can be resolved.

See also CHILDREN AND KIDNEY DISEASE; CHRONIC KIDNEY DISEASE; DEPRESSION; END-STAGE RENAL DISEASE.

Kutner, Nancy G., et al. "Association of Sleep Difficulty with Kidney Disease Quality of Life Cognitive Function Score Reported by Patients Who Recently Started Dialysis." *Clinical Journal of the American Society of Nephrology* 2 (2007): 284–289.

**smoking** Cigarette smoking increases the risk of the development of many diseases, such as RHEUMATOID ARTHRITIS, and also worsens the course of many other diseases and disorders, including kidney diseases and END-STAGE RENAL DISEASE (ESRD). Smoking is perhaps the most preventable cause of death, as well as of many chronic diseases in the United States. A large majority of people who abuse or depend on alcohol, an estimated 80 percent according to Mark S. Gold, M.D., in *The Encyclopedia of Alcoholism and Alcohol Abuse*, also are smokers. The combined use of nicotine and alcohol has a compounded and more harmful effect on the kidneys.

In a study by Melanie K. Haroun and colleagues and published in the *Journal of the American Society of Nephrology* in 2003, the researchers showed that

> Current smoking is associated with a 2.5 times greater risk of later developing CKD [chronic kidney disease] in the population as a whole and when stratified by gender. Possible mechanisms for smoking-related renal injury include the following: an increase in BP [blood pressure] and heart rate; alteration of diurnal [daytime] BP rhythm; an increase in sympathetic nerve activity, an increase in renal vascular resistance leading to a decrease in GFR [glomerular filtration rate]; arteriosclerososis of renal and intrarenal arteries and arterioles; tubulotoxicity; a direct toxic effect on endolethial cells; [and] increased clotting of platelets.

In another study by Anoop Shanker, Ronald Klein, and Barbara E. K. Klein, published in 2006 in the *American Journal of Epidemiology*, the researchers studied the association of smoking and heavy drinking and chronic kidney disease. They made two separate analyses, including an analysis of 324 people with chronic kidney disease and a longitudinal analysis of 3,392 people who did not have chronic kidney disease but who developed it within five years. The researchers found that smoking and heavy drinking (four or more drinks of alcohol per day) were associated with the development of chronic kidney disease, and increased the risk of kidney disease by nearly five times.

In looking at smoking alone, the researchers found that 3.6 percent of those who had never smoked developed chronic kidney disease, compared to 5.8 percent of former smokers. Among those who were current smokers, 15.1 percent developed chronic kidney disease. The researchers also analyzed the effect of stopping smoking on the onset of kidney disease, and they found that the longer the time in years since ending smoking, the more favorable the outcome; for example, if the person had stopped smoking 15 or more years ago, the prevalence of chronic kidney disease was 2.9 percent. If the time when smoking had ended was 5–14 years ago, the prevalence of kidney disease was 3.6 percent. Among those who had quit smoking less than five years ago, 17.1 percent developed chronic kidney disease.

The researchers also looked at gender differences and found that among males who were current smokers, the odds ratio for having chronic kidney disease was more than three-fold or 3.33. This means that the men who continued to smoke had more than a three times greater risk for developing kidney disease than the men who never smoked or who had smoked in the past but had ended the habit. Among women, the risk was lower, or 1.38 times greater for current smokers.

The researchers said:

> In a population-based sample consisting predominantly of older adults, smoking was found to be associated with chronic kidney disease independent of body mass index, NSAID [nonsteroidal anti-inflammatory drug] use, alcohol consumption, hypertension, diabetes and other confounders. The association between smoking and CKD [chronic kidney disease] was supported by evidence of a dose-response trend. We also found an independent association between heavy drinking (≤ [equal to or greater than] 4 servings of alcohol per day) and CKD. Further, joint exposure to smoking and heavy alcohol consumption was associated with almost fivefold odds of developing CKD than was their absence.

It is abundantly clear that individuals who smoke should end this habit as soon as possible to avoid increasing their risk for kidney disease as well as many other health hazards, such as heart disease and cancer. Most physicians will readily educate their patients on medications and other means to end the smoking habit.

See also CHRONIC KIDNEY DISEASE.

Haroun, Melanie, et al. "Risk Factors for Chronic Kidney Disease: A Prospective Study of 23,534 Men and Women in Washington County, Maryland." *Journal of the American Society of Nephrology* 14 (2003): 2,934–2,941.

Shankar, Anoop, Ronald Klein, and Barbara E. K. Klein. "The Association among Smoking, Heavy Drinking, and Chronic Kidney Disease." *American Journal of Epidemiology* 164, no. 3 (2006): 263–271.

**sodium**  An important chemical that is found in salt (sodium chloride) and many other foods, particularly foods that are canned or processed. About 90 percent of the sodium that is consumed by Americans is in the form of salt. Too much sodium in the body can elevate the blood pressure, while too low a sodium level can lead to low blood pressure. However, sufficient sodium deficiency to cause low blood pressure is rare in the absence of conditions that cause excessive sodium losses, such as the excessive use of DIURETICS or prolonged vomiting or diarrhea. Individuals with kidney disease should limit their overall consumption of sodium and eat foods that are low in (or have no) sodium, particularly people who have END-STAGE RENAL DISEASE (ESRD) or who are on DIALYSIS. Salt substitutes should be avoided because they often contain POTASSIUM, which is not healthy for a person with kidney disease. An increased salt intake in a patient with CHRONIC KIDNEY DISEASE increases the risk for PROTEINURIA and is also known to increase the risk and the rate of progression to end-stage renal disease.

Some types of KIDNEY STONES may be indirectly caused by excessive sodium consumption in the diet because higher sodium excretion rates increase the level of uric acid excretion, and some stones are formed of uric acid. Increasing salt intake also leads to increased urinary calcium excretion; because most kidney stones contain calcium, an increased salt consumption can then lead to the development of increased numbers as well as larger size of recurrent kidney stones.

According to the Rand Corporation in 2009, the average American adult consumes about 3,400 mg of sodium per day, and reducing sodium consumption could eliminate a minimum of 11 million cases of hypertension in the United States. The Institute of Medicine recommends that no more than 2,300 mg of sodium be consumed each day by adults, and some groups should consume lower amounts, such as individuals at risk for high blood pressure or who already have high blood pressure. According to the Centers for Disease Control and Prevention (CDC), only about 180 mg of sodium is actually needed each day for health.

Many Americans obtain their sodium from processed foods or from restaurant foods, both of which are high in sodium. The amount of sodium in processed foods can vary dramatically; for example, according to the CDC, one slice of frozen cheese pizza can contain from 450 mg to 1,200 mg of sodium, depending on the brand, and some breakfast sausage brands have twice the sodium content as other brands. Thus, it is important to read food labels, particularly among those who are watching their sodium consumption. It is not possible to read labels when eating out, and the CDC says that some restaurant salads have more than 900 mg of sodium. Thus, it cannot be assumed that salads are invariably healthy foods. (The sodium may be in the dressing that is provided. Individuals can request that their salad dressing be provided on the side so that they can limit the amount of dressing used.) An increasing number of restaurants provide information on "heart healthy foods" which should have a lower amount of sodium.

See also CALCIUM; MAGNESIUM; PHOSPHORUS; VITAMIN D.

Centers for Disease Control and Prevention, National Center for Chronic Disease Prevention and Health Promotion, Division for Heart Disease and Stroke Prevention. "Sodium: The Facts." November 2009.

Rand Corporation. *Hold the Salt: Lowering Sodium Intake Would Improve Health and Save Money.* Santa Monica, Calif.: Rand Corporation, 2009. Available online. URL: http://www.rc.rand.org/pubs/research_briefs/2009/RAND_RB9479.pdf. Accessed March 17, 2010.

**solitary kidney** The condition of having only one kidney. The person may be born with one kidney, which is called renal agenesis, and not discover that there is only one kidney unless imaging or surgery is performed. Others have a kidney removed because of KIDNEY CANCER or other severe kidney disease of one kidney. In addition, some people donate a kidney to a relative or friend with END-STAGE RENAL DISEASE (ESRD) so that person can have a KIDNEY TRANSPLANTATION. Studies have shown that donating a kidney does not affect the individual's life span. The solitary kidney handles all the work of filtering waste and extra fluid from the body, maintaining a normal blood pressure, creating hormones to keep the blood and bones healthy, and maintaining the balance of CALCIUM, PHOSPHORUS, SODIUM, and POTASSIUM in the blood.

Individuals who know that they have one kidney should be careful to maintain a healthy blood pressure that is below 130/80. If the person has HYPERTENSION, then medications can be used, such as ANGIOTENSIN-CONVERTING ENZYME INHIBITORS (ACEIs) or ANGIOTENSIN II RECEPTOR BLOCKERS (ARBs). Sometimes DIURETICS are needed to remove extra fluid. People with one kidney should also be careful to avoid injury, and if they participate in contact sports such as football or hockey, then wearing protective gear is important.

In general, people with only one kidney as a result of the surgical removal of the other kidney, whether from kidney donation, trauma, or cancer surgery, are not at significantly increased risk of disease that results from impaired kidney function.

See also CHRONIC KIDNEY DISEASE.

**stenosis, renal artery**   See RENAL ARTERY STENOSIS.

**streptococcus**   See   POSTSTREPTOCOCCAL GLOMERULONEPHRITIS.

**systemic sclerosis**   See SCLERODERMA/SCLERODERMA RENAL CRISIS.

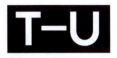

**tubular necrosis, acute**   See MEDICATIONS THAT CAN HARM THE KIDNEYS.

**uremia**   A term that is loosely used to describe the illness accompanying kidney failure, and in particular refers to the nitrogenous waste products that are associated with kidney failure. According to the American Association of Kidney Patients, the word *uremia* was first used in 1847 to indicate the symptoms of kidney failure. At that time, it was mistakenly believed that the urine was going into the blood. A. Brent Alper, Jr., M.D., and colleagues say that it was Piorry who first diagnosed this condition.

Symptoms of uremia can include worsening fatigue, nausea, and vomiting, particularly in the morning, as well as difficulty sleeping and decreased levels of concentration. Because the symptoms are indirectly related to the presence of urea and other nitrogenous waste products in the blood, conditions which increase their level can precipitate or worsen uremia. These conditions include bleeding into the intestinal tract, eating too much protein, and using certain medications, such as glucocorticoids (such as prednisone). In addition, conditions which worsen renal function, such as dehydration or exposure to medications which decrease kidney function, can precipitate or worsen uremia.

### Symptoms and Diagnostic Path

The primary symptoms of uremia are nausea and vomiting, headache, fatigue, appetite loss (which is so severe it could lead to malnutrition or starvation), mental confusion, and weakness.

Electrolyte abnormalities are common. Other symptoms may include muscle cramps, severe itching of the skin, and muscle twitches.

Uremia can affect nearly every organ in the body, such as causing palpitations in the heart or causing the lungs to fill with fluid. The sleepiness and fatigue is a result of the effect of uremia on the brain. Uremic encephalopathy refers to uremia that causes seizures, coma, and then, if it still not treated in time, death. Patients with uremia may also have uremic frost, a condition commonly observed over the lips and around the mouth in which the skin has a very fine residue of a whitish substance believed to be excreted urea. The skin may feel unusually velvety, especially in patients with high levels of pigment, such as African Americans.

Uremia is diagnosed by laboratory tests, such as testing for blood urea nitrogen (BUN). However, there is no specific level of BUN or other laboratory test that definitively diagnoses uremia. Instead, the diagnosis requires taking into account both the level of BUN in the blood and the extent and severity of the patient's symptoms. It is very important to diagnose uremia quickly and treat it because the patient could develop complications such as seizures and coma and in the worst case, could die.

### Treatment Options and Outlook

If the kidney has irreversibly failed, the treatment for uremia is either DIALYSIS or KIDNEY TRANSPLANTATION. If there is a reversible component to the kidney function, then the underlying cause should be found and treated.

### Risk Factors and Preventive Measures

Individuals with CHRONIC KIDNEY DISEASE are at risk for uremia. African Americans and Native Americans with diabetes are at risk for uremia. Kidney function should be regularly and routinely tested in all patients with kidney disease as well as patients without kidney disease, since many individuals with kidney disease have not been diagnosed. Alper et al. noted that the highest prevalence in the world for treated end-stage renal disease (ESRD) is in Japan, then Taiwan and the United States. Patients with ESRD are very likely to have uremia.

See also SLEEP PROBLEMS.

Alper, A. Brent, Jr., M.D., Rajesh G. Shenava, M.D., and Bessie A. Young, M.D. "Uremia." Available online to subscribers at eMedicine Nephrology. URL: http://emedicine.medscape.com/article/245926-overview. Accessed March 18, 2010.

Klinger, Alan, M.D. American Association of Kidney Patients. "What Are the Symptoms of Uremic Poisoning?" Tampa, Fla., 2004. Available online. URL: http://www.aakp.org/aakp-library/symptoms-of-uremic poisoning. Accessed March 18, 2010.

**uremic frost**   See UREMIA.

**urine/urinalysis/urine culture**   Urine is the waste fluid that is produced and excreted by the kidney. A urinalysis is a laboratory examination and analysis of a urine sample to detect infection and disease or to identify other abnormalities. There are many aspects of the urine that may be analyzed; for example, the urine can be studied for whether it is clear or cloudy. Cloudy urine may indicate that an infection is present. With a urinalysis, the urine is also analyzed for white blood cells (indicating an infection) and for blood in the urine (hematuria), which may indicate an infection or a KIDNEY STONE.

The urine may also be analyzed for the presence of protein (PROTEINURIA), an indicator of kidney disease, or be checked for glucose or other signs of disease. The presence of glucose in the urine indicates the likelihood that the patient has DIABETES MELLITUS, and, depending on the severity of the urinary glucose, will indicate the severity of the lack of blood glucose control.

Urine ketones can be identified by standard urinalysis. At present, in conjunction with urinary glucose, this can indicate the presence of diabetic ketoacidodis (DKA), a serious complication of diabetes. In the absence of urinary glucose, this may indicate the presence of starvation or other etiologies for inadequate nutritional intake.

The urinary specific gravity indicates the degree of concentration of the urine. If the urinary specific gravity is low, this can indicate the presence of excessive oral fluid intake. On the other hand, if the urinary specific gravity is very high, this can indicate the presence of dehydration.

Many employers require a urinalysis to detect the presence of illegal drugs before they will hire a new employee.

A urine culture is a laboratory test in which a sterile urine sample is collected by the patient in a small cup that is provided by the physician or laboratory. The laboratory will determine whether bacteria are present in the urine, and if so, the quantitative number of bacteria and the specific type of bacteria. If the urine culture is positive (indicating an infection), then the culture will help the physician to determine which ANTIBIOTICS to prescribe. A urine culture is more accurate than a simple urinalysis in which dipsticks are used to detect possible infection.

### Procedure

Two procedures are used for testing urine: urinalysis and urine culture.

*Urinalysis*   The individual is instructed to urinate in a small cup after cleansing of either the end of the penis for men, or for women, the perineum, with one or more sterile wet towels that are provided. In some cases, the individual is directed to urinate a small amount into the toilet and then to urinate in the cup. In other cases, the individual is instructed to simply urinate in the cup after cleansing the area. Generally the doctor's office uses dipsticks to test for the presence of nitrates and/or white blood cells. If either is present, this suggests the likelihood of a bacterial infection.

*Urine culture*  The patient is usually advised to provide a clean-catch specimen of urine in a provided container. The patient wipes the genital area with a sterile wet towel provided by the physician's staff or the laboratory, as described above in the procedure for urinalysis. The patient may be advised to begin urinating, and then to stop and then to urinate into the container provided for the urine collection.

### Risks and Complications

There are no risks or complications with either a urinalysis or a urine culture.

### Outlook and Lifestyle Modifications

The urinalysis or urine culture will determine if infection is present, and if infection is identified, then most patients will be prescribed antibiotics to treat it. One common lifestyle modification is that the patient with an infection is often advised to markedly increase their intake of fluids, particularly water. Patients with recurrent infections may be advised to drink cranberry juice.

See also CYSTITIS; PYELONEPHRITIS.


**urine microscopy**  See CYSTITIS; URINE/URINALYSIS/URINE CULTURE.


**urolithiasis**  See KIDNEY STONES.

# V

**vesicoureteric reflux**   See REFLUX NEPHROPATHY.

**vitamin D**   A fat-soluble vitamin that is critically important in boosting levels of blood CALCIUM as well as in the absorption of PHOSPHORUS in the intestines. Vitamin D also modulates immune function and reduces inflammation. In 2010, Danish immunologists reported in *Nature Immunology* that vitamin D is crucial to helping the T cells of the immune system to fight infections. In fact, when a foreign pathogen invades the body, the T cells actually seek out vitamin D. Vitamin D is also important for bone growth, and insufficient levels of vitamin D cause rickets in children and osteomalacia in adults. Vitamin D is present in some foods, and it is also produced in the human body when sunlight strikes the skin and causes vitamin D synthesis. Synthetic vitamin D can be taken by individuals who need supplementation. The optimal daily dose of vitamin D is about 25–50 micrograms. However, the vitamin D that is either produced naturally or that comes through dietary sources requires further processing to convert it from an inactive to an active form. This processing essentially occurs only in the kidneys in the normal individual. As a result, as kidney function declines, the occurrence of active vitamin D deficiency increases. Treating these individuals may require the use of prescription vitamin D analogues, such as calcitriol, paricalcitol, or doxercalciferol, that do not require processing in the kidneys.

The best sources of vitamin D in foods are found in the skin of fish such as tuna, salmon, or mackerel, and small amounts of vitamin D are also found in cheese, beef liver, and egg yolks. However, most Americans gain their vitamin D from foods that are fortified with this substance, such as milk and breakfast cereals. Infant formulas are also fortified with vitamin D and other vitamins and minerals.

Vitamin D deficiencies may occur among individuals with CHRONIC KIDNEY DISEASE, especially those with kidney failure, because the kidneys are unable to convert vitamin D to an active form. People who have undergone gastric bypass surgery in order to combat OBESITY may become deficient in vitamin D.

It is also possible to have excessively *high* levels of vitamin D, which is referred to as vitamin D toxicity. Symptoms of vitamin D toxicity are poor appetite, constipation, nausea and vomiting, and weight loss. Vitamin D toxicity can lead to high blood levels of calcium (HYPERCALCEMIA), causing confusing and abnormalities of the heart rhythms. High levels of vitamin D can also cause deposits of phosphate (phosphorus) in the kidneys.

Vitamin D supplements can interact with some medications, particularly corticosteroids such as prednisone, as well as cholesterol-lowering medications such as cholestyramine (Questran, LoCholest, and Prevalite). In addition, phenytoin (Dilantin), a medication prescribed to treat seizures, increases the liver metabolism of vitamin D supplements and reduces the absorption of calcium.

See also MAGNESIUM; POTASSIUM; SODIUM.

Lapp, Julia L. "Vitamin D: Bone Health and Beyond." *American Journal of Lifestyle Medicine* 3 (2009): 386–393.

Von Essen, Marina Rode, et al. "Vitamin D Controls T Cell Antigen Receptor Signaling and Activation of Human T Cells." *Nature Immunology* 11, no. 4 (2010): 344–349.

**Wegener's granulomatosis** A rare systemic autoimmune disease that causes inflammation and damage to the blood vessels of the lungs, sinuses, upper respiratory tract, and kidneys. In the worst case of kidney damage, the kidneys may fail altogether. The cause of Wegener's granulomatosis is unknown; it is not believed to be an inherited disease, nor is it contagious. About 75 percent of individuals with Wegener's granulomatosis have kidney disease, according to the National Institute of Allergy and Infectious Diseases (NIAID); however, many individuals have no symptoms of kidney disease, and kidney disease is detected only with laboratory blood and urine tests.

In 1950, the disorder was named after Dr. Friedrich Wegener, a German pathologist who discovered the nasal aspect of the disorder in 1936; however, there has been a movement to change the name of the disorder because Dr. Wegener has been linked to the Nazi party during World War II and at least one experiment on deceased concentration camp prisoners who had been experimented on. It has been proposed that the disorder be renamed ANCA-associated systemic vasculitis, although Wegener's granulomatosis remains a commonly used term as of this writing.

### Symptoms and Diagnostic Path

The most common first signs of Wegener's granulomatosis are frequent bouts of a runny nose and sinusitis, as well as fever, fatigue, and night sweats. Weight loss and poor appetite are also common. It may also present slowly with renal involvement. This may be manifested as hematuria (blood in the urine), which may appear as bloody appearing, cola-colored, or tea-colored urine. Frequently, hematuria is identified only in screening urinalysis obtained for other reasons. Also, rarely, patients are relatively asymptomatic and are identified solely because of decreased renal function identified in laboratory testing.

Other symptoms may include the following:

- coughing with or without blood
- joint pain
- shortness of breath
- chest pain
- night sweats
- generalized malaise

Often the diagnosis takes some time, as the disorder is often confused with other common disorders, such as sinusitis (which is often present). If Wegener's granulomatosis is suspected, the doctor may order a blood test to check for the presence of antineutrophil cytoplasmic antibodies (ANCA). If these are found in the bloodstream, this is a strong indicator for the diagnosis of Wegener's granulomatosis. However, only a biopsy of the affected organ can definitively prove the presence of this disorder. Because patients may have circulating ANCA antibodies without disease, a biopsy to prove actual disease is necessary before beginning treatment for Wegener's granulomatosis.

A urinalysis is also checked for the presence of blood in the urine or protein in the urine (PROTEINURIA). A computerized tomography (CT) scan of the chest may be performed, as may a routine chest X-ray.

### Treatment Options and Outlook

Medications are used to treat this disorder, including such drugs as cyclophosphamide (Cytoxan) and mycophenolate Mofetil (Cell-Cept). Corticosteroids are also often prescribed, such as prednisone. These medications can cause major side effects, and the individual needs regular checks of kidney function to make sure that the kidneys are functioning properly. It is very important to treat the disease, because without treatment, irreversible renal failure, pulmonary hemorrhage, or death can occur. However, with treatment, the outlook is favorable for most people. The individual may also experience a remission, with the disease returning again about two years later, when treatment becomes imperative again.

### Risk Factors and Preventive Measures

There are no known risk factors to this disease, nor are there any preventive measures to avoid its development. If the disease develops, then the symptoms should be treated and monitored.

Feder, Barnaby J. "A Nazi Past Casts a Pall on Name of a Disease." *New York Times.* January 22, 2008. Available online. URL: http://www.nytimes.com/2008/01/22/health/22dise.html?_r=3&oref=slogin&p agewanted =print. Accessed February 21, 2010.

# APPENDIXES

Appendix I: Organizations
  A. National Organizations
  B. International Kidney Disease Organizations
  C. End-Stage Renal Disease Networks

Appendix II: State Organizations and Programs
  A. State and Territorial Health Insurance Programs
  B. State Health Departments
  C. State Affiliates of the National Kidney Foundation
  D. State and Territorial Diabetes Prevention
      Programs in the United States
  E. Transplant Centers by Home State
  F. State Vocational Rehabilitation Agencies

Appendix III: Canadian Organizations

Appendix IV: Number of Dialysis and Transplant
              Facilities: By State and Territory,
              2001–2006

Appendix V: Abnormalities of Selected Clinical and
            Biochemical Parameters in the NHANES
            1999–2006 Population

Appendix VI: Worldwide Incidence of End-Stage Renal
             Disease

Appendix VII: Worldwide Incidence of End-Stage Renal
              Disease due to Diabetes, 2003–2007

Appendix VIII: Donor Designation Status by State

Appendix IX: Statewide Drug Assistance Programs

# APPENDIX I
## ORGANIZATIONS

## A. National Organizations

### AARP
601 East Street NW
Washington, DC 20049
(888) 687-2277
http://www.aarp.org

### Abledata (Assistive Devices/Rehabilitation)
8630 Fenton Street
Suite 930
Silver Spring, MD 20910
(800) 227-0216
(301) 608-8958 (fax)
http://www.abledata.com

### Administration on Aging
U.S. Department of Health and Human Services
200 Independence Avenue SW
Washington, DC 20201
(202) 619-0724
(202) 357-3555 (fax)
http://www.aoa.gov

### AIDSinfo
P.O. Box 6303
Rockville, MD 20849-6303
(800) HIV-0440 (800-448-0440)
(301) 315-2818 (fax)
http://www.aidsinfo.nih.gov

### Alport Syndrome Foundation
1608 East Briarwood Terrace
Phoenix, AZ 85048
(480) 460-0621
http://www.alportsyndrome.org

### American Academy of Family Physicians
P.O. Box 11210
Shawnee Mission, KS 66207
(800) 274-2237
(913) 906-6075 (fax)
http://www.aafp.org

### American Academy of Neurology
1080 Montreal Avenue
St. Paul, MN 55116
(800) 879-1960
(651) 695-2717
(651) 695-2791 (fax)
http://www.aan.com

### American Association for Marriage and Family Therapy
112 South Alfred Street
Alexandria, VA 22314
(703) 838-9808
(703) 838-9805 (fax)
http://www.aamft.org

### American Association of Clinical Urologists
Two Woodfield Lake
1100 East Woodfield Road
Suite 520
Schaumburg, IL 60173
(847) 517-7225
(847) 517-7229 (fax)
http://www.aacuweb.org

### American Association of Diabetes Educators (AADE)
200 West Madison Avenue
Suite 800
Chicago, IL 60606
(800) 338-3633
http://www.diabeteseducator.org

## American Association of Genitourinary Surgeons

Department of Urology
3875 Taubman Center SPC 5330
1500 East Medical Center Drive
Ann Arbor, MI 48109
(734) 232-4943
(734) 936-8037 (fax)
http://www.aagus.org

## American Association of Kidney Patients

3505 East Frontage Road
Suite 315
Tampa, FL 33607
(800) 749-AAKP
(813) 636-8122 (fax)
http://www.aakp.org

## American Association of People with Disabilities

1629 L Street NW
Suite 950
Washington, DC 20006
(202) 457-0046
(800) 840-8844
(202) 457-0473 (fax)
http://www.aapd.com

## American Autoimmune Related Diseases Association (AARDA)

22100 Gratiot Avenue
East Detroit, MI 48021
(586) 776-3900
http://www.aarda.org

## American Board of Urology

2216 Ivy Road
Suite 210
Charlottesville, VA 22903
(434) 979-0059
(434) 979-0266 (fax)

## American Cancer Society

1599 Clifton Road NE
Atlanta, GA 30329-4251
(404) 320-3333
http://www.cancer.org

## American Chronic Pain Association

P.O. Box 850
Rocklin, CA 95677-0850
(800) 533-3231
(916) 632-3208 (fax)
http://www.theacpa.org

## American College of Emergency Physicians

1125 Executive Circle
Irving, TX 75038-2522
Mailing: P.O. Box 619911
Dallas, TX 75261-9911
(800) 798-1822 or (972) 550-0911
(972) 580-2816 (fax)
http://www.acep.org

## American College of Health Care Administrators

300 North Lee Street
Alexandria, VA 22314
(703) 739-7900
http://www.achca.org

## American College of Medical Genetics

9650 Rockville Pike
Bethesda, MD 20814-3998
(301) 634-7127
http://www.acmg.net//AM/Template.
    cfm?Section=Home3

## American College of Physicians

190 North Independence Mall West
Philadelphia, PA 19106
(800) 523-1546
http://www.acponline.org

## American College of Surgeons

633 North Saint Clair Street
Chicago, IL 60611
(312) 202-5000
(312) 202-5001 (fax)
http://www.facs.org

## American Counseling Association

5999 Stevenson Avenue
Alexandria, VA 22304
(800) 347-6647
(800) 473-2329 (fax)
http://www.counseling.org

**American Diabetes Association (ADA)**
1701 North Beauregard Street
Alexandria, VA 22314
(800) 342-2383
http://www.diabetes.org

**American Dietetic Association**
120 South Riverside Plaza
Suite 2000
Chicago, IL 60606
(800) 877-1600
http://www.eatright.org

**American Foundation for Donation &
   Transplantation**
8154 Forest Hill Avenue
Suite 3
Richmond, VA 23235
(804) 323-9890
(804) 323-1300 (fax)
http://www.scopf.org

**American Geriatrics Society**
The Empire State Building
New York, NY 10118
(212) 308-1414
(212) 832-8646 (fax)
http://www.americangeriatrics.org

**American Health Assistance Foundation**
22512 Gateway Center Drive
Clarksburg, MD 2081
(800) 437-2423
(301) 948-4403 (fax)
http://www.ahaf.org

**American Health Care Association (AHCA)**
1201 L Street NW
Washington, DC 20005
(202) 842-4444
http://www.ahca.org

**American Health Quality Association**
1155 21st Street NW
Suite 202
Washington, DC 20036
(202) 331-5790
(202) 331-9334 (fax)
http://www.ahqa.org

**American Heart Association/American
   Stroke Association**
7272 Greenville Avenue
Dallas, TX 75231-4596
For Heart Association: (800) 242-8721
For Stroke Association: (888) 478-7653
http://www.americanheart.org

**American Hospice Foundation**
2120 L Street NW
Suite 200
Washington, DC 20037
(202) 223-0204
(202) 223-0208 (fax)
http://americanhospice.org

**American Hospital Association**
One North Franklin
Chicago, Illinois 60606-3421
(312) 422-3000
http://www.aha.org

**American Kidney Fund**
6110 Executive Boulevard
Suite 1010
Rockville, MD 20852
(800) 638-8299
(301) 881-0898 (fax)
http://www.kidneyfund.org

**American Kidney Stone Management, Ltd.**
797 Thomas Lane
Columbus, OH 43214
(800) 637-5188
http://www.aksm.com

**American Medical Association**
515 North State Street
Chicago, IL 60610
(800) 621-8335
http://www.ama-assn.org

**American Nephrology Nurses' Association**
East Holly Avenue
Box 56
Pitman, NJ 08071
(888) 600-2662
(856) 589-7463 (fax)
http://www.annanurse.org

**American Nurses Association**
8515 Georgia Avenue
Suite 400
Silver Spring, MD 20910
(800) 274-4262
(301) 628-5001 (fax)
http://www.nursingworld.org

**American Occupational Therapy Association**
4720 Montgomery Lane
Bethesda, MD 20824
(301) 652-2682
(301) 652-7711 (fax)
http://www.aota.org

**American Osteopathic Association**
142 East Ontario Street
Chicago, IL 60611
(800) 621-1773
http://www.osteopathic.org

**American Pharmacists Association**
1100 15th Street NW
Suite 400
Washington, DC 20005
(800) 237-2742
http://www.pharmacist.com

**American Physical Therapy Association**
1111 North Fairfax Street
Alexandria, VA 22314
(800) 999-2782
http://www.apta.org

**American Psychiatric Association**
1000 Wilson Boulevard
Suite 1825
Arlington, VA 22209
(703) 907-7300
http://www.psych.org

**American Psychological Association**
750 First Street NE
Washington, DC 20002-4242
(800) 374-2721
http://www.apa.org

**American Red Cross**
2025 E Street NW

Washington, DC 20006
(800) 435-7669
http://www.redcross.org

**American Renal Associates**
66 Cherry Hill Drive
Beverly, MA 01915
(978) 922-3080
(978) 750-4740 (fax)
http://www.americanrenal.com

**American Society for Artificial Internal Organs**
980 North Federal Highway
Suite 212
Boca Raton, FL 33432
(561) 391-8589
(561) 368-9153 (fax)
http://www.asaio.com

**American Society for Histocompatibility and Immunogenetics**
15000 Commerce Parkway
Suite C
Mt. Laurel, NJ 08054
(856) 638-0428
(856) 439-0525 (fax)
http://www.ashi-hia.org

**American Society for Parenteral and Enteral Nutrition (A.S.P.E.N.)**
8630 Fenton Street
Suite 412
Silver Spring, MD 20910
(301) 587-6315
http://www.nutritioncare.org/

**American Society of Diagnostic and Intervention Nephrology**
c/o Mary Lea Nations
134 Fairmont Street
Suite B
Clinton, MS 39056
(601) 924-2220
(601) 924-0720 (fax)
http://www.asdin.org

**American Society of Hypertension**
148 Madison Avenue, Fifth Floor

New York, NY 10016
(212) 696-9099
http://www.ash-us.org

## American Society of Nephrology
1725 I Street NW
Suite 510
Washington, DC 20006
(202) 659-0599
(202) 659-0709 (fax)
http://www.asn-online.org

## American Society of Pediatric Nephrology
3400 Research Forest Drive
Suite B7
The Woodlands, TX 77381
(281) 419-0052
(281) 419-0082 (fax)
http://www.aspneph.com

## American Society of Transplantation
15000 Commerce Parkway
Suite C
Mt. Laurel, NJ 08054
(856) 439-9986
(856) 439-9982 (fax)
http://www.a-s-t.org

## American Society of Transplant Surgeons
2461 South Clark Street
Suite 640
Arlington, VA 22202
(703) 414-7870
(703) 414-7874 (fax)
http://www.asts.org

## American Urogynecologic Society
2025 M Street NW
Suite 800
Washington, DC 20036
(202) 367-1167
(202) 367-2167 (fax)
http://www.augs.org

## American Urological Association
1000 Corporate Boulevard
Suite 410
Linthicum, MD 21090

(866) 746-4282
(410) 689-3800 (fax)
http://www.auanet.org

## American Urological Association Foundation, Inc.
1000 Corporate Boulevard
Suite 410
Linthicum, MD 21090
(410) 689-3700
(410) 689-3800 (fax)
http://www.urologyhealth.org

## ARCH National Respite Network and Resource Center
800 Eastowne Drive
Suite 105
Chapel Hill, MD 27514
http://www.archrespite.org

## Arthritis Foundation
1330 West Peachtree Street
Suite 100
Atlanta, GA 30309
(800) 568-4045
http://www.arthritis.org

## Association for the Advancement of Medical Instrumentation
1110 North Glebe Road
Suite 220
Arlington, VA 22201
(703) 525-4890
http://www.aami.org

## Association of Organ Procurement Organizations
1364 Beverly Road
Suite 100
McLean, VA 22101
(703) 556-4242
(703) 556-4852 (fax)
http://www.aopo.org

## Association of State and Territorial Health Officials
1275 K Street NW
Suite 800
Washington, DC 20005

(202) 371-9090
http://www.astho.org

**Autosomal Recessive Polycystic Kidney Disease & Congenital Hepatic Fibrosis Alliance (ARPKD/CHF Alliance)**
P.O. Box 70
Kirkwood, PA 17536
(800) 708-8892 or (717) 529-5555
(800) 807-9110 (fax)
http://www.arpkd.org

**Canadian Kidney Foundation**
National Office
300-5165 Sherbrooke Street West
Montreal, QC H4A 1T6
(514) 369-4806
http://www.kidney.ca/

**CancerCare**
275 Seventh Avenue
Floor 22
New York, NY 10001
(800) 813-4673
http://www.cancercare.org

**Cancer Information Service**
National Cancer Institute Public Inquiries Office
6116 Executive Boulevard, Room 3036A, MSC 8322
Bethesda, MD 20892-8322
(800) 422-6237
http://www.cancer.gov

**Centers for Disease Control and Prevention**
1600 Clifton Road
Atlanta, GA 30333
(404) 639-3311
(800) 232-4636
http://www.cdc.org

**Centers for Medicare and Medicaid Services (CMS)**
7500 Security Boulevard
Baltimore, MD 21244
(410) 786-3000
(877) 267-2323
(410) 786-8532 (fax)

http://www.cms.hhs.gov
http://www.medicare.gov

**Chronic Disease Research Group**
914 South Eighth Street
Suite S-206
Minneapolis, MN 55404
(612) 347-3903
http://www.cdrg.org

**Chronic Kidney Disease Initiative**
Centers for Disease Control and Prevention
4770 Buford Highway
Mail Stop K-10
Atlanta, GA 30341
(800) CDC-INFO
(770) 488-1148 (fax)
http://www.cdc.gov/diabetes/projects/kidney.htm

**Clearinghouse on Disability Information**
Office of Special Education and Rehabilitative Services
United States Department of Education
550 12th Street SW, Room 5133
Washington, DC 20202-2550
(202) 245-7307
http://www.ed.gov/about/offices/list/osers/codi.htm.

**Coalition on Donation**
700 North Fourth Street
Richmond, VA 23219
(804) 782-4920
http://www.shareyourlife.org

**Council of Nephrology Social Workers of the National Kidney Foundation**
30 East 33rd Street
New York, NY 10016
(800) 622-9010, ext. 130
http://www.kidney.org/professionals/CNSW

**Department of Health and Human Services**
200 Independence Avenue SW
Washington, D.C. 20201
(202) 619-0257
http://www.hhs.gov

**Diabetes Insipidus and Related Disorders Network**
535 Echo Court
Saline, MI 48176

**Diabetes Insipidus Foundation**
c/o Mike Gandrud
1232 24th Street
Ames, IA 50010
http://www.diabetesinsipidus.org

**Dialysis Patient Citizens**
900 Seventh Street NW
Suite 670
Washington, DC 20001
(888) 423-5002
(202) 789-6935 (fax)
http://www.dialysispatients.org

**Disabled American Veterans (DAV)**
P.O. Box 14301
Cincinnati, OH 45250
(877) 426-2838
http://www.dav.org

**Employee Benefits Security Administration**
Department of Labor
Frances Perkins Building
200 Constitution Avenue NW
Washington, DC 20210
http://www.dol.gov/ebsa

**Endocrine Society**
8401 Connecticut Avenue
Suite 900
Chevy Chase, MD 20815
(888) 363-6274
http://www.endo-society.org

**Endourological Society**
Long Island Jewish Medical Center
Department of Urology
270-05, 76th Avenue
New Hyde Park, NY 11040
(718) 470-3900
(718) 643-8126 (fax)
http://www.endourology.org

**Family Caregiver Alliance**
180 Montgomery Street
Suite 1100
San Francisco, CA 94104
(800) 445-8106
http://www.caregiver.org

**Food and Drug Administration (FDA)**
5600 Fishers Lane
Rockville, MD 20857
(888) 463-6332
http://www.fda.gov

**Food and Nutrition Information Center**
Agricultural Research Service
United States Department of Agriculture
National Agricultural Library
10301 Baltimore Avenue, Room 105
Beltsville, MD 20705-2351
(301) 504-5414
http://www.nal.usda.gov/fnic

**Forum of End-Stage Renal Disease Networks**
P.O. Box 70835
Richmond, VA 23255
(804) 418-7990
http://www.esrdnetworks.org

**Foundation for Biomedical Research**
818 Connecticut Avenue NW
Suite 900
Washington, DC 20006
(202) 457-0654
http://www.fbresearch.org

**Genetic and Rare Diseases Information Center**
P.O. Box 8126
Gaithersburg, MD 20898-8126
(888) 205-2311
http://rarediseases.info.nih.gov/GARD

**Glaucoma Research Foundation**
251 Post Street
Suite 600
San Francisco, CA 94108
(800) 826-6693
http://www.glaucoma.org

**Health Resources and Services
    Administration Information Center**
P.O. Box 2910
Merrifield, VA 22116
(888) 275-4772
http://www.hrsa.gov

**Hereditary Nephritis Foundation**
1390 West 6690 South
Suite 202H
Murray, UT 84123
(801) 262-5901
http://www.cc.utah.edu/~cla6202/HNF.htm

**Hospice Association of America**
228 Seventh Street SE
Washington, DC 20003
(202) 546-4759
http://www.hospice-america.org

**Hospice Foundation of America**
2001 S Street NW
Suite 300
Washington, DC 20009
(800) 854-3402
http://www.hospicefoundation.org

**IgA Nephropathy Support Network**
89 Ashfield Road
Shelburne Falls, MA 01370
(413) 625-9339
http://www.igansupport.org/index.html

**Indian Health Service**
The Reyes Building
Rockville, MD 20852
(301) 443-3593
http://www.ihs.gov

**Institute for Cancer Prevention**
One Dana Road
Valhalla, NY 10595
(914) 592-6317
http://www.ahf.org

**International Myeloma Foundation**
12650 Riverside Drive
Suite 206
North Hollywood, CA 91607

(800) 452-2873
http://www.myeloma.org

**International Pediatric Nephrology
    Association**
Treasurer's Office
Isidro B. Salusky, M.D.
David Geffen School of Medicine at UCLA
10833 Le Conte Avenue
CHS 27-066, MC 169717
Los Angeles, CA 90095
(310) 206-9295
http://www.ipna-online.org

**International Society of Nephrology**
300 Avenue de Teervuren
B-1150 Brussels
Belgium
+32-2-743-1546
+32-2-743-1550 (fax)
http://www.nature.com/isn

**International Transplant Nurses Society**
1739 East Carson Street
Box 351
Pittsburgh, PA 15203
(412) 343-4867
(412) 343-3959 (fax)
http://www.itns.org

**Juvenile Diabetes Research Foundation
    International**
26 Broadway, 14th Floor
New York, NY 10004
(800) 533-2873
(212) 785-9595 (fax)
http://www.jdf.org

**Kidney & Urology Foundation of America,
    Inc.**
152 Madison Ave, Suite 201
New York, NY 10016
(212) 629-9770 or (800) 633-6628
http://www.kidneyurology.org

**Kidney Cancer Association**
1234 Sherman Avenue
Suite 203
Evanston, IL 60202-1378

(800) 850-9132 or (847) 332-1051
(847) 332-2978 (fax)
http://www.curekidneycancer.org

**Kidney Care Partners**
2550 M Street NW
Washington, DC 20037
(703) 830-9192
http://www.kidneycarepartners.org

**Kidney Disease: Improving Global Outcomes (KDIGO)**
30 East 33rd Street
Suite 900
New York, NY 10016
(212) 889-3427
http://www.kdigo.org/

**Life Options/Rehabilitation Resource Center**
c/o Medical Education Institute, Inc.
414 D'Onofrio Drive
Suite 200
Madison, WI 53719
(800) 468-7777
http://www.lifeoptions.org

**Lower Extremity Amputation Prevention Program**
Health Resources and Services Administration
5600 Fishers Lane
Rockville, MD 20857
(888) 275-4772
http://www.hrsa.gov/leap

**Lupus Foundation of America, Inc.**
2000 L Street NW
Suite 710
Washington, DC 20036
(800) 558-0121
http://www.lupus.org

**March of Dimes**
1275 Mamaroneck Avenue
White Plains, NY 10605
(914) 997-4488
http://www.marchofdimes.com

**Maternal and Child Health Information Resource Center**
1200 18th Street NW
Suite 700
Washington, DC 20036
(202) 842-2000
http://www.mchb.hrsa.gov/mchirc

**Maternal and Child Health Library**
National Center for Education in Maternal and Child Health
P.O. Box 571272
Washington, DC 20057
(202) 784-9770
http://www.nchlibrary.info

**Meals on Wheels Association of America**
203 South Union Street
Alexandria, VA 22314
(703) 548-5558
http://www.mowaa.org

**Medical Education Institute**
414 D'Onofrio Drive
Suite 200
Madison, WI 53719
(608) 833-8033
(608) 833-8366 (fax)
http://www.meiresearch.org

**MedicAlert Foundation**
2323 Colorado Avenue
Turlock, CA 95382
(888) 633-4298
http://www.medicalert.org

**Medicare Rights Center**
1460 Broadway, 17th Floor
New York, NY 10036
(212) 869-3850
http://www.medicarerights.org

**The Medicine Program**
P.O. Box 1089
Poplar Bluff, MO 63902
(866) 694-3893
http://www.themedicineprogram.com

## National Aging Information and Referral Support Center
National Association of State Units on Aging
1201 15th Street NW
Suite 350
Washington, DC 20005
(202) 898-2578
http://www.nasua.org/issues/tech_assist_
    resources/national_aging_ir_support_ctr /
    index.html

## National Alliance for Hispanic Health
1501 16th Street NW
Washington, DC 20036
(202) 387-5000
http://www.hispanichealth.org

## National Association for Healthcare Quality
4700 West Lake Avenue
Glenview, IL 60025
(847) 375-4720
(847) 375-6320 (fax)
http://www.nahq.org

## National Association for Home Care
228 Seventh Street SE
Washington, DC 20003
(202) 547-7424
http://www.nahc.org

## National Association of Community Health Centers
7200 Wisconsin Avenue
Suite 210
Bethesda, MD 20814
(301) 347-0459
http://www.nachc.com

## National Association of Nephrology Technicians/Technologists
P.O. Box 2307
Dayton, OH 45401
(877) 607-6268
(937) 586-3699 (fax)
http://www.dialysistech.org

## National Association of Social Workers
750 First Street NE
Suite 700
Washington, DC 20002
(800) 638-8799
http://www.naswdc.org

## National Cancer Institute
6116 Executive Boulevard
Bethesda, MD 20892
(800) 422-6237
http://www.nci.nih.gov

## National Center for Health Statistics
Presidential Building, Room 1064
6525 Belcrest Road
Hyattsville, MD 20782
(301) 458-4636
http://www.cdc.gov/nchs

## National Center on Minority Health and Health Disparities
National Institutes of Health
6707 Democracy Boulevard
Suite 800, MSC 5465
Bethesda, MD 20892
(301) 402-1366
http://www.ncmhd.nih.gov

## National Diabetes Education Program
One Diabetes Way
Bethesda, MD 20892
(800) 438-5383
(703) 738-4929 (fax)
http://www.ndep.nih.gov

## National Diabetes Information Clearinghouse
One Information Way
Bethesda, MD 20892
(800) 860-8747
(703) 738-4929 (fax)
http://www.diabetes.niddk.nih.gov

## National Eye Institute
National Institutes of Health
Department of Health and Human Services
31 Center Drive
Room 6A32, MSC 2510
Bethesda, MD 20892
(301) 496-5248
http://www.nei.nih.gov

**National Foundation for the Treatment of Pain**
P.O. Box 70045
Houston, TX 77270
(713) 862-9332
http://www.paincare.org

**National Foundation for Transplants (formerly the Organ Transplant Fund)**
1102 Brookfield Road, Suite 200
Memphis, TN 38119
(800) 489-3863 or (901) 684-1697
http://www.transplants.org

**National Health Information Center**
P.O. Box 1133
Washington, DC 20013-1133
(800) 336-4797
http://www.health.gov/nhic

**National Heart, Lung, and Blood Institute Health Information Center**
P.O. Box 30105
Bethesda, MD 20824
(301) 592-8573
http://www.nhlbi.nih.gov

**National Hospice and Palliative Care Organization**
1700 Diagonal Road
Suite 625
Alexandria, VA 22315
(800) 658-8898
http://www.nhpco.org

**National Information Center on Health Services Research and Health Care Technology**
National Library of Medicine
Building 38A, Room 4S-410
8000 Rockville Pike, MSC 3833
Bethesda, MD 20894
(301) 496-0176
http://www.nlm.nih.gov/nichsr

**National Injury Information Clearinghouse**
U.S. Consumer Product Safety Commission
4330 East West Highway, Room 504

Bethesda, MD 20814
(301) 504-7921
http://www.cpsc.gov/about/clrnghse.html

**National Institute for Occupational Safety and Health Information**
4676 Columbia Parkway, C-19
Cincinnati, OH 45226
(800) 232-4636
http://www.cdc.gov/niosh

**National Institute of Child Health and Human Development**
Information Resource Center
P.O. Box 3006
Rockville, MD 20847
(800) 370-2943
http://www.nichd.nih.gov

**National Institute of Diabetes and Digestive and Kidney Diseases (NIDDK)**
National Institutes of Health
Building 31, Room 9A06
31 Center Drive
MSC 2560
Bethesda, MD 20892
(301) 496-3583
http://www.niddk.nih.gov

**National Institute of Diabetes & Digestive & Kidney Diseases (NIDDK)**
NIDDK Clearinghouse
One Information Way
Bethesda, MD 20892
(800) 860-8747
(703) 738-4929 (fax)
http://www.niddk.nih.gov

**National Institute of Mental Health**
6001 Executive Boulevard, Room 8184, MSC 9663
Bethesda, Md. 20892
(866) 615-6464
http://www.nimh.nih.gov

**National Institute on Aging Information Center**
P.O. Box 8057
Gaithersburg, MD 20898-8057

(800) 222-2225
http://www.nia.nih.gov

## National Institute on Alcohol Abuse and Alcoholism (NIAAA)
5365 Fishers Lane, MWC 9304
Bethesda, MD 20892
(301) 443-3860
http://www.niaaa.nih.gov

## National Kidney and Urologic
Diseases Information Clearinghouse (NKUDIC)
Three Information Way
Bethesda, MD 20892-3580
(800) 891-5390 or (301) 654-4415
http://www.kidney.niddk.nih.gov

## National Kidney Disease Education Program (NKDEP)
Three Kidney Information Way
Bethesda, MD 20892
(866) 4-KIDNEY
http://www.nkdep.nih.gov

## National Kidney Foundation (NKF)
30 East 33rd Street
New York, NY 10016
(800) 622-9010 or (212) 889-2210
(212) 689-9261 (fax)
http://www.kidney.org

## National Mental Health Association
2000 North Beauregard Street, Sixth Floor
Alexandria, VA 22311
(703) 684-7722
http://www.nmha.org

## National Organization for Rare Disorders
55 Kenosia Avenue
Danbury, CT 06813
(203) 744-0100
(203) 798-2291 (fax)
http://www.rarediseases.org

## National Osteoporosis Foundation
1232 22nd Street NW
Washington, DC 20037
(202) 223-2226
http://www.nof.org

## National Patient Safety Foundation
268 Summer Street
Sixth Floor
Boston, MA 02210
(617) 391-9900
(617) 391-9999 (fax)
http://www.npsf.org

## National Quality Forum
601 13th Street NW
Suite 500 North
Washington, DC 20005
(202) 783-1300
(202) 783-3434 (fax)
http://www.qualityforum.org

## National Rehabilitation Information Center
200 Forbes Boulevard
Suite 202
Lanham, MD 20706
(800) 346-2742
http://www.naric.com

## National Renal Administrators Association
100 North 20th Street
Fourth Floor
Philadelphia, PA 19103
(215) 320-4655
(215) 564-2175 (fax)
http://www.nraa.org

## National Resource Center on Supportive Housing & Home Modifications
USC Andrus Gerontology Center
Los Angeles, CA 90089
(213) 740-1364
http://www.homemods.org

## National Rural Health Association
521 East 63rd Street
Kansas City, MO 64111
(816) 756-3140
http://www.nrharural.org

## National Sleep Foundation
1522 K Street NW
Suite 500

Washington, DC 20005
(202) 347-3471
http://www.sleepfoundation.org

**National Women's Health Information
    Center**
8270 Willow Oaks Corporate Drive
Fairfax, VA 22031
(800) 994-9662
http://www.womenshealth.gov

**The NephCure Foundation**
15 Waterloo Avenue, Suite 200
Berwyn, PA 19312
(866) 637-4287 (NEPHCURE)
(610) 540-0190 (fax)
http://www.nephcure.org

**Nephrogenic Diabetes Insipidus
    Foundation**
Main Street
P.O. Box 1390
Eastsound, WA 98245
(888) 376-6343
(888) 376-6356 (fax)
http://www.ndif.org

**Network 8 Inc.**
660 Katherine Drive
Suite 306
Flowood, MS 39232
(601) 936-9260
http://www.esrdnetwork8.org/

**North American Society for Dialysis and
    Transplantation**
4010 Bentley Drive
Pearland, TX 77584
(281) 997-1944
(281) 997-0518 (fax)
http://www.nasdat.org

**North American Transplant Coordinators
    Organization (NATCO)**
P.O. Box 15384
Lenexa, KS 66285
(913) 492-4612
(913) 895-4652 (fax)
http://www.natco1.org

**Northwest Renal Network**
4702 42nd Avenue SW
Seattle, WA 98116
(206) 923-0714
http://www.nwrenalnetwork.org/

**Office of Minority Health Resource
    Center**
Office of Minority Health
P.O. Box 37337
Washington, DC 20013-7337
(800) 444-6472
http://www.omhrc.gov

**Office on Smoking and Health**
National Center for Chronic Disease Prevention
    and Health Promotion
Centers for Disease Control and Prevention
Mail Stop K-50
4770 Buford Highway NE
Atlanta, GA 30341-3717
(800) 232-4636
http://www.cdc.gov/tobacco

**Oxalosis and Hyperoxaluria Foundation**
201 East 19th Street
Suite 12 E
New York, NY 10003
(212) 777-0470
(212) 777-0471 (fax)
http://www.ohf.org

**Pharmaceutical Research and
    Manufacturers of America**
1100 15th Street NW
Washington, DC 20005
http://www.pparx.org

**Polycystic Kidney Disease Foundation**
9221 Ward Parkway
Suite 400
Kansas City, MO 64114
(800) 753-2873
(816) 931-8655 (fax)
http://www.pkdcure.org

**The Renal Network, Inc.**
911 East 86th Street, Suite 202
Indianapolis, IN 46240

(317) 257-8265
http://www.therenalnetwork.org

**Renal Physicians Association**
1700 Rockville Pike
Suite 220
Rockville, MD 20852
(301) 468-3515
(301) 468-3511 (fax)
http://www.renalmd.org

**Renal Support Network**
1311 North Maryland Avenue
Glendale, CA 91207
(818) 543-0896
(818) 244-9540 (fax)
http://www.rsnhope.org

**Scientific Registry of Transplant Recipients**
315 West Huron Street
Suite 360
Ann Arbor, MI 48103
(800) 830-9664
http://wwwl.ustransplant.org

**Scleroderma Research Foundation**
220 Montgomery Street
Suite 1411
San Francisco, CA 94104
(800) 441-CURE (2873)
http://www.srfcure.org/contact

**Sjögren's Syndrome Foundation**
6707 Democracy Boulevard
Suite 325
Bethesda, MD 20817
(800) 475-6473
http://www.sjogrens.org

**Social Security Administration**
Office of Public Inquiries
6401 Security Boulevard
Baltimore, MD 21235
(800) 772-1213
http://www.socialsecurity.gov

**Society for Urodynamics and Female Urology**
1100 East Woodfield Road

Suite 520
Schaumburg, IL 60173
(847) 517-7225
(847) 517-7229 (fax)
http://www.sufuorg.com

**Society of Government Service Urologists**
P.O. Box 681965
San Antonio, TX 78268
(210) 681-5800
(210) 680-7725 (fax)
http://www.sgsu.org

**Society of University Urologists**
1111 North Plaza Drive
Suite 520
Schaumburg, IL 60173
(847) 517-7225
(847) 517-7229 (fax)
http://www.suunet.org

**The Southeastern Kidney Council**
1000 Saint Albans Drive, Suite 270
Raleigh, NC 27609
(919) 855-0882
http://www.esrdnetwork6.org/

**Southern California Renal Disease Council**
6255 Sunset Boulevard, Suite 2211
Los Angeles, CA 90028
(323) 962-2020
http://www.esrdnetwork18.org

**Substance Abuse and Mental Health Services Administration**
1 Choke Cherry Road
Rockville, MD 20850
(800) 729-6686
http://www.samhsa.gov

**Transatlantic Renal Council**
Cranbury Gates Office Park
109 South Main Street
Suite 21
Cranbury, New Jersey 08512
(609) 490-0310

**The Transplantation Society**
International Headquarters

1255 University Street
Suite 325
Montreal, Quebec
Canada H3B 3B4
(514) 874-1717
(514) 874-1716 (fax)
http://www.transplantation-soc.org

**Transplant Recipients International
Organization (TRIO)**
2100 M Street NW
Suite 602
Washington, DC 20036
(800) TRIO-386 or (202) 293-0980
http://www.trioweb.org

**United Network for Organ Sharing**
P.O. Box 2484
Richmond, VA 23218
(888) 894-6361
(804) 782-4817 (fax)
http://www.unos.org

**United States Renal Data System (USRDS)
Coordinating Center**
914 South Eighth Street
Suite D206
Minneapolis, MN 55404
(888) 008-7737
(612) 347-5878 (fax)
http://www.usrds.org

**Urology Society of America**
305 Second Avenue
Suite 200
Waltham, MA 02451
(781) 895-9078
(781) 895-9088 (fax)
http://www.urologysocietyofamerica.org

**Vasculitis Foundation**
P.O. Box 28660
Kansas City, MO 64188-8660
(800) 277-9474
http://www.vasculitisfoundation.org

**Visiting Nurse Association of America**
900 19th Street NW
Suite 200

Washington, DC 20006
(202) 384-1420
http://www.vnaa.org

**Weight-Control Information Network**
National Institute of Diabetes and Digestive and
    Kidney Diseases
One WIN Way
Bethesda, MD 20892-3665
(877) 946-4627
http://win.niddk.nih.gov

**Women in Government**
Kidney Health Policy Resource Center
2600 Virginia Avenue
Suite 709
Washington, DC 20037
(888) 333-0164

# B. International Kidney Disease Organizations

Kidney disease is a serious problem worldwide. This appendix includes some key international kidney disease organizations.

**Australian and New Zealand Society of
    Nephrology**
145 Macquarie Street
Sydney, NSW 2000
Australia
+612 9256 5461
+612 9241 4083 (fax)
http://www.nephrology.edu/au

**Canadian Association of Nephrology
    Nurses and Technologists**
336 Younge Street
Suite 322
Barrie, ON L4N 4C8
(877) 720-2819
http://www.cannt.ca/en

**International Transplant Nurses Society**
1739 East Carson Street Box 351
Pittsburgh, PA 15203
(412) 343-4867
(412) 343-3959 (fax)
http://www.itns.org

**Kidney Health Australia**
GPO Box 9993
Melbourne VIC 3001
03 9674 4300
http://www.kidney.org/au

## C. End-Stage Renal Disease Networks

There are eighteen end-stage renal disease networks nationwide as of this writing in 2010, and they are all umbrellaed under the Forum of ESRD Networks. These networks provide information on treatment for kidney failure. All ESRD Networks are listed in this appendix. Some networks also list a toll-free number for patients only, and some list their fax numbers.

### NETWORK 1

(Connecticut, Maine, Massachusetts, New Hampshire, Rhode Island, Vermont)

**ESRD Network of New England**
30 Hazel Terrace
Suite 14
Woodbridge CT 06525
(203) 387-9332
(203) 389-9902 (fax)
http://www.networkofnewengland.org/

### NETWORK 2

(New York)

**ESRD Network of New York**
1979 Marcus Avenue
Lake Success, NY 11042
(516) 209-5578
(516) 326-8929 (fax)
Patients only: (800) 238-3773
http://esrd.ipro.org/

### NETWORK 3

(New Jersey, Puerto Rico, Virgin Islands)

**Quality Insights Renal Network 3**
Cranbury Gates Office Park
109 South Main Street
Suite 21

Cranbury, NJ 08512
(609) 490-0310
(609) 490-0835 (fax)
Toll free patients' line: (888) 877-8400
http://www/tarcweb.org

### NETWORK 4

(Delaware, Pennsylvania)

**ESRD Network 4, Inc.**
40 24th Street
Suite 410
Pittsburgh, PA 15222
(412) 325-2250
(412) 325-1811 (fax)
Patient only toll-free number: (800) 548-9205
http://www.esrdnetwork4.org/

### NETWORK 5

(Virginia, West Virginia, Maryland, District of Columbia)

**Mid-Atlantic Renal Coalition**
ESRD Network 5
1527 Huguenot Road
Midlothian, VA 23113
(804) 794-3757
(804) 794-3793 (fax)
Patients only: (866) 651-6272
http://www.esrdnet5.org

### NETWORK 6

(Georgia, North Carolina, South Carolina)

**Southeastern Kidney Council, Inc.**
1000 St. Albans Drive
Suite 270
Raleigh, NC 27609
(919) 855-0882
(919) 855-0753 (fax)
Patients only: (800) 524-7139
http://www.esrdnetwork6.org

### NETWORK 7

(Florida)

**Florida ESRD Network**
5201 West Kennedy Boulevard

Suite 900
Tampa, FL 33609-1812
(813) 383-1530
(813) 354-1513 (fax)
http://www.fmqai.com/ESRD/esrd.htm

### NETWORK 8

(Alabama, Mississippi, Tennessee)

**Network 8, Inc.**
1755 Lelia Drive
Suite 400
Jackson, MS 39216
(601) 936-9260
(601) 932-4446 (fax)
Patients only: (877) 936-9260
http://www.esrdnetwork8.org

### NETWORK 9/10

(Illinois, Indiana, Kentucky, Ohio)

**The Renal Network, Inc.**
911 East 86th Street
Suite 202
Indianapolis IN 46240
(317) 257-8265
(317) 257-8291 (fax)
For patients: (800) 456-6919
http://www.therenalnetwork.org/

### NETWORK 11

(Minnesota, Michigan, North Dakota, South
Dakota, Wisconsin)

**Renal Network of the Upper Midwest, Inc.**
1360 Energy Park Drive
Suite 200
Saint Paul, Minnesota 55108
(651) 644-9877
(651) 644-9853 (fax)
http://www.esrdnet11.org/

### NETWORK 12

(Iowa, Kansas, Missouri, Nebraska)

**Heartland Kidney Network**
7505 Northwest Tiffany Springs Parkway
Suite 230

Kansas City, MO 64153
(816) 880-9990
(816) 880-9088
Patients only: (800) 444-9965
http://www.heartlandkidney.org/

### NETWORK 13

(Arkansas, Louisiana, Oklahoma)

**ESRD Network 13**
4200 Perimeter Center Drive
Suite 102
Oklahoma City, OK 73112
(405) 942-6000
(405) 942-6884 (fax)
For patients: (800) 472-8664
http://www.network13.org/

### NETWORK 14

(Texas)

**ESRD Network of Texas, Inc.**
4040 McEwen
Suite 350
Dallas, TX 75244
(972) 503-3215
(972) 503-3219 (fax)
Patients only: (877) 886-4435
http://www.esrdnetwork.org/

### NETWORK 15

(Arizona, Colorado, Nevada, New Mexico, Utah,
Wyoming)

**Intermountain ESRD Network, Inc.**
165 South Union Boulevard
Suite 466
Lakewood, CO 80228
(303) 831-8818
(303) 860-8392 (fax)
Patients only: (800) 783-8818
http://www.esrdnet15.org/

### NETWORK 16

(Alaska, Idaho, Montana, Oregon, Washington)

**Northwest Renal Network**
4702 42nd Avenue SW

Seattle, WA 98116
(206) 923-0714
(206) 923-0716 (fax)
Patients only: (800) 262-1514
http://www.nwrenalnetwork.org

## NETWORK 17

(Amerian Samoa, Guam, Mariana Islands, Hawaii, Northern California)

### Western Pacific Renal Network, LLC

505 San Marin Drive, Building A
Suite 300
Novato, CA 94945
(415) 897-2400
(415) 897-2422 (fax)

Patients only: (800) 232-3773
http://www.esrdnet17.org

## NETWORK 18

(Southern California)

### Southern California Renal Disease Council, Inc.

6255 Sunset Boulevard
Suite 2211
Los Angeles, CA 90028
(323) 962-2020
(323) 962-2891 (fax)
Patients only: (800) 637-4767
http://www.esrdnetwork18.org

# APPENDIX II
## STATE ORGANIZATIONS AND PROGRAMS

### A. State and Territorial Health Insurance Programs

State Health Insurance Programs (SHIP) provide assistance to individuals who cannot afford their Medicare copayments for kidney dialysis or kidney transplantation (as well as for other diseases). Each state or territory receives a federal grant. States provide assistance through their elderly services program, state insurance program, or other offices.

### ALABAMA

**State Health Insurance Assistance Program**
Alabama Department of Senior Services
770 Washington Avenue RSA Plaza
Suite 470
Montgomery, AL 36130
(800) 243-5463
(334) 242-5743
http://www.alabamaageline.gov
Open 8 AM–5 PM

### ALASKA

**Alaska State Health Insurance Assistance Program (SHIP)**
3601 C Street
Suite 310
Anchorage, AK 99503
(909) 269-3680 (In-state only)
(800) 478-6065 (Out of state)
http://medicare.alaska.gov
Hours: 9 AM–5 PM

### ARIZONA

**State Health Insurance Assistance Program**
Arizona Aging and Adult Administration
1717 West Jefferson
Suite 010A
Phoenix, AZ 85007
(800) 432-4040. Spanish available upon request.
http://www.de.state.az.us/aaa/programs/ship/
default.asp
Hours: 8 AM–4 PM

### ARKANSAS

**Seniors Health Insurance Information Program (SHIP)**
Arkansas State Insurance Department
1200 West Third Street
Little Rock, AR 72201
(800) 224-6330
http://www.insurance.arkansas.gov/seniors/
homepage.htm
Hours: 8 AM–4:30 PM

### CALIFORNIA

**Health Insurance Counseling and Advocacy Program (HICAP)**
California Department of Aging
1300 National Drive
Suite 200
Sacramento, CA 95834
(800) 434-0222 (In-state calls only)
(916) 231-5110
http://www.aging.ca/gov/HICAP
Hours: 9 AM–4 PM

### COLORADO

**Senior Health Insurance Assistance Program (SHIP)**
Division of Insurance
1560 Broadway
Suite 850

Denver, CO 80202
(800) 544-9181 (In-state)
(888) 696-7213 (Out of state)

## CONNECTICUT

**Connecticut Program for Health Insurance Assistance**
Division of Social Services
25 Sigourney Street
Hartford, CT 06106
(800) 994-9422 (In-state only)
http://www.ct.gov/agingservices
Hours: 8:30 AM–4 PM

## DELAWARE

**ELDERinfo**
Delaware Insurance Department
Rodney Building
841 Silver Lake Boulevard
Dover, DE 19904
(800) 336-9500 (In-state only)
(302) 739-6266
http://delawareinsurance.gov/departments/
   elder/eldindex.shtml
Hours: 8 AM–4:30 PM

## DISTRICT OF COLUMBIA

**Health Insurance Counseling Project**
George Washington University
National Law Center
Building A-B, First Floor
2136 Pennsylvania Avenue
Washington, DC 20052
(202) 739-0668
http://www.gwhospital.com/Senior-Advantage/
   Want-to-Lower-Your-Medicare-Costs-

## FLORIDA

**Serving Health Insurance Needs of Elders (SHINE)**
Florida Department of Elder Affairs
4040 Esplanade Way
Suite 280 South
Tallahassee, FL 32399
(800) 963-5337

http://www.floridaSHINE.org
Hours: 8 AM–5 PM

## GEORGIA

**Georgia Cares**
Division of Aging Services
Two Peachtree Street, North West
Atlanta, GA 30303
(800) 669-8387
http://www.mygeorgiacares.org

## GUAM

**Division of Senior Citizens**
Department of Public Health and Social Services
P.O. Box 2816
Hagatna, Guam 96932
(671) 735-7393

## HAWAII

**SAGE Plus**
Hawaii Executive Office on Aging
250 South Hotel Street
Fourth Floor
Honolulu, HI 96813
(888) 875-9229
http://www2.state.hi.us/eoa/programs/sage_plus/

## IDAHO

**Senior Health Insurance Benefits Advisors (SHIBA)**
Idaho Department of Insurance
700 West State
Third Floor
Boise, ID 83720
(800) 247-4422
http://www.doi.idaho.gov/shiba/shwelcome.
   aspx

## ILLINOIS

**Senior Health Insurance Information Program (SHIP)**
Illinois Department of Insurance
320 West Washington Street
Springfield, IL 62767
(800) 548-9034 (In-state only)
(217) 785-9021
http://www.idfpr.com/DOI/Ship/ship_help.asp

## INDIANA

**Senior Health Insurance Information Program (SHIP)**
Community Healthcare System
St. Catherine Hospital
4321 Fir Street
East Chicago, IN 46312
(219) 392-7777
http://www.comhs.org/stcatherine/shiip.asp

## IOWA

**Senior Health Insurance Information Program (SHIP)**
Iowa Insurance Division
339 Maple Street
Des Moines, IA 50319
(800) 351-4664
http://www.shiip.state.ia.us/

## KANSAS

**Senior Health Insurance Counseling for Kansas (SHICK)**
Kansas Department on Aging
New England Building
503 South Kansas Avenue
Topeka, KS 66003
(800) 860-5260
http://agingkansas.org/shick/shick_index.html

## KENTUCKY

**State Health Insurance Program (SHIP)**
Office on Aging
Kentucky Cabinet for Health and Family Services
275 East Main Street, 5C-D
Frankfort, KY 40621
(877) 293-7447 (In-state only)
(502) 564-6930
http://www.chfs.ky.gov/dail/ship.htm

## LOUISIANA

**Senior Health Insurance Information Program (SHIP)**
Louisiana Department of Insurance
1702 North Third Street
P.O. Box 94214
Baton Rouge, LA 70804
(800) 259-5301
http://www.ldi.state.la.us/

## MAINE

**Maine Health Insurance Counseling Program**
Bureau of Elder and Adult Services
35 Anthony Avenue
State House Station 11
Augusta, ME 04333
(877) 353-3771 (In-state only)
(207) 621-0087
http://www.familiesusa.org/resources/program-locator/resources/maine/page-29153496.html.

## MARYLAND

**Senior Health Insurance Assistance Program (SHIP)**
Department of Aging
301 West Preston Street
Baltimore, MD 21201
(800) 243-3425 (In-state only)
(410) 767-1100
http://www.mdoa.state.md.us.ship.html

## MASSACHUSETTS

**Serving Health Information Needs of Elders (SHINE)**
Executive Office of Elder Affairs
One Ashburton Place
Fifth Floor
Boston, MA 02108
(800) 243-4636, option 2
http://www.medicareoutreach.org

## MICHIGAN

**Medicare/Medicaid Assistance Project (MMAP)**
6105 West St. Joseph
Lansing, MI 48917
(800) 803-7174
http://www.mymmap.org/

## MINNESOTA

**Senior LinkAge Line**
Minnesota Board on Aging
Minnesota Department of Human Services
540 Cedar Street
P.O. Box 64976
St. Paul, MN 55164
(800) 333-2433
http://www.mnaging.org/aedvisor/SLL.htm

## MISSISSIPPI

**Insurance Counseling and Assistance
    Program**
Division of Aging and Adult Services
750 North State Street
Jackson, MS 39202
(800) 948-3090
http://www.mdhs.state.ms.us/aas_info.
    html#MICAP

## MISSOURI

**Community Leaders Assisting Insured of
    Missouri (CLAIM)**
Primaris
3425 Constitution Court
Jefferson City, MO 65109
(800) 390-3330
http://www.primaris.org/beneficiaries/medicare_
    help.asp

## MONTANA

**State Health Insurance Counseling
    Program (SHIC)**
State Office on Aging
111 North Sanders Street
Helena, MT 59604
(800) 551-3191
http://www.dphhs.mt.gov/sltc/services/aging/
    ship.shtml

## NEBRASKA

**Nebraska Health Insurance Information
    Counseling and Assistance Program
    (NICA)**
Department of Insurance
Terminal Building
941 O Street

Suite 400
Lincoln, NE 68508
(800) 234-7119
http://www.doi.ne.gov/shiip/index.htm

## NEVADA

**State Health Insurance Advisory Program
    (SHIP)**
Nevada Division of Aging Services
3100 West Sahara
Suite 103
Las Vegas, NV 89102
(800) 307-4444
http://nvaging.net/ship/ship_main.htm

## NEW HAMPSHIRE

**Health Insurance Counseling, Education,
    Assistance Service (HICEAS)**
Division of Elderly & Adult Services
P.O. Box 2338
State Office Park Street South
Concord, NH 03301
(800) 852-3388 (In-state only)
http://www.familiesusa.org/resources/program-
    locator/resources/new-hampshire/page-
    29153986.html

## NEW JERSEY

**Senior Health Insurance Assistance
    Program (SHIP)**
Division of Aging and Community Services
New Jersey Department of Health and Senior
    Services
P.O. Box 807
Trenton, NJ 08625
(877) 222-3737
http://www.state.nj.us/health/senior/ship.shtml

## NEW MEXICO

**Benefits Counseling**
New Mexico State Agency on Aging
2550 Cerrillos Road
Santa Fe, NM 87505
(800) 432-2080 (In-state only)
(505) 476-4799
https://www.shiptalk.org/shiptalk/shiptalkinfo
    lib/PromotionalProfiles/NMSHIPpr ofile.pdf

## NEW YORK

### Health Insurance Information Counseling and Assistance Program (HIICAP)

New York State Office for the Aging
Two Empire State Plaza
Agency Building 2
Albany, NY 12223
(800) 333-4114
http://hiicap.state.ny.us/home/welcome.htm

## NORTH CAROLINA

### North Carolina Seniors' Health Insurance Information Program (SHIIP)

Department of Insurance
111 Seaboard Avenue
Raleigh, NC 27604
(800) 443-9354 (In-state only)
(919) 733-0111
http://wwwl.ncdoi.com/Consumer/Shiip/Shiip.
asp

## NORTH DAKOTA

### Senior Health Insurance Counseling (SHIC)

North Dakota Department of Insurance
600 East Boulevard, Department 401
Bismarck, ND 58505
(800) 247-0560
http://www.nd.gov/ndins/consumer/shic/

## OHIO

### Ohio Senior Health Insurance Information Program (OSHIP)

Ohio Department of Insurance
50 West Town Street
Third Floor—Suite 300
Columbus, OH 43215
(800) 686-1578
http://www.insurance.ohio.gov/aboutodi/
ODIDiv/Pages/ContactOSHIIP.aspx

## OKLAHOMA

### Oklahoma Insurance Department

Senior Health Insurance Counseling Program
(SHICP)
P.O. Box 53408
2401 North West 23rd Street
Suite 28

Oklahoma City, OK 73107
(800) 763-2828 (In-state only)
(405) 521-6628
http://www.oid.state.ok.us/consumer/shicp.html

## OREGON

### Senior Health Insurance Benefits Assistance (SHIBA)

Oregon Division of Insurance
350 Winter Street, North East
Room 440
Salem, OR 97301
(800) 722-4134 (In-state only)
(503) 947-7979
http://www.oregon.gov/DCBS/SHIBA/

## PENNSYLVANIA

### Pennsylvania Department of Aging

555 Walnut Street
Fifth Floor
Harrisburg, PA 17101
(800) 783-7067
http://www.aging.state.pa.us/portal/server.pt/
community/department_of_aging_home/
18206

## PUERTO RICO

### Puerto Rico Governor's Office of Elderly Affairs

Cobias Plaza Building
Unlevel Stop 23
Ponce de Leon
San Juan, PR 00902
(877) 725-4300

## RHODE ISLAND

### Senior Health Insurance Program (SHIP)

Department of Elderly Affairs
160 Pine Street
Providence, RI 02903
(401) 462-3000 (Ask for SHIP)
http://www.dea.ri.gov/insurance

## SOUTH CAROLINA

### Insurance Counseling Assistance and Referrals for Elders (I-CARE)

Department of Health and Human Services

1801 Main Street
Columbia, SC 29202
(800) 868-9095
http://www.aging.sc.gov/Seniors/ICARE.htm

## SOUTH DAKOTA

**Senior Health Information and Insurance
  Education (SHIINE)**
Center for Active Generations
2300 West 46th Street
Sioux Falls, SD 57104
(800) 536-8197
http://www.shiine.net/

## TENNESSEE

**State Health Insurance Assistance
  Program (SHIP)**
Commission on Aging and Disability
Andrew Jackson Building
Eighth Floor
500 Deaderick Street
Nashville, TN 37243
(877) 801-0044
http://www.state.tn.us/comaging/ship.html

## TEXAS

**Health Insurance Information, Counseling,
  and Advocacy Program (HICAP)**
Texas Department on Aging
4900 North Lamar
P.O. Box 12786
Austin, TX 78751
(800) 252-9240 (Ask for HICAP)
http://www.tdi.state.tx.us/consumer/hicap/
  hicaphme.html

## UTAH

**Health Insurance Information Program
  (HIIP)**
Utah Division of Aging and Adult Services
Department of Social Services
120 North 200 West Street
Box 45500
Salt Lake City, UT 84103
(800) 541-7735 (In-state only)
(801) 538-3910 (Ask for Health Insurance
  information)

## VERMONT

**State Health Insurance Assistance
  Program (SHIP)**
Northeastern Vermont Area Agency on Aging
1161 Portland Street
St. Johnsbury, VT 05819
(800) 642-5119 (In-state only)
(802) 751-0428
http://www.medicarehelpvt.net/

## VIRGINIA

**Virginia Insurance Counseling Assistance
  Project (VICAP)**
Department for the Aging
1600 Forest Avenue
Suite 102
Richmond, VA 23229
(800) 552-3402
http://www.aging.state.va.us/vicap.htm

## VIRGIN ISLANDS

**State Health Insurance Assistance
  Program (VISHIP)**
Governor Juan F. Luis Hospital Medical Center
4007 Estate Diamond
St. Croix, VI 00820
(340) 772-7368

## WASHINGTON

**Statewide Health Insurance Benefits
  Advisors (SHIBA)**
Washington State Office of the Insurance
  Commissioner
810 Third Avenue
Suite 650
Seattle, WA 98104
(800) 397-4422
http://www.insurance.wa.gov/shiba/index.shtml

## WEST VIRGINIA

**Senior Health Insurance Network (SHINE)**
West Virginia Bureau of Senior Services
1900 Kanawha Boulevard
East Building 10
Charleston, WV 25305
(800) 987-4463
http://www.state.wv.us/seniorservices/shine/

## WISCONSIN

### Elderly Benefits Specialists

Bureau of Aging and Long Term Care Resources
One West Wilson Street
Room 450
P.O. Box 7850
Madison, WI 53707
(800) 242-1060
http://dhfs.wisconsin.gov/aging/genage/
    benspecs.htm

## WYOMING

### Wyoming State Health Insurance Assistance Program (WYSHIIP)

Wyoming Senior Citizens, Inc.
P.O. Box BD
Riverton, WY 82501
(800) 856-4398
http://www.wyomingseniors.com/WSHIIP.htm

## B. State Health Departments

State health organizations often coordinate health services for kidney patients. They also manage state Medicaid programs for low-income disabled people.

## ALABAMA

### Alabama Department of Public Health

The RSA Tower
201 Monroe Street
Montgomery, AL 36104
(334) 206-5300
http://www.adph.org

## ALASKA

### Office of the Commissioner

Health and Social Services
350 Main Street, Room 404
P.O. Box 110601
Juneau, AK 99811
(907) 465-3030
http://health.hss.state.ak.us/commissioner

## ARIZONA

### Arizona Department of Health Services

150 North 18th Avenue
Phoenix, AZ 85007
(602) 542-1000
http://www.azdhs.gov

## ARKANSAS

### Department of Health

4815 West Markham
Little Rock, AR 72203
(501) 661-2000
http://www.healthyarkansas.com/health.html

## CALIFORNIA

### California Department of Health

714 P Street, Room 1253
Sacramento, CA 95899
(916) 440-7400
http://www.dhs.ca.gov

## COLORADO

### Colorado Department of Public Health and Environment

4300 Cherry Creek Drive South
Denver, CO 80246
(303) 692-2000
http://www.cdphe.state.co.us/ic/infohom.html

## CONNECTICUT

### Connecticut Department of Public Health

410 Capitol Avenue
P.O. Box 340308
Hartford, CT 06134
(860) 509-8000
http://www.ct.gov/dph/site/default.asp

## DELAWARE

### Delaware Health and Social Services

1901 North DuPont Highway
New Castle, DE 19720
(302) 255-9040
http://www.state.de.us/dhss

## DISTRICT OF COLUMBIA

### Department of Health

825 North Capitol Street NE
Washington, DC 20002
(202) 671-5000
http://doh.dc/gov/doh/site/default.asp

## FLORIDA

**Department of Health**
4052 Bald Cypress Way
Tallahassee, FL 32399
(850) 245-4147
http://esetappsdoh.doh.state.fl.us

## GEORGIA

**Georgia Department of Community Health**
Two Peachtree Street, 40th Floor
Atlanta, GA 30303
(404) 656-4507
http://dch.georgia.gov

## HAWAII

**Hawaii State Department of Health**
1250 Punchbowl Street
Honolulu, HI 96813
(808) 586-4400
http://www.hawaii.gov/health

## IDAHO

**Idaho Department of Health and Welfare**
450 West State Street
Boise, ID 83720
(208) 334-5500
http://www.healthandwelfare.idaho.gov

## ILLINOIS

**Illinois Department of Public Health**
535 West Jefferson Street
Springfield, IL 62761
(217) 782-4977
http://www.idph.state.il.us

## INDIANA

**Indiana State Department of Health**
Two North Meridian Street
Indianapolis, IN 46204
(317) 233-1325
http://www.in.gov/isdh

## IOWA

**Iowa Department of Public Health**
321 East 12th Street
Des Moines, IA 50319
(515) 281-7689
http://www.idph.state.is.us/

## KANSAS

**Kansas Department of Health and Environment**
Curtis State Office Building
1000 Southwest Jackson
Topeka, KS 66612
(785) 296-1500
http://www.kdheks.gov

## KENTUCKY

**Cabinet for Health and Family Services**
Office of the Secretary
275 East Main Street
Frankfort, KY 40621
http://chfs.ky.gov/dph/

## LOUISIANA

**Louisiana Department of Health & Hospitals**
628 North Fourth Street
P.O. Box 629
Baton Rouge, LA 70821
(225) 342-5568
http://www.dhh.louisiana.gov

## MAINE

**Maine Center for Disease Control and Prevention**
286 Water Street
State House Station 11
Augusta, ME 04333
(207) 287-8016
http://www.maine.gov/dhhs/boh/index.shtml

## MARYLAND

**Maryland Department of Health & Mental Hygiene**
201 West Preston Street
Baltimore, MD 21201
(410) 767-8500
http://www.dhmh.state.md.us/

## MASSACHUSETTS

**Massachusetts Department of Public Health**
250 Washington Street
Boston, MA 02108
(617) 624-6000
http://www.mass.gov/dph/dphhome.htm

## MICHIGAN

**Michigan Department of Community Health**
Capitol View Building
201 Townsend Street
Lansing, MI 48913
(517) 373-3740
http://www.michigan.gov/mdch

## MINNESOTA

**Minnesota Department of Health**
P.O. Box 64975
St. Paul, MN 55164
(651) 201-5000
http://www.health.state.mn.us

## MISSISSIPPI

**Mississippi Department of Health**
570 East Woodrow Wilson Drive
Jackson, MS 39216
(601) 576-7400
http://www.msdh.state.ms.us

## MISSOURI

**Missouri Department of Health & Senior Services**
P.O. Box 570
Jefferson City, MO 65102
(573) 751-6400
http://www.dhss.mo.gov

## MONTANA

**Montana Department of Public Health and Human Services**
1400 Broadway
Helena, MT 59620
(406) 444-1861

## NEBRASKA

**Nebraska Department of Health and Human Services**
P.O. Box 95944
Lincoln, NE 68509
(402) 471-2306
http://www.hhs.state.ne.us

## NEVADA

**Nevada Department of Health and Human Services**
505 East King Street, Room 600
Carson City, NV 89710
(775) 684-4000
http://www.hr.state.nv.us/

## NEW HAMPSHIRE

**New Hampshire Department of Health and Human Services**
State Office Park South
129 Pleasant Street
Concord, NH 03301
(603) 271-4688
http://www.dhhs.state.nh.us

## NEW JERSEY

**Department of Health and Senior Services**
P.O. Box 360
Trenton, NJ 08625
(609) 292-7837
http://www.state.nj.us/health/

## NEW MEXICO

**New Mexico Department of Health**
1190 South St. Francis Drive
Santa Fe, NM 87502
(505) 827-2613
http://www.health.state.nm.us

## NEW YORK

**New York State Department of Health**
Corning Tower
Empire State Plaza
Albany, NY 12237
(866) 881-2809
http://www.health.state.ny.us

## NORTH CAROLINA

**North Carolina Department of Health and Human Services**
2001 Mail Service Center
Raleigh, NC 27699
(919) 733-4534
http://www.dhhs.state.nc.us

## NORTH DAKOTA

**North Dakota Department of Health**
600 East Boulevard Avenue
Bismarck, ND 58505
(701) 328-2372
http://www.ndhan.gov

## OHIO

**Ohio Department of Health**
246 North High Street
Columbus, OH 43126
(614) 644-8562
http://www.odh.ohio.gov

## OKLAHOMA

**Oklahoma Health Care Authority**
4545 North Lincoln Boulevard
Suite 124
Oklahoma City, OK 73105
(405) 522-7300
http://www.ohca.state.ok.us

## OREGON

**Oregon Public Health Division**
800 Northeast Oregon Street
Portland, OR 97232
(503) 731-4000
http://oregon.gov/DHS/ph

## PENNSYLVANIA

**Pennsylvania Department of Health**
Health and Welfare Building
Seventh and Forster Streets
Harrisburg, PA 17120
(877) 724-3258
http://www.portal.health.state.pa.us/portal/
   server.pt/community/department_of_
   health_home/17457

## RHODE ISLAND

**Rhode Island Department of Health**
Three Capitol Hill
Providence, RI 02908
(401) 222-2231
http://www.health.state.ri.us

## SOUTH CAROLINA

**South Carolina Department of Health and Human Services**
P.O. Box 8206
Columbia, SC 29202
(803) 898-2500
http://www.dhhs.state.sc.us

## SOUTH DAKOTA

**South Dakota Department of Health**
600 East Capitol Avenue
Pierre, SD 57501
(605) 773-3361
http://www.state.sd.us/doh

## TENNESSEE

**Tennessee Department of Health**
Cordell Hull Building, Third Floor
Nashville, TN 37247
(615) 741-3111
http://state.tn.us/health

## TEXAS

**Texas Department of State Health Services**
1100 West 49th Street
Austin, TX 78756
(512) 458-7111
http://www.dshs.state.tx.us

## UTAH

**Utah Department of Health**
288 North 1460 West
Salt Lake City, UT 84114
(801) 538-6101
http://www.health.utah.gov

## VERMONT

**Vermont Department of Health**
108 Cherry Street
Burlington, VT 05402

(802) 863-7200
http://healthvermont.gov

## VIRGINIA

**Virginia Department of Health**
P.O. Box 2448
Richmond, VA 23218
(804) 864-7001
http://www.vdh.state.va.us

## WASHINGTON

**Washington Department of Social and Health Services**
P.O. Box 45010
Olympia, WA 98504
(360) 902-7800
http://www.dshs.wa.gov

## WEST VIRGINIA

**Office of Community Health Systems**
350 Capitol Street, Room 515
Charleston, WV 25301
(304) 558-3210
http://www.wvochs.org

## WISCONSIN

**Department of Health and Family Services**
One West Wilson Street
Madison, WI 53702
(608) 266-1865
http://www.shfs.state.wi.us

## WYOMING

**Wyoming Department of Health**
117 Hathaway Building
2300 Capitol Avenue
Cheyenne, WY 82002
(307) 777-7656
http://wdh.state.wy.us

## C. State Affiliates of the National Kidney Foundation

The National Kidney Foundation is a national nonprofit organization which has many affiliates nationwide. Some affiliates cover several states; for example the affiliate in Massachu-

settes covers five New England states: Maine, Massachusetts, Rhode Island, New Hampshire, and Vermont. (Connecticut has its own site.)

## ARIZONA

**NKF of Arizona, Inc.**
4203 East Indian School Road
Suite 140
Phoenix, AZ 85018
(602) 840-1644
(602) 840-2360 (fax)
http://www.azkidney.org

## ARKANSAS

**National Kidney Foundation of Arkansas, Inc.**
4942 West Markham
Suite 1
Little Rock, AR 72205
(501) 664-4343
(501) 664-7145 (fax)

## CALIFORNIA

**NKF of North California & North Nevada, Inc.**
131 Steuart Street
Suite 520
San Francisco, CA 94105
(415) 543-3303
(415) 543-3331 (fax)
http://www.kidneynca.org

**NKF of Southern California, Inc.**
15490 Centura Boulevard
Suite 210
Sherman Oaks, CA 91403
(800) 747-5527
http://www.kidneysocal.org

## COLORADO

**NKF of CO, MT & WY, Inc.**
3151 South Vaughn Way
Suite 505
Aurora, CO 80014
(720) 748-9991
(720) 748-1273 (fax)
http://www.kidneycimw.org

## CONNECTICUT

**National Kidney Foundation of Connecticut, Inc.**
2139 Silas Deane Highway
Suite 208
Rocky Hill, CT 06067
(800) 441-1280
http://www.kidneyct.org

## DISTRICT OF COLUMBIA

**NKF Serving the National Capital Area, Inc.**
5335 Wisconsin Avenue NW
Suite 300
Washington, DC 20015
(202) 244-7900
http://www.kidneywdc.org

## FLORIDA

**NKF of Florida, Inc.**
1040 Woodcock Road
Suite 119
Orlando, FL 32803
(407) 894-7325
(800) 927-9659
(407) 895-0051 (fax)
http://www.kidneyfla.org

## GEORGIA

**NKF Serving Georgia**
2951 Flowers Road South
Suite 211
Atlanta, GA 30341
(770) 452-1539, extension 18
(800) 633-2339
(770) 452-7564 (fax)
http://www.kidneyga.org

## HAWAII

**NKF of Hawaii, Inc.**
1314 South King Street
Suite 305
Honolulu, HI 96814
(808) 593-1515
http://www.kidneyhi.org

## ILLINOIS

**NKF of Illinois, Inc.**
215 West Illinois St.
Suite 1C
Chicago, IL 60654
(312) 321-1500
(312) 321-1505 (fax)
http://www.nkfi.org

## INDIANA

**NKD of Indiana, Inc.**
911 East 86th Street
Suite 100
Indianapolis, IN 46240
(800) 382-9971
http://www.kidneyindiana.org

## KANSAS

**NKF Serving Kansas & Western Missouri**
6405 Metcalf Avenue
Suite 204
Overland Park, KS 66202
(800) 444-8113
(913) 722-4841 (fax)
http://www.kidneyksmo.org

## KENTUCKY

**NKF of Kentucky, Inc.**
250 East Liberty Street
Suite 710
Louisville, KY 40202
(800) 737-5433
http://www.nkfk.org

## LOUISIANA

**NKF of Louisiana, Inc.**
8200 Hampson Street
Suite 425
New Orleans, LA 70118
(800) 462-3694
(504) 861-1976 (fax)
http://www.kidneyla.org

## MARYLAND

**NKF of Maryland, Inc.**
1107 Kenilworth Drive
Suite 202

Baltimore, MD 21204
(410) 494-8545
(410) 494-8549 (fax)
http://www.kidneymd.org

## MASSACHUSETTS

### NKF Serving New England

85 Astor Avenue
Suite 2
Norwood, MA 02062
(781) 278-0222
(800) 542-4001
(781) 278-0333 (fax)
http://www.kidneyhealth.org

## MICHIGAN

### NKF of Michigan, Inc.

1169 Oak Valley Drive
Ann Arbor, MI 48108
(734) 222-9800
(800) 482-1455
(734) 222-9801 (fax)
http://www.nkfm.org

## MINNESOTA

### NKF Serving Minnesota, the Dakotas and Iowa

1970 Oakcrest Avenue
Suite 208
Saint Paul, MN 55413
(651) 636-7300
(800) 596-7943
(651) 636-9700 (fax)

## MISSISSIPPI

### Mississippi Kidney Foundation

3000 Old Canton
Suite 110
Jackson, MS 39216
(800) 232-1592
(601) 981-3612 (fax)
http://www.kidneyms.org

## MISSOURI

### NKF Serving E. Missouri, Metro East and Nebraska

10803 Olive Boulevard

Suite 200
Creve Coeur, MO 63141
(314) 961-2828
(800) 489-9585
(314) 961-0888 (fax)
http://www.kidneyemo.org

## NEVADA

### NKF Serving Southern Nevada

2550 East Desert Inn Road
Suite 444
Las Vegas, NV 89121
(702) 735-9222
(800) 282-0190
(816) 221-7984 (fax)

## NEW MEXICO

### NKF Serving New Mexico

3167 San Mateo Boulevard NE
Suite 162
Albuquerque, NM 87110
(505) 830-3542
(800) 282-0190
(913) 722-4841 (fax)

## NEW YORK

### NKF of Central New York, Inc.

731 James Street
Suite 200
Syracuse, NY 13203
(315) 476-0311
(877) 8-KIDNEY
(315) 476-3707 (fax)
http://www.cnykidney.org

### NKF of Northeast New York, Inc.

99 Troy Road
Suite 200
East Greenbush, NY 12061
(518) 458-9697
http://www.nkfneny.org

### NKF of Western New York

300 Delaware Avenue
Suite 100
Buffalo, NY 14202

(716) 835-1323
(716) 835-2281 (fax)
http://www.nkfofwny.org

**NKF Serving Greater New York**
30 East 33rd Street, Floor 3
New York, NY 10016
(212) 889-2210
(800) 622-9010
(212) 779-8056 (fax)
http://www.kidneygny.org

**NKF Serving Upstate New York**
15 Prince Street
Rochester, NY 14607
(585) 697-0874
(800) 724-9421
(585) 697-0895 (fax)
http://www.kidneynyup.org

## NORTH CAROLINA

**NKF of North Carolina, Inc.**
4819 Park Road
Charlotte, NC 28209
(704) 552-7870
(877) 858-3808
(704) 519-0022 (fax)
http://www.kidneync.org

## OHIO

**NKF Serving Ohio**
1373 Grandview Avenue
Suite 200
Columbus, OH 43212
(614) 481-4030
(614) 481-4038 (fax)
http://www.nkfofohio.org

## OKLAHOMA

**NKF Serving Oklahoma**
10600 South Pennsylvania Avenue
Suite 16-144
Oklahoma City, OK 73170
(800) 282-0190
(913) 722-4841 (fax)
http://www.kidney.org/site/index.cfm?ch=405

## PENNSYLVANIA

**NKF Serving the Alleghenies**
700 Fifth Avenue, Floor 4
Pittsburgh, PA 15210
(412) 261-4115
(800) 261-4115
(412) 261-1405 (fax)
http://www.kidneyall.org

**NKF Serving the Delaware Valley**
111 South Independence Mall East
Suite 411
The Philadelphia Bourse Building
Philadelphia, PA 19106
(215) 923-8611
(800) 697-7007
(215) 923-2199 (fax)
http://www.nkfdv.org

## SOUTH CAROLINA

**NKF of South Carolina, Inc.**
500 Taylor Street
Suite 101
Columbia, SC 29201
(803) 799-3870
(800) 488-2277
http://www.kidneysc.org

## TENNESSEE

**National Kidney Foundation of Middle Tennessee, Inc.**
2120 Crestmoor Road
Nashville, TN 37215
(615) 383-3887
http://www.nkfmdtn.org

**NKF of West Tennessee, Inc.**
857 Mount Mariah Road
Suite 201
Memphis, TN 38117
(901) 683-6185
(800) 273-3869
(901) 683-6189 (fax)
http://www.nkfwtn.org

## TEXAS

**NKF of Southeast Texas, Inc.**
2400 Augusta Drive
Suite 252
Houston, TX 77057
(713) 952-5499
(800) 961-5693
(713) 952-5497 (fax)
http://www.nkfset.org

**NKF Serving North Texas**
5429 Lyndon B. Johnson Freeway
Suite 250
Dallas, TX 75240
(877) 543-6397
http://www.nkft.org

## UTAH

**NKF of Utah & Idaho, Inc.**
3707 North Canyon Road
Suite 1D
Provo, UT 84604
(800) 869-5277
http://www.kidneyut.org

## VIRGINIA

**NKD Serving Virginia**
1742 East Parham Road
Richmond, VA 23228
(888) 543-6398
http://www.kidneyva.org

## WISCONSIN

**NKF of Wisconsin, Inc.**
16655 West Bluemound Road
Suite 240
Brookfield, WI 53005
(800) 543-6393
http://www.kidneywi.org

# D. State and Territorial Diabetes Prevention Programs in the United States

Diabetes is the foremost cause of chronic kidney disease and of kidney failure in the United States. For this reason, an appendix on state and territorial diabetes prevention programs is provided. Some prevention programs are within the department of health, while others are within other state organizations.

## ALABAMA

**Alabama Diabetes Prevention and Control Program**
Bureau of Health Promotion & Chronic Disease
State of Alabama Department of Public Health
201 Monroe Street
Suite 976
Montgomery, AL 36104
(334) 206-5300
(334) 206-5609 (fax)
http://www.adph.org/diabetes

## ALASKA

**Alaska Diabetes Prevention and Control Program**
P.O. Box 240249
3601 C Street
Suite 722
Anchorage, AK 99524-0249
(907) 269-8035
(907) 269-5446 (fax)
http://www.hss.state.ak.us/dph/chronic/
    diabetes/default.htm

## ARIZONA

**Arizona Diabetes Control and Prevention**
Arizona Department of Health Services
150 North 18th Avenue
Suite 310
Phoenix, AZ 85007
(602) 542-1214
(602) 542-6412 (fax)
http://www.azdiabetes.gov

## ARKANSAS

**Arkansas Department of Health**
4815 West Markham, Slot 3
Little Rock, AR 72205
(501) 661-2093
(501) 661-2009 (fax)
http://www.healtharkansas.com/services/
    services_diabetes.html

## CALIFORNIA

**California Department of Public Health**
Diabetes Prevention and Control Program,
  MS 7211
P.O. Box 997377
Sacramento, CA 95899-7377
(916) 552-9942
(916) 552-9988 (fax)
http://www.caldiabetes.org

## COLORADO

**Colorado Diabetes Prevention and Control
  Program**
Colorado Department of Public Health and
  Environment
4300 Cherry Creek Drive South, A-5
Denver, CO 80246
(303) 692-2577
(303) 691-7900 (fax)
http://www.cdphe.state.co.us/pp/diabetes

## CONNECTICUT

**Connecticut Department of Public Health**
Health Information Systems and Reporting
  Section
410 Capitol Avenue
Hartford, CT 06134-0308
(860) 509-7711
(860) 509-8403 (fax)
http://www.ct.gov/dph

## DELAWARE

**Delaware Diabetes Prevention and
  Control Program**
Tomas Collins Building
Suite 10
540 South DuPont Highway
Dover, DE 19901
(302) 744-1020
(302) 739-2544 (fax)
http://www.dhss.delaware.gov/dph/

## DISTRICT OF COLUMBIA

**District of Columbia Diabetes Prevention
  and Control Program**
825 North Capitol Street NE, Third Floor

Washington, DC 20002
(202) 671-5000
(202) 442-4825 (fax)

## FLORIDA

**Florida Diabetes Prevention and Control
  Program**
Bureau of Chronic Disease Prevention and
  Health Promotion
Department of Health
4052 Bald Cypress Way
Bin A-18
Tallahassee, FL 32399-1744
(850) 245-4330
(850) 245-4391 (fax)
http://www.floridadiabetes.org

## GEORGIA

**Georgia Diabetes Prevention and Control**
DIIR-Chronic Disease Prevention and Health
  Promotion Branch
2 Peachtree Street
Suite 16-293
Atlanta, GA 30303
(404) 657-6313

## HAWAII

**Hawaii State Department of Health**
Diabetes Prevention and Control Program
601 Kamokila Boulevard, Room 344
Kapolei, HI 96707
(808) 692-7462
(808) 692-7461 (fax)

## IDAHO

**Idaho Diabetes Control and Prevention
  Program**
Bureau of Health Promotion, Division of
  Health
Department of Health and Welfare
450 West State Street
P.O. Box 83720
Boise, ID 83720-0036
(208) 334-4928
(208) 334-6573 (fax)
http://www.diabetesprogram.idaho.gov

## ILLINOIS

**Illinois Department of Human Services**
Bureau of Family Nutrition
Diabetes Prevention and Control Program
35 West Jefferson Street
Springfield, IL 62702-5058
(217) 782-2166
(217) 785-5247 (fax)
http://www.dhs.state.il.us/page.aspx?item=33873

## INDIANA

**Indiana Diabetes Prevention and Control Program**
Indiana State Department of Health
Two North Meridian Street 6B
Indianapolis, IN 46204
(317) 233-7634
(317) 233-7127 (fax)

## IOWA

**Iowa Diabetes Prevention and Control Program**
Iowa Department of Public Health
321 East Twelfth Street Lucas Building
Des Moines, IA 50319-0075
(515) 242-6204
(515) 281-6475
http://www.idph.state/a.us/hpcdp/diabetes

## KANSAS

**Kansas Diabetes Prevention and Control Program**
Office of Health Promotion
Kansas Department of Health and Environment
1000 Southwest Jackson
Suite 230
Topeka, KS 66612
(785) 291-3739
(785) 296-8059
http://www.kdheks.gov/diabetes/index.htm

## KENTUCKY

**Kentucky Diabetes Prevention and Control Program**
Chronic Disease Prevention and Control Branch
275 East Main Street, HS2W-E
Frankfort, KY 40621-0001
(502) 564-7996
(502) 564-4667 (fax)
http://chfs.ky.gov/dph/ach/cd/diabetes.htm

## LOUISIANA

**Louisiana Diabetes Program**
628 North Fourth Street, Second Floor
Bienville Building
Baton Rouge, LA 70802
(225) 342-2663
(225) 342-2652 (fax)
http://www.dhh.louisiana.gov

## MAINE

**Maine Diabetes Prevention and Control Program**
Division of Chronic Disease
286 Water Street, Fifth Floor
11 State House Station
Augusta, ME 04333-0011
(207) 287-5380
(207) 287-7213 (fax)
http://www.maine.gov/dhhs/bohdcfh/dcp

## MARYLAND

**Maryland Diabetes Prevention and Control**
201 West Preston Street, Third Floor
Baltimore, MD 21201
(410) 767-3608
(410) 333-5030 (fax)
http://www.fha.state.md.us/cphs/diabetes.cfm

## MASSACHUSETTS

**Massachusetts Diabetes Prevention and Control Program**
Massachusetts Department of Public Health
250 Washington Street, Fourth Floor
Boston, MA 02108
(617) 624-5429
(617) 624-5075 (fax)
http://www.mass.gov.dph (Search "diabetes")

## MICHIGAN

**Michigan Department of Community Health Diabetes and Other Chronic Diseases Section**
109 West Michigan Avenue
Lansing, MI 48913
(517) 335-8789

(517) 335-9461 (fax)
http://www.michigan.gov/diabetes

## MINNESOTA

**Minnesota Diabetes Program**
Minnesota Department of Health
P.O. Box 64882
St. Paul, MN 55164-0882
(651) 201-5423
(651) 201-5800 (fax)
http://www.health.state.mn.us/diabetes

## MISSISSIPPI

**Mississippi Diabetes Prevention and
Control Program**
570 East Woodrow Wilson Drive
Osborne Building
Suite 200
Jackson, MS 39215-1700
(601) 576-7781
(601) 576-7444 (fax)
http://www.msdh.state.ms.us/msdhsite/_
    static/43,0,296.html

## MISSOURI

**Missouri Diabetes Prevention and Control
Program**
Bureau of Cancer and Chronic Disease Control
Section for Chronic Disease Prevention and
    Nutrition Services
Missouri Department of Health and Senior
    Services
930 Wildwood
P.O. Box 570
Jefferson City, MO 65102
(573) 522-2861
(573) 522-2898 (fax)
http://www.dhss.mo.gov/diabetes

## MONTANA

**Montana Diabetes Project**
1400 Broadway, Room C314B
P.O. Box 202951
Helena, MT 59620-2951
(406) 444-6677
(406) 444-7465 (fax)
http://www.diabetes.mt.gov

## NEBRASKA

**Nebraska Diabetes Prevention and
Control Program**
Nebraska Department of Health and Human
    Services
301 Centennial Mall South
P.O. Box 95026
Lincoln, NE 68509-5026
(800) 745-9311
(402) 471-6446 (fax)
http://www.dhhs.ne.gov/dpc/ndcp.htm

## NEVADA

**Nevada Diabetes Prevention and Control
Program**
Nevada State Health Division
4150 Technology Way
Suite 101
Carson City, NV 89706
(775) 684-5996
(775) 684-5998 (fax)
http://health.nv.gov/

## NEW HAMPSHIRE

**New Hampshire Diabetes Education
Program**
NH Department of Health and Human
    Services
29 Hazen Drive
Concord, NH 03301
(603) 271-5173
(603) 271-5199 (fax)
http://www.dhhs.state.nh.us/DHHS/CDPC/dep.
    htm

## NEW JERSEY

**New Jersey Department of Health &
Senior Services**
Wellness and Chronic Disease Prevention
    Program
50 East State Street
P.O. Box 364
Trenton, NJ 08625
(609) 984-6137
(609) 292-9288 (fax)
http://www.state.nj.us/health/fhs/diabetes/
    index.shtml

## NEW MEXICO

**New Mexico Diabetes Prevention and Control Program**
New Mexico Department of Health
810 West San Mateo Road
Suite 200E
Santa Fe, NM 87505
(505) 476-7615
(505) 476-7622 (fax)
http://www.diabetesnm.org

## NEW YORK

**New York State Department of Health**
Bureau of Chronic Disease Services
Diabetes Prevention and Control Program
150 Broadway, Room 350
Albany, NY 12204-0678
(518) 474-1222
(518) 473-0642 (fax)
http://www.nyhealth.gov/diseases/conditions/
   diabetes

## NORTH CAROLINA

**North Carolina Diabetes Prevention and Control Program**
5505 Six Forks Road, Third Floor
Raleigh, NC 27609
(919) 707-5340
(919) 870-4801 (fax)
http://www.ncdiabetes.org

## NORTH DAKOTA

**North Dakota Diabetes and Prevention Program**
North Dakota Department of Health
600 East Boulevard Avenue, Department 301
Bismarck, ND 58505-0200
(701) 328-2367
(701) 328-2036 (fax)
http://www.diabetesnd.org

## OHIO

**Ohio Diabetes Prevention and Control Program**
Ohio Department of Health
Diabetes Unit Eighth Floor

246 North High Street
Columbus, OH 43266-0588
(614) 466-2144
(614) 644-7740 (fax)
http://www.odh.ohio.gov/odhprograms/hprr/
   diabete/diab1.aspx

## OKLAHOMA

**Oklahoma State Department of Health**
Diabetes Prevention and Control Program
1000 Northeast 10th Street
Oklahoma City, OK 73117-1299
(405) 271-4072
(405) 271-6315 (fax)

## OREGON

**Oregon Diabetes Prevention and Control Program**
Health Promotion and Chronic Disease Prevention Program
Oregon Department of Human Services
Public Health Division
800 Northeast Oregon Street
Suite 730
Portland, OR 97232-2162
(971) 673-0984
(971) 673-0994 (fax)
http://oregon.gov/DHS/ph/diabetes

## PENNSYLVANIA

**Pennsylvania Department of Health**
Division of Nutrition and Physical Activity
Health & Welfare Building, Room 1000
Seventh and Forster Streets
Harrisburg, PA 17120
(717) 787-5876
(717) 783-5498 (fax)
http://www.health.state.pa.us/diabetes

## RHODE ISLAND

**Rhode Island Diabetes Prevention and Control Program**
Rhode Island Department of Health
Three Capitol Hill, Room 409
Providence, RI 02908
(401) 222-6957

(401) 222-4415 (fax)
http://www.health.ri.gov/disease/diabetes/
   index.php

## SOUTH CAROLINA

**South Carolina Diabetes Prevention &
Control Program**
Bureau of Chronic Disease Prevention and
   Home Health Services
South Carolina Department of Health and
   Environmental Control
1800 St. Julian Place
Columbia, SC 29204
(803) 545-4471
(803) 545-4921 (fax)
http://www.scdhec.gov/health/chcdp/diabetes

## SOUTH DAKOTA

**South Dakota Diabetes Prevention &
Control Program**
South Dakota Department of Health
615 East Fourth Street
Pierre, SD 57591
(605) 773-7046
(605) 773-5509 (fax)
http://diabetes.sd.gov

## TENNESSEE

**Diabetes Prevention and Control Program**
Tennessee Department of Health, Nutrition and
   Wellness
425 Fifth Avenue North
Cordell Hull Building, Fifth Floor
Nashville, TN 37247
(615) 532-8192
(615) 532-7189 (fax)
http://health.state.tn.us

## TEXAS

**Texas Diabetes Prevention and Control
Program**
Texas Department of State Health Services
MC 1965 P.O. Box 149347
Austin, TX 78714-9347
(512) 458-7490
(512) 458-7408 (fax)
http://www.dshs.state.tx.us/diabetes/

## UTAH

**Utah Diabetes Prevention and Control
Program**
Utah Department of Health
P.O. Box 142107
Salt Lake City, UT 84114
(801) 538-6141 or (888) 222-2542
http://www.health.utah.gov/diabetes

## VERMONT

**Vermont Diabetes Prevention and Control
Program**
Vermont Department of Health
108 Cherry Street
P.O. Box 70
Burlington, VT 05402-0070
(802) 865-7708
(802) 651-1634 (fax)
http://healthvermont.gov/prevent/diabetes/
   diabetes.aspx

## VIRGINIA

**Virginia Department of Health**
Division of Chronic Disease Control and
   Prevention
Diabetes Prevention and Control Project
109 Governor Street, 10th Floor
Richmond, VA 23219
(804) 864-7877
(804) 864-7880 (fax)
http://www.vahealth.org/cdpc/diabetes

## WASHINGTON

**Washington State Diabetes Prevention
and Control Program**
Washington State Department of Health
P.O. Box 47855
Olympia, WA 98504-7855
(360) 236-3963
(360) 236-3708 (fax)
http://www.doh.wa/gov/cfh/diabetes

## WEST VIRGINIA

**West Virginia Diabetes Prevention and
Control Program**
350 Capitol Street, Room 206

Charleston, WV 25301
(304) 558-0644
(304) 558-1553 (fax)
http://www.wvdiabetes.org/

## WISCONSIN

**Wisconsin Diabetes Prevention and Control Program**
One West Wilson
P.O. Box 2659
Madison, WI 53701-2659
(608) 261-9422
(608) 266-8925 (fax)

## WYOMING

**Wyoming Department of Health**
Diabetes Prevention & Control Program
6101 Yellowstone Road
Suite 259A
Cheyenne, WY 82002
(307) 777-3579
(307) 777-8604 (fax)
http://wdh.state.wy.us/PHSD/DIABETES/
index

# TERRITORIES

## AMERICAN SAMOA

**American Samoa Diabetes Prevention & Control Program**
American Samoa Government
P.O. Box 5061
Pago Pago, AS 96799
(684) 633-2186
(684) 633-5379 (fax)

## FEDERATED STATES OF MICRONESIA

**Department of Health, Education and Social Affairs**
FSM Diabetes Prevention & Control Program
P.O. Box 70, PS
FMS National Government
Palikir, Pohnpei, FM 96941
(0-11-691) 320-2619/2643
Fax: (0-11-691) 320-5263 (fax)

## GUAM

**Guam Diabetes Control and Prevention Program**
Department of Public Health and Social Services
P.O. Box 2816
Agana, GU 96910
(0-11-671) 475-0282
(0-11-671) 477-7945 (fax)

## MARIANA ISLANDS

**Diabetes Control and Prevention Program**
Government of Northern Mariana
P.O. Box 409 CK
Saipan, Commwealth Northern Mariana Islands 96950
(0-11-670) 234-8950, extension 2005
(0-11-670) 234-8930 (fax)

## MARSHALL ISLANDS

**Republic of the Marshall Islands Diabetes Control and Prevention Program**
Ministry of Health Services
P.O. Box 16
Republic of the Marshall Islands 96960
(011-692) 625-3355
(011-692) 625-3432 (fax)

## REPUBLIC OF PALAU

**Palau Diabetes Prevention and Control Program Coordinator**
Director of Public Health
P.O. Box 6027
Ministry of Health
Koror, Palau PW 96940
(0-11-680) 488-6262
(0-11-680) 488-8667 (fax)

## PUERTO RICO

**Puerto Rico Diabetes Control and Prevention Program**
Puerto Rico Department of Health
Secretaria Auxiliar de Promocioón y Proteción de la Salud
División de Prevención y Control de Enfermedades Transmisibles

P.O. Box 70184
San Juan, PR 00936
(787) 274-5634
(787) 274-5523 (fax)
http://www.salud.gov.pr

## VIRGIN ISLANDS

**Virgin Islands Department of Health**
Bureau of Health Education & Promotion
Diabetes Prevention & Control Program
3500 Estate Richmond
Charles Harwood Complex
Christiansted, St Croix, VI 00820-4370
(340) 773-1311, extension 3144
(340) 773-8354 (fax)
http://www.usvidiabetes.org

# E. Transplant Centers by Home State

This general listing provides the central authority for transplants in each state (some states have more than one central authority, such as California), as well as a list of medical centers where transplants of all types are performed. (The kidney transplant is the most common form of transplant.) Centers in one state may provide services to individuals from other states.

## ALABAMA

*Alabama Organ Center (ALOB)*
University of South Alabama Medical Center, Mobile, AL
Baptist Medical Center Princeton, Birmingham, AL
Children's Hospital of Alabama, Birmingham, AL
University of Alabama Hospital, Birmingham, AL

## ARIZONA

*Donor Network of Arizona (AZOB)*
Phoenix Children's Hospital, Phoenix, AZ
Banner Good Samaritan Medical Center, Phoenix, AZ
Phoenix Regional Medical Center, Phoenix, AZ
Mayo Clinic Hospital, Phoenix, AZ

St. Joseph's Hospital and Medical Center, Phoenix, AZ
Scottsdale Healthcare Osborn, Scottsdale, AZ
Veterans Administration Medical Center Tucson, Tucson, AZ
University Medical Center, University of Arizona, Tucson, AZ

## ARKANSAS

*Arkansas Regional Organ Recovery Agency (AROR)*
Baptist Medical Center, Little Rock, AR
Arkansas Children's Hospital, Little Rock, AR
The University Hospital of Arkansas, Little Rock, AR
John L. McClellan Veterans Administration Hospital, Little Rock, AR

## CALIFORNIA

*California Transplant Donor Network (CADN)*
Alta Bates Medical Center, Berkeley, CA
El Camino Hospital, Mountain View, CA
Kaiser Permanente, Hospital Oakland, Oakland, CA
Kaiser Permanente, San Francisco Medical Center, San Francisco, CA
Lucile Salter Packard Children's Hospital at Stanford, Palo Alto, CA
California Pacific Medical Center, San Francisco, CA
University of California San Francisco Medical Center, San Francisco, CA
Stanford University Medical Center, Stanford, CA

*Golden State Donor Services (CAGS)*
Summit Medical Center, Oakland, CA
Santa Rosa Memorial Hospital, Santa Rosa, CA
Sutter Memorial Hospital, Sacramento, CA
University of California Davis Medical Center, Sacramento, CA

*OneLegacy (CAOP)*
Saint Bernardine Medical Center, San Bernardino, CA
Childrens Hospital Los Angeles, Los Angeles, CA

Cedars-Sinai Medical Center, Los Angeles, CA

City of Hope National Medical Center, Duarte, CA

University of California Irvine Medical Center, Orange, CA

Harbor UCLA Medical Center, Torrance, CA

St. Mary Medical Center, Long Beach, CA

Loma Linda University Medical Center, Loma Linda, CA

Riverside Community Hospital, Riverside, CA

Arrowhead Regional Medical Center, Colton, CA

St. Joseph Hospital, Orange, CA

St. Vincent Medical Center, Los Angeles, CA

University of California at Los Angeles Medical Center, Los Angeles, CA

University of Southern California University Hospital, Los Angeles, CA

Western Medical Center, Santa Ana, CA

*Lifesharing—A Donate Life Organization (CASD)*
Rady Children's Hospital and Health Center, San Diego, CA

Scripps Green Hospital, La Jolla, CA

University of California San Diego Medical Center, San Diego, CA

Sharp Memorial Hospital, San Diego, CA

## COLORADO

*Donor Alliance (CORS)*
Children's Hospital, Aurora, CO

Memorial Hospital, Colorado Springs, CO

Centura Porter Adventist Hospital, Denver, CO

Poudre Valley Hospital, Fort Collins, CO

Presbyterian/St. Luke's Medical Center, Denver, CO

University of Colorado Hospital/Health Science Center, Aurora, CO

## CONNECTICUT (SEE ALSO MASSACHUSETTS)

*LifeChoice Donor Services (CTOP)*
Hartford Hospital, Hartford, CT

Baystate Medical Center, Springfield, MA

## DELAWARE (SEE PENNSYLVANIA)

## DISTRICT OF COLUMBIA

*Washington Regional Transplant Community (DCTC)*
Children's National Medical Center, Washington, DC

Georgetown University Medical Center, Washington, DC

George Washington University Medical Center, Washington, DC

Howard University Hospital, Washington, DC

Providence Hospital, Washington, DC

Washington Hospital Center, Washington, DC

Walter Reed Army Medical Center, Washington, DC

Warren Grant Magnuson Clinical Center, Bethesda, MD

Shady Grove Adventist Hospital, Rockville, MD

Inova Fairfax Hospital, Falls Church, VA

## FLORIDA

*TransLife (FLFH)*
Bert Fish Medical Center, New Smyrna Beach, FL

Florida Hospital Medical Center, Orlando, FL

Halifax Medical Center, Daytona Beach, FL

*Life Alliance Organ Recovery Agency (FLMP)*
Broward General Medical Center, Ft. Lauderdale, FL

Cleveland Clinic Hospital Florida, Weston, FL

Jackson Memorial Hospital, University of Miami School of Medicine, Miami, FL

Miami Children's Hospital, Miami, FL

*LifeQuest Organ Recovery Services (FLUF)*
Shands Jacksonville, Jacksonville, FL

Mayo Clinic, Jacksonville, Jacksonville, FL

Tallahassee Memorial Hospital, Tallahassee, FL

Shands Hospital at the University of Florida, Gainesvile, FL

University Medical Center, Jacksonville, FL

*LifeLink of Florida (FLWC)*
All Children's Hospital, St. Petersburg, FL

Southwest Florida Regional Medical Center, Ft. Myers, FL
St. Joseph's Hospital, Tampa, FL
Tampa General Hospital, Tampa, FL

### GEORGIA

*LifeLink of Georgia (GALL)*
Children's Healthcare of Atlanta at Egleston, Atlanta, GA
Emory University Hospital, Atlanta, GA
Medical College of Georgia, Augusta, GA
Piedmont Hospital, Atlanta, GA
Saint Joseph's Hospital of Atlanta, Atlanta, GA

### HAWAII

*Organ Donor Center of Hawaii (HIOP)*
Hawaii Medical Center East, Honolulu, HI

### ILLINOIS

*Gift of Life Organ & Tissue Donor Network (OLIP)*
Advocate Christ Medical Center, Oak Lawn, IL
Children's Memorial Hospital, Chicago, IL
Evanston Hospital, Evanston, IL
Loyola University Medical Center, Maywood, IL
Hines Veterans Administration Medical Center, Maywood, IL
Memorial Medical Center, Springfield, IL
Northwestern Memorial Hospital, Chicago, IL
Rush University Medical Center, Chicago, IL
OSF Saint Francis Medical Center, Peoria, IL
St. John's Hospital, Springfield, IL
University of Chicago Medical Center, Chicago, IL
University of Illinois Medical Center, Chicago, IL

### INDIANA

*Indiana Organ Procurement Organization (INOP)*
Clarian Health/Methodist/Indiana U/Riley, Indianapolis, IN
Indiana University Medical Center, Indianapolis, IN

Lutheran Hospital of Fort Wayne, Ft. Wayne, IN
St. Vincent Hospital and Health Care Center, Indianapolis, IN

### IOWA

*Iowa Donor Network (IAOP)*
Iowa Methodist Medical Center, Des Moines, IA
University of Iowa Hospitals and Clinics, Iowa City, IA
Iowa City VA Medical Center, Iowa City, IA
Mercy Medical Center—Des Moines, Des Moines, IA

### KANSAS (SEE ALSO MISSOURI)

*Midwest Transplantation Network (MWOB)*
Via Christi Regional Medical Center, St. Francis Campus, Wichita, KS
University of Kansas Hospital, Kansas City, KS
Children's Mercy Hospital, Kansas City, MO
St. Luke's Hospital of Kansas City, Kansas City, MO
Menorah Medical Center, Kansas City MO
Research Medical Center, Kansas City, MO
St. John's Regional Medical Center, Joplin, MO
University of Missouri Hospital and Clinics, Columbia, MO

### KENTUCKY

*Kentucky Organ Donor Affiliates (KYDA)*
Columbia Audubon Hospital, Louisville, KY
Jewish Hospital, Louisville, KY
Kosair Children's Hospital, Louisville, KY
University of Kentucky Medical Center, Lexington, KY

### LOUISIANA

*Louisiana Organ Procurement Agency (LAOP)*
Children's Hospital, New Orleans, LA
Kenner Regional Medical Center, Kenner, LA
Lakeview Regional Medical Center, Covington, LA
University Medical Center, Lafayette, LA

University Hospital, New Orleans, LA

Ochsner Foundation Hospital, New Orleans, LA

Lindy Boggs Medical Center, New Orleans, LA

Schumpert Health System, Shreveport, LA

Louisiana State University Medical Center, Shreveport, LA

Tulane Medical Center, New Orleans, LA

Willis Knighton Medical Center, Shreveport, LA

### MAINE (SEE MASSACHUSETTS)

### MARYLAND (SEE ALSO DISTRICT OF COLUMBIA)

*The Living Legacy Foundation of Maryland (MDPC)*

Johns Hopkins Bayview Medical Center, Baltimore, MD

Johns Hopkins Hospital, Baltimore, MD

University of Maryland Medical System, Baltimore, MD

### MASSACHUSETTS (SEE ALSO CONNECTICUT)

*New England Organ Bank (MAOB)*

Yale New Haven Hospital, New Haven, CT

Beth Israel Deaconess Medical Center, Boston, MA

Boston Medical Center, Boston, MA

Boston Veterans Administration Medical Center, Boston, MA

Children's Hospital, Boston, MA

New England Deaconess Hospital, Boston, MA

Lahey Clinic Medical Center, Burlington, MA

Massachusetts General Hospital, Boston, MA

Tufts Medical Center, Boston, MA

Brigham and Women's Hospital, Boston, MA

University of Massachusetts Memorial Medical Center, Worcester, MA

Maine Medical Center, Portland, ME

Mary Hitchcock Memorial Hospital, Lebanon, NH

Rhode Island Hospital, Providence, RI

### MICHIGAN

*Gift of Life Michigan (MIOP)*

William Beaumont Hospital, Royal Oak, MI

Children's Hospital of Michigan, Detroit, MI

Helen DeVos Children's Hospital, Grand Rapids, MI

Henry Ford Hospital, Detroit, MI

Harper University Hospital—Detroit Medical Center, Detroit, MI

Hurley Medical Center, Flint, MI

Borgess Medical Center, Kalamazoo, MI

Grace Hospital, Detroit, MI

St. John Hospital and Medical Center, Detroit, MI

St. Mary's Health Care—Main Hospital, Grand Rapids, MI

University of Michigan Medical Center, Ann Arbor, MI

### MINNESOTA

*LifeSource Upper Midwest Organ Procurement Organization (MNOP)*

Abbott Northwestern Hospital, Minneapolis, MN

Childrens Health Care—Minneapolis, Minneapolis, MN

Hennepin County Medical Center, Minneapolis, MN

Rochester Methodist Hospital (Mayo Clinic), Rochester, MN

Metropolitan Mount Sinai Medical Center, Minneapolis, MN

Veterans Administration Medical Center Minneapolis, Minneapolis, MN

Saint Marys Hospital (Mayo Clinic), Rochester, MN

University of Minnesota Medical Center, Fairview, Minneapolis, MN

Dakota Heartland Health System, Fargo, ND

Medcenter One Health Systems, Bismarck, ND

MeritCare Hospital, Fargo, ND

Avera McKennan Hospital, Sioux Falls, SD

Sanford Health/YSD Medical Center, Sioux Falls, SD

### MISSISSIPPI

*Mississippi Organ Recovery Agency (MSOP)*

University of Mississippi Medical Center, Jackson, MS

## MISSOURI (SEE ALSO KANSAS)

*Mid-America Transplant Services (MOMA)*
St. Francis Hospital and Medical Center, Topeka, KS
Barnes-Jewish Hospital, St. Louis, MO
Cardinal Glennon Children's Hospital, St. Louis, MO
John Cochran Veterans Administration Hospital, St. Louis, MO
DePaul Health Center, Bridgeton, MO
St. John's Mercy Medical Center, St. Louis, MO
Saint Louis University Hospital, St. Louis, MO

## NEBRASKA

*Nebraska Organ Recovery System (BEOR)*
BryanLGH Medical Center East, Lincoln, NE
Nebraska Health System Clarkson Hospital, Omaha, NE
Saint Joseph Hospital at Creighton University Medical Center, Omaha, NE
Nebraska Medical Center, Omaha, NE

## NEVADA

*Nevada Donor Network (NVLV)*
Sunrise Hospital and Medical Center, Las Vegas, NV
University Medical Center of Southern Nevada, Las Vegas, NV

## NEW HAMPSHIRE (SEE MASSACHUSETTS)

## NEW JERSEY

*New Jersey Organ and Tissue Sharing Network OPO (NJTO)*
Newark Beth Israel Medical Center, Newark, NJ
Hackensack University Medical Center, Hackensack, NJ
Our Lady of Lourdes Medical Center, Camden, NJ
Robert Wood Johnson University Hospital, New Brunswick, NJ
Saint Barnabas Medical Center, Livingston, NJ
University Hospital, Newark, NJ

## NEW MEXICO

*New Mexico Donor Services (NMOP)*
University Hospital, Albuquerque, NM
Presbyterian Hospital, Albuquerque, NM

## NEW YORK

*Center for Donation and Transplant (NYAP)*
Albany Medical Center Hospital, Albany, NY
Fletcher Allen Health Care, Burlington, VT

*Finger Lakes Donor Recovery Program (NYGL)*
Strong Memorial Hospital, Rochester, NY
State University of New York Upstate Medical University, Syracuse, NY

*New York Organ Donor Network (NYRT)*
NY Presbyterian Hospital/Columbia University Medical Center, New York, NY
State University of New York, Downstate Medical Center, Brooklyn, NY
Montefiore Medical Center, Bronx, NY
Mount Sinai Medical Center, New York, NY
North Shore University Hospital, Manhasset, NY
NY Presbyterian Hospital/Cornell/Rogosin, New York, NY
University Hospital of SUNY, Stony Brook, NY
St. Luke's Roosevelt Hospital Center, New York, NY
Westchester Medical Center, Valhalla, NY

*Upstate New York Transplant Services Inc (NYWN)*
Children's Hospital of Buffalo, Buffalo, NY
Buffalo General Hospital/Children's Hospital, Buffalo, NY
Buffalo Veterans Administration Medical Center, Buffalo, NY
Erie County Medical Center, Buffalo, NY

## NORTH CAROLINA

*Lifeshare of the Carolinas (NCCM)*
Carolinas Medical Center, Charlotte, NC

*Carolina Donor Services (NCNC)*
North Carolina Baptist Hospital, Winston Salem, NC
Duke University Medical Center, Durham, NC
Durham VA Medical Center, Durham, NC

Pitt County Memorial Hospital, Greenville, NC

University of North Carolina Hospitals, Chapel Hill, NC

## NORTH DAKOTA (SEE MINNESOTA)

## OHIO

*LifeBanc (OHLB)*

Akron City Hospital, Akron, OH

Children's Hospital Medical Center of Akron, Akron, OH

The Cleveland Clinic Foundation, Cleveland, OH

St. Elizabeth Health Center, Youngstown, OH

University Hospitals of Cleveland, Cleveland, OH

*Life Connection of Ohio (OHLC)*

University of Toledo Medical Center, Toledo, OH

Miami Valley Hospital, Dayton, OH

*Lifeline of Ohio (OHLP)*

Nationwide Children's Hospital, Columbus, OH

Ohio State University Medical Center, Columbus, OH

*LifeCenter Organ Donor Network (OHOV)*

Children's Hospital Medical Center, Cincinnati, OH

The Christ Hospital, Cincinnati, OH

University of Cincinnati/University Hospital, Cincinnati, OH

## OKLAHOMA

*LifeShare Transplant Donor Services of Oklahoma (OKOP)*

Integris Baptist Medical Center, Oklahoma City, OK

Children's Hospital of Oklahoma, Oklahoma City, OK

Hillcrest Medical Center, Tulsa, OK

OU Medical Center, Oklahoma City, OK

St. Anthony Hospital, Oklahoma City, OK

Saint Francis Hospital, Tulsa, OK

St. John Medical Center, Tulsa, OK

## OREGON

*Pacific Northwest Transplant Bank (ORUO)*

Legacy Good Samaritan Hospital and Medical Center, Portland, OR

Providence Portland Medical Center, Portland, OR

St. Vincent Hospital and Medical Center, Portland, OR

Oregon Health & Sciences University, Portland, OR

Portland Veterans Administration Medical Center, Portland, OR

## PENNSYLVANIA

*Gift of Life Donor Program (PADV)*

Alfred I. DuPont Hospital for Children, Wilmington, DE

Christiana Care Health Services, Newark, DE

Albert Einstein Medical Center, Philadelphia, PA

Children's Hospital of Philadelphia, Philadelphia, PA

Geisinger Medical Center, Danville, PA

Penn State Milton S. Hershey Medical Center, Hershey, PA

Pinnacle Health System at Harrisburg Hospital, Harrisburg, PA

Hahnemann University Hospital, Philadelphia, PA

The Lankenau Hospital, Wynnewood, PA

Lehigh Valley Hospital, Allentown, PA

St. Christopher's Hospital for Children, Philadelphia, PA

Thomas Jefferson University Hospital, Philadelphia, PA

Temple University Hospital, Philadelphia, PA

Hospital of the University of Pennsylvania, Philadelphia, PA

Geisinger Wyoming Valley Medical Center, Wilkes-Barre, PA

*Center for Organ Recovery and Education (PATF)*

Allegheny General Hospital, Pittsburgh, PA

Children's Hospital of Pittsburgh, Pittsburgh, PA

University of Pittsburgh Medical Center, Pittsburgh, PA

Oalkand Veterans Administration Medical Center, Pittsburgh, PA

VA Pittsburgh Healthcare System, Pittsburgh, PA

Charleston Area Medical Center, Charleston, WV

West Virginia University Hospital, Morgantown, WV

## RHODE ISLAND (SEE MASSACHUSETTS)

## SOUTH CAROLINA

*LifePoint (SCOP)*
Medical University of South Carolina, Charleston, SC
Richland Memorial Hospital, Columbia, SC

## SOUTH DAKOTA (SEE MINNESOTA)

## TENNESSEE

*Tennessee Donor Services (TNDS)*
Eerlander Medical Center, Chattanooga, TN
Johnson City Medical Center Hospital, Johnson City, TN
Centennial Medical Center, Nashville, TN
Saint Thomas Hospital, Nashville, TN
University of Tennessee Medical Center of Knoxville, Knoxville, TN
Vanderbilt University Medical Center, Nashville, TN
Nashville Veterans Administration Hospital, Nashville, TN

*Mid-South Transplant Foundation (TNMS)*
Baptist Memorial Hospital, Memphis, TN
Le Bonheur Children's Medical Center, Memphis, TN
Methodist University Hospital, Memphis, TN
University of Tennessee Medical Center, Memphis, TN

## TEXAS

*LifeGift Organ Donation Center (TXOC)*
Baylor All Saints Medical Center, Fort Worth, TX

Cook Children's Medical Center, Fort Worth, TX
Harris Methodist Fort Worth Hospital, Fort Worth, TX
Baylor Medical Center Grapevine, Grapevine, TX
Memorial Hermann Hospital, University of Texas at Houston, Houston, TX
St. Luke's Episcopal Hospital, Houston, TX
University Medical Center, Lubbock, TX
Covenant Medical Center, Lubbock, TX
The Methodist Hospital, Houston, TX
Texas Children's Hospital, Houston, TX
Michael E. DeBakey VA Medical Center, Houston, TX

*Texas Organ Sharing Alliance (TXSA)*
Brackenridge Hospital, Austin, TX
Broke Army Medical Center, Fort Sam Houston, TX
University Hospital, San Antonio, TX
Methodist Children's Hospital of South Texas, San Antonio, TX
Seton Medical Center, Austin, TX
North Austin Medical Center, Austin, TX
Methodist Specialty and Transplant Hospital, San Antonio, TX
McAllen Medical Center, McAllen, TX
Christus Santa Rosa Medical Center, San Antonio, TX
Wilford Hall Medical Center, Lackland AFB, TX

*Southwest Transplant Alliance (TXSB)*
Children's Medical Center of Dallas, Dallas, TX
Driscoll Children's Hospital, Corpus Christi, TX
Medical City Dallas Hospital, Dallas, TX
University of Texas Medical Branch at Galveston, Galveston, TX
Methodist Dallas Medical Center, Dallas, TX
Parkland Memorial, Hospital, Dallas, TX
Sierra Medical Center, El Paso, TX
University Hospital—St. Paul, Dallas, TX
Scott and White Memorial Hospital, Temple, TX

Baylor University Medical Center, Dallas, TX

East Texas Medical Center, Tyler, TX

### UTAH

*Intermountain Donor Services (UTOP)*

Intermountain Medical Center, Murray, UT

University of Utah Medical Center, Salt Lake City, UT

Salt Lake City Veterans Administration Medical Center, Salt Lake City, UT

Primary Children's Medical Center, Salt Lake City, UT

### VERMONT (SEE NEW YORK)

### VIRGINIA (SEE ALSO DISTRICT OF COLUMBIA)

*LifeNet Health (VATH)*

Children's Hospital of the King's Daughters, Norfolk, VA

Henrico Doctors Hospital, Richmond, VA

Medical College of Virginia Hospitals, Richmond, VA

Hunter Holmes McGuire Veterans Administration Medical Center, Richmond, VA

Sentara Norfolk General Hospital, Norfolk, VA

University of Virginia Health Sciences Center, Charlottesville, VA

### WASHINGTON

*LifeCenter Northwest Organ Donation Network (WALC)*

Children's Hospital & Regional Medical Center, Seattle, WA

Sacred Heart Medical Center, Spokane, WA

Swedish Medical Center, Seattle, WA

University of Washington Medical Center, Seattle, WA

Virginia Mason Medical Center, Seattle, WA

### WEST VIRGINIA (SEE PENNSYLVANIA)

### WISCONSIN

*Wisconsin Donor Network (WISE)*

Children's Hospital of Wisconsin, Milwaukee, WI

John I. Doyne Hospital, Milwaukee, WI

Froedtert Memorial Lutheran Hospital, Milwaukee, WI

Zablocki Veterans Administration Medical Center, Milwaukee, WI

Aurora St. Luke's Medical Center, Milwaukee, WI

*Organ Procurement Organization at the University of Wisconsin (WIUW)*

Source: U.S. Department of Health and Human Services. *2008 Annual Report of the U.S. Organ Procurement and Transplantation Network and the Scientific Registry of Transplant Recipients: Transplant Data 1998–2007.* Health Resources and Services Administration, Healthcare Systems Bureau, Division of Transplantation, Rockville, Md., October 2009.

The data and analyses reported in the 2008 Annual Report of the U.S. Organ Procurement and Transplantation Network and the Scientific Registry of Transplant Recipients have been supplied by UNOS and Arbor Research under contract with HHS/HRSA. The authors alone are responsible for reporting and interpreting these data; the views expressed herein are those of the authors and not necessarily those of the U.S. Government.

## F. State Vocational Rehabilitation Agencies

Vocational rehabilitation agencies help disabled people with training and other services that they need to return to work.

### ALABAMA

**Alabama Department of Rehabilitation Services**

602 South Lawrence Street

Montgomery, AL 36104

(334) 293-7500

(800) 441-7607

(334) 293-7383 (fax)

http://www.rehab.state.al.us/Home/default. aspx?url=/Home/Main

### ALASKA

**Alaska Division of Vocational Rehabilitation**

801 West 10th Street

Suite A

Juneau, AK 99801
(907) 465-2814
(800) 478-2815
(907) 465-2856 (fax)
http://www.labor.state.ak.us/dvr/home.htm

## ARIZONA

**Arizona Rehabilitation Services Administration**
1789 West Jefferson 2 NW
Phoenix, AZ 85007
(602) 542-3332
(800) 563-1221
(602) 542-3778 (fax)
http://www.azdes.gov/rsa

## ARKANSAS

**Arkansas Rehabilitation Services**
1616 Brookwood Drive
P.O. Box 3781
Little Rock, AR 72203
(501) 296-1600
(800) 330-0632
(501) 296-1655 (fax)
http://www.arsinfo.org

## CALIFORNIA

**California Health and Human Service Agency**
Department of Rehabilitation
721 Capitol Mall
Sacramento, CA 95814
(916) 324-1313
http://www.rehab.cahwnet.gov

## COLORADO

**Colorado Division of Vocational Rehabilitation**
1575 Sherman Street
Denver, CO 80203
(303) 866-5700
(303) 866-4047 (fax)
http://www.cdhs.state.co.us/dvr

## CONNECTICUT

**Bureau of Rehabilitation Services**
Department of Social Services
25 Sigourney Street, 11th Floor
Hartford, CT 06106
(860) 424-4844
http://www.brs.state.ct.us

## DELAWARE

**Delaware Division of Vocational Rehabilitation**
4425 North Market Street
P.O. Box 9969
Wilmington, DE 19809
(302) 761-8275
http://www.delawareworks.com/dvr/welcome.
  shtml

## DISTRICT OF COLUMBIA

**DC Rehabilitation Services Administration**
810 First Street NE, 10th Floor
Washington, DC 20002
(202) 442-8663
(202) 442-8742 (fax)

## FLORIDA

**Division of Vocational Rehabilitation**
2002-A Old Saint Augustine Road
Tallahassee, FL 32301
(850) 245-3399
(800) 451-4327
http://rehabworks.org

## GEORGIA

**Georgia Department of Labor**
Rehabilitation Services
148 Andrew Young International Boulevard
Suite 510, Sussex Place
Atlanta, GA 30303
(404) 232-3910
http://www.vocrehabga.org

## HAWAII

**Hawaii Vocational Rehabilitation & Services for the Blind**
The State Kakuhihewa Building
601 Kamokila Boulevard, Room 515
Kapolei, HI 96707
(808) 692-7715
http://www.hawaii.gov/dhs/self-sufficiency/vr/

## IDAHO

**Idaho Division of Vocational Rehabilitation**
Agency of the State Board of Education
650 West State Street
Room 150
P.O. Box 83720
Boise, ID 83720
(208) 334-3390
(800) 856-2720
(208) 334-5305 (fax)
http://www.vr.idaho.gov/

## ILLINOIS

**Department of Human Services**
Office of Rehabilitation Services
623 East Adams Street
P.O. Box 19429
Springfield, IL 62794
(800) 843-6154
http://www.dhs.state.il.us/ors/

## INDIANA

**Division of Disability & Rehabilitative Services**
402 West Washington Street, C-453
P.O. Box 7083
Indianapolis, IN 46207
(317) 232-1252
(317) 232-6478 (fax)
http://www.in.gov/fssa/2328.htm

## IOWA

**Iowa Vocational Rehabilitation Services (IVRS)**
510 East 12th Street
Des Moines, IA 50319
(515) 281-4211
(515) 281-7645 (fax)
http://www.ivrs.iowa.gov/

## KANSAS

**Department of Social and Rehabilitation Services**
915 Harrison Street Office Building

Topeka, KS 66612
(785) 296-3959
(785) 296-2173 (fax)
http://www.srskansas.org

## KENTUCKY

**Kentucky Office of Vocational Rehabilitation**
275 East Main Street
Frankfort, KY 40621
(502) 564-4440
(800) 372-7172
http://ovr.ky.gov/

## LOUISIANA

**Louisiana Rehabilitation Services**
627 North Fourth Street
Baton Rouge, LA 70802
(225) 219-2225
(800) 737-2958
(225) 219-4993 (fax)

## MAINE

**Maine Bureau of Rehabilitation Services**
Division of Vocation Rehabilitation
150 State House Station
Augusta, ME 04333
(800) 698-0150
(207) 287-5292 (fax)
http://www.maine.gov/rehab/

## MARYLAND

**Maryland State Department of Education**
Division of Rehabilitation Services
2301 Argonne Drive
Baltimore, MD 21218
(410) 554-9442
(888) 554-0334
(410) 554-9412 (fax)
http://www.dors.state.md.us/dors/

## MASSACHUSETTS

**Massachusetts Rehabilitation Commission**
Fort Point Place
Suite 600

27 Wormwood Street
Boston, MA 02210
(617) 204-3600
(800) 245-6543
(617) 727-1354 (fax)
http://www.mass.gov/mrc/

### MICHIGAN

**Michigan Department of Labor and
    Economic Growth**
Rehabilitation Services
201 North Washington Square, Fourth Floor
P.O. Box 30010
Lansing, MI 48909
(517) 373-4026
(800) 605-6722
(517) 335-7277 (fax)

### MINNESOTA

**Department of Employment and
    Economic Development**
Rehabilitation Services Branch
332 Minnesota Street
Suite E200
Saint Paul, MN 55101
(651) 259-7366
(800) 328-9095
(651) 297-5159 (fax)
http://www.deed.state.mn.us/rehab/vr/
    main_vr.htm

### MISSISSIPPI

**Mississippi Department of Rehabilitation
    Services**
1281 Highway S1
Madison, MS 39110
(800) 443-1000
http://www.mdrs.state.ms.us/

### MISSOURI

**Missouri Division of Vocational
    Rehabilitation**
3024 Dupont Circle
Jefferson City, MO 65109

(573) 751-3251
(877) 222-8963
(573) 751-1441 (fax)
http://dese.mo.gov/vr/

### MONTANA

**Montana Vocational Rehabilitation**
111 North Sanders
P.O. Box 4210
Helena, MT 59604
(406) 444-2590
(877) 296-1197
(406) 444-3632 (fax)
http://www.dphhs.mt.gov/dsd/mvr.shtml

### NEBRASKA

**Nebraska Department of Education**
Vocational Rehabilitation
P.O. Box 94987
301 Centennial Mall South
Lincoln, NE 68509
(402) 471-3644
(800) 742-7594
(402) 471-0788 (fax)
http://www.vocrehab.state.ne.us/

### NEVADA

**Department of Employment, Training and
    Rehabilitation**
1370 South Curry Street
Carson City, NV 89703
(775) 684-4070
(775) 684-4184 (fax)
http://detr.state.nv.us/rehab/reh_index.htm

### NEW HAMPSHIRE

**Department of Education**
Bureau of Vocational Rehabilitation
21 South Fruit Street
Suite 20
Concord, NH 03301
(603) 271-3471
(800) 299-1647
(603) 271-7095 (fax)

## NEW JERSEY

**New Jersey Division of Vocational Rehabilitation Services**
LWD Building, 10th Floor
John Fitch Plaza
P.O. Box 398
Trenton, NJ 08625
(609) 292-5987
(609) 292-8347 (fax)
http://lwd.dol.state.nj.us/labor/dvrs/DVRIndex.
  html

## NEW MEXICO

**New Mexico Division of Vocational Rehabilitation**
435 St. Michael's Drive, Building D
Santa Fe, NM 87505
(505) 954-8500
(800) 224-7005
(505) 954-8562 (fax)
http://www.dvrgetsjobs.com/

## NEW YORK

**Vocational and Educational Services for Individuals with Disabilities**
One Commerce Plaza
Albany, NY 12234
(800) 222-JOBS
(518) 486-4154 (fax)
http://www.vesid.nysed.gov/

## NORTH CAROLINA

**North Carolina Division of Vocational Rehabilitation Services**
2801 Mail Services Center
Raleigh, NC 27699
(919) 855-3579
(800) 689-9090
(919) 733-7968 (fax)
http://dvr.dhhs.state.nc.us/

## NORTH DAKOTA

**North Dakota Disability Services Division**
Vocational Rehabilitation
1237 West Divide Avenue
Suite 1B
Bismarck, ND 58501
(701) 328-8950
(800) 755-2745
(701) 328-8969 (fax)
http://www.nd.gov/dhs/services/disabilities/
  index.html

## OHIO

**Ohio Rehabilitation Services Commission**
400 East Campus View Boulevard
Columbus, OH 43235
(614) 438-1200
(800) 282-4536
(614) 438-1257 (fax)
http://www.rsc.ohio.gov

## OKLAHOMA

**Department of Rehabilitation Services**
3535 Northwest 58th Street
Suite 500
Oklahoma City, OK 73112
(405) 951-3400
(800) 845-8476
(405) 951-3529 (fax)
http://www.okrehab.org/

## OREGON

**Office of Vocational Rehabilitation Services**
Department of Human Services
500 Summer Street NE, E-87
Salem, OR 97301
(503) 945-5880
(503) 947-5010 (fax)
http://www.oregon.gov/DHS/vr/

## PENNSYLVANIA

**Department of Labor and Industry**
Office of Vocational Rehabilitation
1521 North Sixth Street
Harrisburg, PA 17102
(717) 787-5244
(800) 442-6351

## RHODE ISLAND

**Department of Human Services**
Office of Rehabilitation Services
40 Fountain Street
Providence, RI 02903
(401) 421-7005
(401) 222-3574 (fax)
http://www.ors.ri.gov/

## SOUTH CAROLINA

**South Carolina Vocational Rehabilitation Department**
State Office Building
1410 Boston Avenue
P.O. Box 15
West Columbia, SC 29171
(803) 896-6500
http://www.scvrd.net/

## SOUTH DAKOTA

**Division of Rehabilitation Services**
East Highway 34, Hillsview Plaza
c/o 500 East Capitol
Pierre, SD 57501
(605) 773-3195
(605) 773-5483 (fax)
http://dhs.sd.gov/drs/

## TENNESSEE

**Department of Human Services**
Vocational Rehabilitation Services
Citizens Plaza State Office Building
400 Deaderick Street, Second Floor
Nashville, TN 37248
(615) 313-4891
(615) 741-6508 (fax)
http://www.state.tn.us/humanserv/rehab/vrs.htm

## TEXAS

**Texas Department of Assistive and Rehabilitative Services**
Division for Rehabilitation Services
4800 Lamar Boulevard
Austin, TX 78756

(800) 628-5115
http://www.dars.state.tx.us/drs

## UTAH

**Utah State Office of Rehabilitation**
250 East 500 South
Salt Lake City, UT 84111
(801) 538-7530
(800) 473-7530
(801) 538-7522 (fax)
http://www.usor.utah.gov/

## VERMONT

**Division of Vocational Rehabilitation**
Department of Aging and Disabilities
Agency of Human Services
Weeks 1A, 103 South Main Street
Waterbury, VT 05671
(866) 879-6757
http://www.vocrehabvermont.org

## VIRGINIA

**Virginia Department of Rehabilitation Services**
8004 Franklin Frams Drive
Richmond, VA 23229
(804) 662-7000
(804) 662-9532 (fax)
http://www.vadrs.org/

## WASHINGTON

**Division of Vocational Rehabilitation**
P.O. Box 45340
Olympia, WA 98504
(360) 725-3636
(800) 637-5627
(360) 438-8007 (fax)
http://www.dshs.wa.gov/dvr/

## WEST VIRGINIA

**West Virginia Division of Rehabilitation Services**
P.O. Box 50890, State Capitol
Charleston, WV 25305
(800) 642-8207
http://www.wvdrs.org/

## WISCONSIN

**Wisconsin Division of Vocational Rehabilitation**
201 East Washington Avenue
P.O. Box 7852
Madison, WI 53707
(608) 261-0050
(800) 442-3477
(608) 266-1133 (fax)
http://www.dwd.state.wi.us/dvr/

## WYOMING

**Wyoming Division of Vocational Rehabilitation**
122 West 25th Street
Herschler Building 2E
Cheyenne, WY 82002
(307) 777-8650
(307) 777-5857 (fax)
http://wyomingworkforce.org/vr/

# APPENDIX III
## CANADIAN ORGANIZATIONS

## A. Canadian Kidney Foundation Offices

**National Office**
30-5165 Sherbooke Street West
Montreal, QC H4A 1T6
(514) 369-4806

**British Columbia Branch**
200-4940 Canada Way
Burnaby, BC V5G 4K6
(604) 736-9775, extension 224
http://www.kidney.bc.ca

**Northern Alberta & the Territories Branch**
10642 178 Street
Suite 101
Edmonton, AB T5S 1H4
(780) 451-6900
http://www.kidney.ab.ca

**Southern Alberta Branch**
6007 1A Street SW
Calgary, AB T2H 0G5
(403) 255-6108
http://www.kidneyfoundation.ab.ca

**Saskatchewan Branch**
1-2217 Hanselman Court
Saskatoon, SK S7L 6A8
(306) 664-8588
http://www.kidney.sk.ca

**Manitoba Branch**
1-42 Dovercourt Drive
Winnipeg, MB R3Y 1G4
(204) 989-0800
http://www.kidney.mb.ca

**Ontario Branch**
1599 Hunrontaro Street
Suite 201
Mississauga, ON L5G 4S1
(905) 278-3003
(905) 271-4990 (fax)

**Ontario Branch**
15 Gervais Drive
Suite 700
Toronto, ON M3C 1Y8
(416) 445-0373
http://www.kidney.on.ca

**Quebec Branch**
2300 Rene Levesque Boulevard West
Montreal, QC H3H 2R5
(514) 938-4515
http://www.kidneyquebec.ca

**New Brunswick Branch**
42 Durelle Street
Suite 2
Fredericton, NB E3C 1N8
(506) 453-0533

**Nova Scotia Branch**
15-6960 Mumford Road
Halifax, NS B3L 4P1
(902) 429-9298
(800) 889-5557
(902) 425-5348 (fax)

**Prince Edward Island Branch**
P.O. Box 2324
Charlottetown, PE C1A 8C1
(902) 892-9009

**Newfoundland and Labrador Branch**
66 Kenmount Road
Suite 303
St. John's, NL A1B 3V7
(709) 753-8999

**Saint John Chapter**
215 Wentworth Street
Saint John, NB E2L 2T4
(506) 634-0519
(506) 642-1995 (fax)

## B. Canadian Diabetes Association Branches

Diabetes is a major health risk in Canada, and thus an appendix on territorial programs is offered here, with regional offices of the Canadian Diabetes Association.

### NATIONAL OFFICE

**Canadian Diabetes Association**
1400-522 University Avenue
Toronto, ON M5G 2R5
(800) BANTING

### REGIONAL OFFICES

#### ALBERTA

**Calgary and District Branch**
204-2324 32 Avenue NE
Calgary, AB T2E 6Z3
(403) 266-0620
(403) 269-8927 (fax)

**Medicine Hat and District Branch**
102-73 7 St. SE
Medicine Hat, AB T1A 1J2
(403) 529-1259
(403) 529-1565 (fax)

**Edmonton and District Branch**
1010-10117 Jasper Avenue NW
Edmonton, AB T5J 1W8
(780) 423-1232
(780) 423-3322 (fax)

**Red Deer and District Branch**
#06-5015 48th Street
Red Deer, AB T4N 1S9
(403) 346-4631
(403) 341-3015 (fax)

**Lethbridge and District Branch**
210D 12 A Street North
Lethbridge, AB T1H 2J1
(403) 327-4114
(403) 328-4658 (fax)

#### BRITISH COLUMBIA

**100 Mile House and District Branch**
Box 1676
100 Mile House, BC V0K 2E0

**Dawson Creek and District Branch**
Box 2361
Dawson Creek BC V1G 4T9

**Kamloops and District Branch**
1589 Sutherland Avenue
Kelowna, BC V1Y 5V7
(250) 374-5744

#### MANITOBA

**Brandon (Westman) Branch and District Office**
Westman Branch
727B 10th Street
Brandon, MB R7A 4G7
(204) 728-2382
(204) 726-1603 (fax)

**Canadian Diabetes Association (Manitoba and Nunavut)**
200-310 Broadway
Winnipeg, MB R3C 0S6
(204) 925-3800
(204) 949-0266 (fax)

**Dauphin (Parklands) Branch and District Office**
118 Main Street North
Dauphin, MB R7N 1C2
(204) 638-6248
(204) 638-0423 (fax)

## NEW BRUNSWICK

**Regional Office**
61 Carleton Street
Suite 2
Fredericton, NB E3B 3T2
(506) 452-9009
(800) 884-4232
(506) 455-4728 (fax)

## NEWFOUNDLAND AND LABRADOR

**Newfoundland and Labrador Regional
   Leadership Centre**
29031 Pippy Place
Suite 2007
St. John's, NL A1B 3X2
(709) 754-0953
(709) 754-0734 (fax)

## NORTHWEST TERRITORIES

**Northern Alberta and Northwest
   Territories Regional Leadership Centre**
1010-10117 Hapser Avenue NW
Edmonton, AB T5J 1W8
(780) 423-1232
(780) 423-3322 (fax)

## NOVA SCOTIA

**Regional Leadership Centre**
137 Chain Lake Drive
Suite 101
Halifax, NS B3S 1B3
(902) 453-4232
(902) 453-4440 (fax)
(800) 326-7712

**Cape Breton Branch**
Emergency Services Centre
850 Grand Lake Road
Suite 3
Sydney, NS B1P 5T9
(902) 564-6461
(902) 564-5354 (fax)

**Annapolis Valley Branch**
P.O. Box 2450
Wolfville, NS B4P 2S3
(902) 542-3870 (phone/fax)

## NUNAVUT

**Manitoba and Nunavut Regional
   Leadership Centre**
200-310 Broadway
Winnipeg, MB R3C 0S6
(204) 925-3800
(204) 949-0266 (fax)

## ONTARIO

**Barrie Branch (Simcoe County/Muskokas/
   Perry Sound)**
556 Bryne Drive
Unit #4
Barrie, ON L4N 9P6
(705) 737-3611
(705) 737-4912 (fax)

**Brantford Branch**
St. Joseph Lifecare Centre
99 Wayne Gretsky Parkway
Fifth Floor
Brantford, ON N3S 6T6
(519) 756-9131
(519) 756-4262 (fax)

**Brockville Branch**
42 George Street
P.O. Box 1911
Brockville, ON K6V 6N4
(613) 345-0992
(613) 345-6545 (fax)

**Cambridge and District Branch**
14 Irvin Street
Suite 1
Kitchener, ON N2H 1K8
(519) 742-1481
(519) 742-1282 (fax)

**Chatham and District Branch**
P.O. Box 724
Chatham, ON N7M 5L1
(519) 351-6020
(519) 351-5167 (fax)

**Cornwall and District Branch**
119 Sydney Street
Cornwall, ON K6H 3H1

(613) 938-7497
(613) 938-9782 (fax)

**Oshawa Region Branch**
235 Yorkland Boulevard
Suite 200
Toronto, ON M2J 4YB
(416) 363-0177
(416) 491-8927 (fax)

**Elliot Lake/Blind River Branch**
c/o North East Ontario Regional Leadership
    Centre
2141 Lasalle Boulevard
Unit F
W Sudbury, ON P3A 2A3

## PRINCE EDWARD ISLAND

**Coordinator, Donations & Sponsorships**
Sherwood Business Center
161 St. Peter's Road
Charlottetown, PE C1A 5P7
(902) 894-3195
(902) 368-1928 (fax)

## SASKATCHEWAN

**North Saskatchewan Regional Leadership
    Centre**
104-2301 Avenue C North

Saskatoon, SK S7L 5Z5
(306) 933-1238
(800) 996-4446
(306) 244-2012 (fax)

**South Saskatchewan Regional Leadership
    Centre**
917A Albert St.
Regina, SK S4R 2P6
(306) 584-8445
(800) 297-7488
(306) 586-9704 (fax)

## YUKON

**Northern British Columbia and Yukon
    Regional Office**
103-490 Quebec Street
Prince George, BC V2L 5N5
(250) 561-9284

**Whitehorse & District Branch**
Box 31207
211 Main Street
Whitehorse, YT Y1A 5P7

# APPENDIX IV

## NUMBER OF DIALYSIS AND TRANSPLANT FACILITIES: BY STATE AND TERRITORY, 2001–2006

As can be seen from the table, the number of facilities proving dialysis and transplants has increased in some states, and stayed flat in others. In considering all states and U.S. territories, however, the number of facilities increased from 4,184 in 2001 to 5,062 in 2006.

| State | 2001 | 2002 | 2003 | 2004 | 2005 | 2006 |
|---|---|---|---|---|---|---|
| Alabama | 99 | 101 | 106 | 110 | 110 | 110 |
| Alaska | 2 | 2 | 2 | 4 | 4 | 4 |
| Arizona | 87 | 91 | 94 | 95 | 99 | 102 |
| Arkansas | 64 | 64 | 65 | 64 | 64 | 60 |
| California | 366 | 383 | 408 | 421 | 427 | 440 |
| Colorado | 39 | 42 | 42 | 45 | 52 | 53 |
| Connecticut | 33 | 32 | 32 | 32 | 32 | 34 |
| Delaware | 13 | 15 | 15 | 17 | 17 | 18 |
| District of Columbia | 23 | 23 | 24 | 22 | 23 | 22 |
| Florida | 262 | 264 | 269 | 279 | 288 | 294 |
| Georgia | 199 | 216 | 219 | 222 | 237 | 246 |
| Hawaii | 16 | 18 | 19 | 18 | 18 | 29 |
| Idaho | 7 | 7 | 7 | 9 | 12 | 16 |
| Illinois | 148 | 158 | 172 | 180 | 197 | 198 |
| Indiana | 82 | 93 | 93 | 96 | 98 | 110 |
| Iowa | 49 | 51 | 55 | 57 | 58 | 63 |
| Kansas | 40 | 42 | 43 | 44 | 45 | 46 |
| Kentucky | 51 | 57 | 65 | 67 | 72 | 77 |
| Louisiana | 132 | 135 | 134 | 142 | 153 | 145 |
| Maine | 13 | 15 | 18 | 19 | 19 | 20 |
| Maryland | 106 | 115 | 116 | 115 | 110 | 113 |
| Massachusetts | 70 | 73 | 75 | 77 | 81 | 81 |
| Michigan | 118 | 125 | 139 | 145 | 150 | 156 |
| Minnesota | 69 | 74 | 72 | 75 | 82 | 82 |
| Mississippi | 65 | 66 | 67 | 68 | 68 | 69 |
| Missouri | 102 | 108 | 111 | 113 | 119 | 125 |
| Montana | 15 | 15 | 15 | 15 | 13 | 13 |
| Nebraska | 25 | 31 | 36 | 34 | 35 | 35 |
| Nevada | 19 | 22 | 22 | 25 | 25 | 25 |

| State | 2001 | 2002 | 2003 | 2004 | 2005 | 2006 |
|---|---|---|---|---|---|---|
| New Hampshire | 10 | 11 | 10 | 10 | 12 | 11 |
| New Jersey | 93 | 101 | 108 | 116 | 116 | 118 |
| New Mexico | 30 | 30 | 31 | 32 | 33 | 35 |
| New York | 223 | 239 | 239 | 245 | 249 | 243 |
| North Carolina | 118 | 130 | 138 | 145 | 149 | 153 |
| North Dakota | 13 | 14 | 14 | 14 | 14 | 14 |
| Ohio | 160 | 173 | 186 | 193 | 202 | 211 |
| Oklahoma | 58 | 62 | 62 | 62 | 67 | 68 |
| Oregon | 43 | 46 | 45 | 45 | 47 | 51 |
| Pennsylvania | 223 | 231 | 232 | 232 | 243 | 242 |
| Rhode Island | 13 | 14 | 14 | 17 | 18 | 18 |
| South Carolina | 82 | 86 | 92 | 93 | 100 | 107 |
| South Dakota | 21 | 22 | 22 | 23 | 23 | 26 |
| Tennessee | 116 | 127 | 130 | 128 | 127 | 131 |
| Texas | 309 | 324 | 341 | 366 | 411 | 423 |
| Utah | 23 | 27 | 25 | 24 | 25 | 25 |
| Vermont | 6 | 6 | 6 | 6 | 6 | 7 |
| Virginia | 125 | 126 | 131 | 133 | 137 | 141 |
| Washington | 49 | 53 | 50 | 54 | 58 | 60 |
| West Virginia | 22 | 23 | 22 | 23 | 25 | 26 |
| Wisconsin | 82 | 90 | 98 | 102 | 111 | 112 |
| Wyoming | 9 | 9 | 9 | 9 | 9 | 9 |
| | | | | | | |
| American Samoa | 1 | 1 | 1 | 1 | 1 | 1 |
| Guam | 3 | 3 | 3 | 3 | 3 | 3 |
| Puerto Rico | 34 | 42 | 42 | 41 | 38 | 38 |
| Virgin Islands | 2 | 2 | 3 | 3 | 3 | 3 |
| Total | 4,184 | 4,431 | 4,588 | 4,730 | 4,935 | 5,062 |

Source: Adapted from U.S. Renal Data System. *USRDS 2008 Annual Data Report: Atlas of Chronic Kidney Disease and End-Stage Renal Disease in the United States.* Bethesda, Md.: National Institutes of Health, National Institute of Diabetes and Digestive and Kidney Diseases, 2008. p. 277.

Note: The data reported here have been supplied by the United States Renal Data System (USRDS). The interpretation and reporting of these data are the responsibility of the authors and in no way should be seen as an official policy or interpretation of the U.S. government.

# APPENDIX V

## ABNORMALITIES OF SELECTED CLINICAL AND BIOCHEMICAL PARAMETERS IN THE NHANES 1999–2006 POPULATION: BY CHRONIC KIDNEY DISEASE STAGE IDENTIFIED WITH CREATININE FORMULA (PERCENT OF PARTICIPANTS)

This chart provides data from the National Health and Nutrition Examination Survey (NHANES), an annual study of health data, and clearly shows differences in the measurements of individuals with no chronic kidney disease (CKD) as well as those who are in Stages 1–2, 3, and 4–5. Stage 5 is end-stage renal disease (ESRD), or kidney failure.

| Abnormal Level | No CKD | Stages 1–2 | Stage 3 | Stages 4–5 |
|---|---|---|---|---|
| Potassium ≥ 4/5 mmol/l | 8.3 | 12.1 | 21.3 | 47.5 |
| Bicarbonate ≤ 20.4 mmol/l | 4.9 | 6.6 | 5.2 | 22.3 |
| Uric acid ≥ 7.7 mg/dl | 5.0 | 9.2 | 19.2 | 41.8 |
| Calcium ≤ 8.9 mg/dl | 6.8 | 7.1 | 5.8 | 22.1 |
| Phosphorus ≥ 4.7 mg/dl | 4.6 | 3.9 | 6.2 | 32.1 |
| Systolic blood pressure ≥ 140 mm Hg | 12.2 | 33.7 | 38.9 | 54.4 |
| Diastolic blood pressure ≥ 90 mm Hg | 5.3 | 10.6 | 4.9 | 9.1 |
| Reduced HDL ("good" cholesterol) | 30.4 | 37.2 | 34.9 | 45.2 |
| Elevated triglycerides | 30.9 | 41.7 | 43.5 | 47.4 |
| Elevated fasting glucose | 31.4 | 55.0 | 53.4 | 50.7 |
| Elevated waist circumference | 48.6 | 62.3 | 66.1 | 69.0 |
| World Health Organization (WHO) anemia | 4.3 | 6.9 | 11.9 | 47.8 |

Source: Adapted from *USRDS 2009 Annual Data Report. Volume One: Atlas of Chronic Kidney Disease and End-Stage Renal Disease in the United States*. Bethesda, Md.: National Institutes of Health, National Institute of Diabetes and Digestive and Kidney Diseases, 2009, p. 42.

The data reported here have been supplied by the United States Renal Data System (USRDS). The interpretation and reporting of these data are the responsibility of the authors and in no way should be seen as an official policy or interpretation of the U.S. government.

# APPENDIX VI

## WORLDWIDE INCIDENCE OF END-STAGE RENAL DISEASE

This table, provided by the United States Renal Data System in 2009, compares the incidence (new cases in a year) of end-stage renal disease in many countries worldwide, starting in 2003 and ending in 2007. As can be seen from this table, the rate of ESRD is very high in the United States, and the only higher rates are in Tai-wan and in (Jalisco) Mexico. According to the USRDS, however, it is important to note that an affluent nation may treat older individuals for ESRD while developing nations may restrict such treatment only to younger and healthier patients (and fewer young and healthy patients develop ESRD than elderly patients).

### INCIDENCE OF ESRD, BY YEAR (PER MILLION POPULATION) IN SELECTED COUNTRIES WORLDWIDE, 2003–2007

| Country | 2003 | 2004 | 2005 | 2006 | 2007 |
|---|---|---|---|---|---|
| Argentina | – | 137 | 140 | 141 | 151 |
| Australia | 100 | 97 | 113 | 118 | 110 |
| Austria | 140 | 161 | 154 | 159 | 151 |
| Bangladesh | 8 | 7 | 8 | 8 | 13 |
| Belgium, Dutch speaking | 175 | 181 | 183 | 193 | 186 |
| Belgium, French speaking | 161 | 186 | 177 | 186 | 185 |
| Bosnia & Herzegovina | 106 | 108 | 104 | 133 | 151 |
| Canada | 162 | 163 | 163 | 163 | – |
| Chile | 130 | 157 | 135 | 141 | 144 |
| Croatia | 131 | 155 | 144 | – | – |
| Czech Republic | 167 | 166 | 175 | 186 | 185 |
| Denmark | 132 | 131 | 121 | 119 | 140 |
| Finland | 95 | 97 | 97 | 87 | 92 |
| France | – | – | 139 | 140 | 138 |
| Germany | 186 | 194 | 203 | 213 | – |
| Greece | 180 | 197 | 194 | 197 | 190 |
| Hong Kong | 128 | 141 | 145 | 149 | 147 |
| Hungary | 139 | 139 | 162 | 159 | 165 |
| Iceland | 73 | 79 | 67 | 69 | 81 |
| Iran | 61 | 71 | 72 | 66 | – |
| Israel | 188 | 189 | 186 | 192 | 193 |
| Italy | 133 | 161 | 121 | – | – |

*(table continues)*

**INCIDENCE OF ESRD, BY YEAR (PER MILLION POPULATION) IN SELECTED COUNTRIES WORLDWIDE, 2003–2007**
*(continued)*

| Country | 2003 | 2004 | 2005 | 2006 | 2007 |
|---|---|---|---|---|---|
| Jalisco (Mexico) | 280 | 346 | 302 | 346 | 372 |
| Japan | 263 | 267 | 271 | 275 | 285 |
| Luxembourg | 180 | 188 | 164 | 224 | – |
| Malaysia | 106 | 114 | 121 | 137 | 143 |
| Netherlands | 103 | 106 | 107 | 112 | 118 |
| New Zealand | 115 | 113 | 112 | 119 | 109 |
| Norway | 96 | 101 | 99 | 100 | 113 |
| Pakistan | 32 | – | 22 | 29 | – |
| Philippines | 60 | 75 | 79 | 80 | 92 |
| Poland | 103 | 97 | 120 | 122 | 127 |
| Republic of Korea | 152 | 171 | 173 | 185 | 184 |
| Romania | – | – | 94 | 75 | 90 |
| Russia | 19 | 17 | 24 | 28 | – |
| Scotland | 121 | 115 | 125 | 116 | 114 |
| Shanghai | 232 | 263 | 275 | 282 | – |
| Spain | – | 175 | 126 | 128 | 121 |
| Sweden | 122 | 123 | 121 | 130 | 129 |
| Taiwan | 391 | 405 | 435 | 420 | 415 |
| Thailand | 78 | 123 | 110 | 139 | 159 |
| Turkey | 112 | 121 | 179 | 192 | 229 |
| United Kingdom (England, Wales and Northern Ireland) | – | 91 | 101 | 105 | 106 |
| United States | 343 | 347 | 354 | 365 | 361 |
| Uruguay | 146 | 151 | 146 | 138 | 143 |

Adapted from United States Renal Data System. *USRDS 2009 Annual Data Report: Atlas of Chronic Kidney Disease and End-Stage Renal Disease in the United States.* Bethesda, Md.: National Institutes of Health, National Institute of Diabetes and Digestive and Kidney Diseases, 2009, p. 348.

The data reported here have been supplied by the United States Renal Data System (USRDS). The interpretation and reporting of these data are the responsibility of the authors and in no way should be seen as an official policy or interpretation of the U.S. government.

# APPENDIX VII

## WORLDWIDE INCIDENCE OF END-STAGE RENAL DISEASE DUE TO DIABETES, 2003–2007

This table provides worldwide data for the years 2003–07 on the incidence of kidney failure (end-stage renal disease) caused by diabetes among individuals in selected countries worldwide, including the United States. As can be seen from the table, the United States is fifth after Malaysia, Mexico (Jalisco), Hong Kong, and the Republic of Korea in the high percentage of the incidence (newly diagnosed cases in a year) of end-stage renal disease (ESRD) caused by diabetes mellitus.

In the United States, nearly 44 percent of all new cases of ESRD in 2007 were caused by diabetes. The rate for Malaysia was 58.5 percent, followed by Mexico (55.0 percent), Hong Kong (45.1 percent) and Korea (44.9 percent). Some countries had rates of less than 20 percent of ESRD that was caused by diabetes, such as Romania, Iceland, Norway, Scotland, the Netherlands, the United Kingdom, and Bosnia and Herzegovina. Data is missing for some countries in some years because it was not provided in the original table.

| PERCENTAGE OF INCIDENT PATIENTS WITH ESRD DUE TO DIABETES, BY YEAR | | | | | |
|---|---|---|---|---|---|
| Country | 2003 | 2004 | 2005 | 2006 | 2007 |
| Argentina | – | 31.4 | 34.7 | 33.8 | 31.2 |
| Australia | 26.0 | 30.3 | 31.5 | 32.6 | 30.9 |
| Austria | 33.5 | 32.3 | 33.5 | 33.0 | 31.5 |
| Belgium, Dutch speaking | 24.0 | 24.4 | 23.9 | 22.2 | 23.4 |
| Belgium, French speaking | 25.0 | 21.2 | 23.7 | 22.6 | 22.9 |
| Bosnia & Herzegovina | 22.9 | 20.1 | 20.6 | 21.5 | 19.7 |
| Canada | 34.2 | 34.3 | 34.9 | 34.4 | – |
| Croatia | 26.9 | 29.0 | 30.0 | – | – |
| Denmark | 22.6 | 21.5 | 24.2 | 24.0 | 22.6 |
| Finland | 34.9 | 33.2 | 34.6 | 35.7 | 35.3 |
| France | – | – | 23.3 | 34.7 | 22.2 |
| Germany | 36.3 | 34.2 | 34.9 | 34.4 | – |
| Greece | 28.0 | 28.3 | 29.4 | 29.4 | 27.8 |
| Hong Kong | 39.9 | 40.5 | 41.1 | 40.2 | 45.1 |
| Hungary | 25.5 | 29.5 | 26.2 | 27.5 | 29.2 |
| Iceland | 0.0 | 4.3 | 15.0 | 28.6 | 12.0 |
| Israel | 39.0 | 42.2 | 40.7 | 41.9 | 41.8 |

*(table continues)*

313

**PERCENTAGE OF INCIDENT PATIENTS WITH ESRD DUE TO DIABETES, BY YEAR**
*(continued)*

| Country | 2003 | 2004 | 2005 | 2006 | 2007 |
|---|---|---|---|---|---|
| Italy | 16.2 | 16.2 | 18.0 | – | – |
| Jalisco (Mexico) | 51.0 | 56.0 | 60.0 | 49.9 | 55.0 |
| Japan | 40.6 | 40.9 | 41.6 | 42.5 | 43.2 |
| Luxembourg | – | – | – | 28.2 | – |
| Malaysia | 53.9 | 55.1 | 55.9 | 59.2 | 58.5 |
| Netherlands | 16.6 | 17.4 | 15.6 | 16.0 | 17.9 |
| New Zealand | 41.3 | 40.7 | 42.0 | 42.2 | 41.0 |
| Norway | 15.8 | 17.3 | 12.8 | 16.5 | 13.6 |
| Pakistan | 40.0 | – | 36.3 | 37.7 | – |
| Philippines | 32.8 | 33.5 | 36.9 | 38.5 | 24.1 |
| Poland | 22.6 | 26.9 | 27.2 | 29.6 | 24.1 |
| Republic of Korea | 42.5 | 43.4 | 38.5 | 42.3 | 44.9 |
| Romania | – | – | 10.7 | 12.3 | 11.7 |
| Russia | 10.7 | – | 11.0 | 13.9 | – |
| Scotland | 18.9 | 17.9 | 21.7 | 21.6 | 17.6 |
| Spain | – | 17.5 | 23.2 | 23.3 | 21.5 |
| Sweden | 24.0 | 25.1 | 25.8 | 26.1 | 27.1 |
| Taiwan | 36.8 | 40.1 | 41.8 | 43.0 | 43.1 |
| Turkey | 23.1 | 21.3 | 30.2 | 23.1 | 22.8 |
| United Kingdom (England, Wales and Northern Ireland) | – | 19.1 | 19.0 | 20.6 | 19.6 |
| United States | 44.9 | 45.0 | 44.4 | 44.4 | 43.9 |
| Uruguay | 29.6 | 21.8 | 29.6 | 22.1 | 22.1 |

Adapted from United States Renal Data System. *USRDS 2009 Annual Data Report: Atlas of Chronic Kidney Disease and End-Stage Renal Disease in the United States.* Bethesda, Md.: National Institutes of Health, National Institute of Diabetes and Digestive and Kidney Diseases, 2009, p. 349.

The data reported here have been supplied by the United States Renal Data System (USRDS). The interpretation and reporting of these data are the responsibility of the authors and in no way should be seen as an official policy or interpretation of the U.S. government.

# APPENDIX VIII
## DONOR DESIGNATION STATUS BY STATE

Not enough people plan to donate their organs upon their deaths but some people do make such a plan. In some states, the plan can be overturned by family members, while in others, it is inviolate. Many states have donor registries on which individuals can register well before they become ill. When a person agrees to donate his or her organs after death, this is "first person consent." The following chart provided by the United Network for Organ Sharing (UNOS) shows the laws of each state as of this writing and also provides Web sites for most states so readers can obtain further information. Contact the UNOS or go to their Web site at www.unos.org to find the most recent data. UNOS updates their list on a quarterly basis.

| State | First Person Consent | Comments | Registry |
|---|---|---|---|
| Alabama | Yes | Alabama does not require family consent to carry out your wishes to be an organ, eye, or tissue donor. | alabamalifelegacy.org |
| Alaska | Yes | Life Alaska Donor Services (tissue bank) maintains the official Alaska registry. Law signed in 2004 enables DMV [Department of Motor Vehicles] transfer to Life Alaska's existing registry. The public can also register by mail or directly at the DMV. | www.alaskadonorregistr.org |
| Arizona | Yes | Legislation passed in March 2002. Once registry is in place, Arizona will proceed with first person consent in practice. | www.azdonorregistry.org |
| Arkansas | Yes | Arkansas Senate Bill 35 to develop an organ donor registry passed during the 1997 Regular Session. Donor registration in Arkansas is legally binding. Family consent is not requested before proceeding with donation. | Yes—affiliated with the DMV |
| California | Yes | California's statewide online registry launched on April 4, 2005. | www.donatelifecalifornial.org or www.donevidacalifornia.org |
| Colorado | Yes | Law enacted by Colorado State legislature in 1968 to establish a centralized, confidential donor registry. Recovery agencies enforced law in October 2001. | www.donatelife.colorado.org |
| Connecticut | Yes | Connecticut has a first person consent registry maintained by the DMV that OPO and medical staff can access. It is legally binding. | N/A |
| Delaware | Yes | | www.donatelife-de.org |

*(table continues)*

*(table continued)*

| State | First Person Consent | Comments | Registry |
|-------|----------------------|----------|----------|
| District of Columbia | Yes | | www.donatelifedc.org |
| Florida | Yes | Florida Senate Bill 334 signed into law May 2003. | www.donatelifeflorida.org |
| Georgia | Yes | Went into effect in July 2008. | www.donatelifegeorgia.org |
| Hawaii | Yes | Hawaii's UAGA states that when a person has executed a valid document of gift (donor card, etc.), the consent of no other person is needed in order to proceed with organ removal. | www.donatelifehawaii.com |
| Idaho | Yes | | www.yesidaho.org |
| Illinois | Yes | Families can no longer override an individual's wish to donate. | www.cyberdriveillinois.com or call 800-210-2106. |
| Indiana | Yes | Changed language of the UAGA to indicate that a family could not override a donor's wishes. House enrolled Act 1628, Amended 1C 29-2-16-2-5. Effective July 2001. | www.indianadonationalliance foundation.org |
| Iowa | Yes | Law went into effect July 1, 2002. First Person Consent Bill (Senate File 2195) allows "a written statement attached to or imprinted or noted on a driver's license or nonoperator's ID card, an entry in a donor registry, a donor's will or any other written document used by a donor to make an anatomical gift." | N/A |
| Kansas | No | Updated in 1994, Chapter 65, Article 32, 65-3214 (d) states: "An anatomical gift that is not revoked by the donor before death is irrevocable and does not require the consent or concurrence of any person after the donor's death." | ww.mwtn.org |
| Kentucky | Yes | | www.donatelifeky.org |
| Louisiana | Yes | | www.lopa.org |
| Maine | Yes | Maine has a first person consent registry maintained by the DMV that OPO and medical staff can access. It is legally binding. | www.neob.org/media.htm |
| Maryland | Yes | Maryland has a first person consent registry maintained by the DMVY that the OPO can access. | https://secure.rmv.state.ma.us/ OrganDonor/intro.aspx |
| Massachusetts | Yes | Massachusetts has a first person consent registry maintained by the DMV that OPO and medical staff can access. It is legally binding. | www.neob.org/madia.htm |
| Michigan | Yes | Legislation was passed in August 1998 stating the Secretary of State would provide a donor registry with all driver's license and personal ID applications and renewals. In turn, the Secretary of State scans new registrant information and forwards that information to Gift of Life Michigan. | www.giftoflifemichigan.org |
| Minnesota | Yes | 2002 Darlene Luther Anatomical Gift Act specifies that donor designation is evidence of intent to donate at the time of death and is sufficient authorization where a legally-binding document of gift exists. OPO implemented practice honoring donor designation as authorization for donation on May 1, 2003. | www.DonateLifeMN.org |

| State | First Person Consent | Comments | Registry |
|---|---|---|---|
| Mississippi | Yes | | www.donatelifems.org |
| Missouri | | Bill passed in 1996. In practice, OPOs still obtain family consent before proceeding with donation. | www.Missouriorgandonor.com |
| Montana | Yes | | www.DonateLifeToday.com |
| Nebraska | Yes | | www.nedonation.org |
| Nevada | Yes | Donor registry established through the passage of Assembly Bill 497 in the 2001 legislative session. Also set up an Anatomical Gift account, through the DMV, to collect $1.00 or more to fund a Task Force on Organ and Tissue Donation Education. OPO and Tissue and Eye Bank have stated that they will honor first person consent. Still speak with the family, but have changed their approach and now state they already have consent because of the driver's license. | www.nvdonor.org |
| New Hampshire | Yes | First person consent, DMV-based register legislation passed—awaiting legislation. | www.DonateLifeNewEngland.org |
| New Jersey | Yes | Legislation since 1998 provides that documented intent of a decedent to donate organs or tissues upon death shall not be revoked by any person otherwise designated to consent to such donation. | www.donatelifenj.org |
| New Mexico | Yes | Legislation became effective May 2002. The driver's license will serve as one way to designate first person consent (also on donor card, living will, or durable power of attorney for health care). | http://www.nmdonor.org |
| New York | Yes | Current law requires two witnesses; legislation pending to eliminate requirement to update NY law to UAGA. | www.health.state.ny.us |
| North Carolina | Yes | First-person consent law went into effect on October 1, 2007. Heart on driver's license indicates first person consent for organs and eye, but not tissue. Online registry covering first person consent for organs, eye, and/or tissue launched on April 1, 2008. | www.donatelife.nc.org |
| North Dakota | Yes | 1987 UAGA states the driver's license indication serves as authorization for donation. OPO implemented practice honoring donor designation as authorization for donation on May 1, 2003. | Yes, affiliated with DMV |
| Ohio | Yes | Ohio's first person consent legislation became effective July 2002. In 2005, online registration unveiled. | www.DonateLifeOhio.org |
| Oklahoma | Yes | Online registry officially launched April 2004. | www.lifeshareregistry.org |
| Oregon | Yes | Oregon's statewide registry launched on April 2, 2007. | www.donatelifenw.org |
| Pennsylvania | Yes | First person consent legislation passed in 1994. | www.donatelife-pa.org |
| Rhode Island | Yes | Rhode Island has a first person consent registry maintained by the DMV that OPO and medical staff can access. It is legally binding. | http://www.neob.org/ridla.org |

*(table continues)*

*(table continued)*

| State | First Person Consent | Comments | Registry |
|---|---|---|---|
| South Carolina | Yes | South Carolina does honor first person consent and makes the wishes of the donor paramount to wishes of others. | www.donatelifesc.org |
| South Dakota | Yes | | Yes—affiliated with DMV |
| Tennessee | Yes | | www.tndonorregistry.org |
| Utah | Yes | Online registry launched April 2002. | www.yesutah.org |
| Vermont | No | Has an online advance directive registry wherein individuals may register end-of-life decisions. Donation decisions may be made within this registry. OPO staff have access to this registry of decisions. | http://healthvermont.gov/vadr |
| Virginia | Yes | First person consent and registry legislation adopted July 1, 2000. Registry info from DMV will be transferred monthly. Will proceed with donation if they have legal documentation. Online registry officially launched August 2003. | www.save7lives.org |
| Washington | | Legislation regarding the specifics of the donor registry creation and maintenance approved in the spring of 2003. | www.DonateLifeToday.com |
| Wisconsin | No | A statewide consortium is working to create a first person authorization registry to ensure each donor's wishes are honored. | www.donatelifewisconsin.org |
| West Virginia | Yes | First person consent legislation implemented in 1995. | https://donatelife.wv.gov |
| Wyoming | Yes | Wyoming law is based on Colorado law. | www.donatelifewyoming.org |

Source: United Network for Organ Sharing. "Donor Designation (First Person Consent) Status by State." February 3, 2010. Available online. URL: http://www.transplantliving.org/community/publications/newfactsheets.aspx?fact=consent#. Accessed April 8, 2010.

# APPENDIX IX
## STATEWIDE DRUG ASSISTANCE PROGRAMS

Many people with chronic kidney disease and end-stage renal disease (ESRD) or kidney failure struggle to pay their medication expenses. This table provides a state-by-state listing of information on medication assistance for people with kidney disease as well as other diseases. (Many people with chronic kidney disease also have diabetes and hypertension.) Some states have more than one program and are thus listed several times in the table.

| State | Population Served: E=Elderly* D=Disabled L-Low income M=Medicare | Name of Program | Program Type | Contact Information |
|---|---|---|---|---|
| Alabama | E (55+) D | SeniorRx | Govt. PAP assistance program | 800-AGE-LINE 800-243-5463 |
| Alaska | | No program | | |
| Arizona | All | Arizona CoppeRx Card Prescription Discount Program (RxAmerica) | Govt. drug discount card | 1-888-227-8315 |
| Arkansas | L | Arkansas Health Care Access Foundation, Inc. | Nonprofit prescription assistance program | 1-800-950-8233 or 1-501-221-3033 |
| California | M | Drug Discount Program for Medicare Recipients | Govt. prescription assistance program | Show your Medicare card at participating pharmacies to get drugs at Medi-Cal prices (when paying out of pocket) 1-800-434-0222 |
| Colorado | | No program | | |
| Connecticut | E, D, or M | Connecticut Pharmaceutical Assistance Contract to the Elderly and the Disabled Program (ConnPACE) | Govt. prescription assistance program; will wrap around Medicare Part D | 1-800-423-5026 |
| Delaware | E, D, or M | Delaware Prescription Assistance Program (DPAP) | Govt. prescription assistance program; will wrap around Medicare Part D | 1-800-996-9969 |

*(table continues)*

319

*(table continued)*

| State | Population Served: E=Elderly* D=Disabled L-Low income M=Medicare | Name of Program | Program Type | Contact Information |
|---|---|---|---|---|
| District of Columbia | L (under 64 yrs old) | DC Healthcare Alliance | Govt. health care insurance program | 1-202-842-2810 or 1-866- 842-2810 |
| Florida | E, L | Florida Discount Drug Card Govt. drug discount card | | 1-866-341-8894 |
| Georgia | | | No program | |
| Hawaii | M | State Pharmacy Assistance Program | Govt. prescription assistance program; will wrap around Medicare Part D | 1-808-692-7999 or 1-866-878-9769 |
| Hawaii | E, D, or M | | | |
| Idaho | | No program | | |
| Illinois | E, D or M | Illinois Cares Rx | Govt. prescription assistance program; will wrap around Medicare Part D | 1-800-226-0768 |
| Illinois | L | Illinois Rx Buying Club | Govt. drug discount card | 1-866-215-3462 |
| Indiana | | No program | | |
| Iowa | | No program | | |
| Kansas | | No program | | |
| Kentucky | L | Health Kentucky | Nonprofit prescription assistance program | 1-800-633-8100 |
| Kentucky | | Kentucky Pharmacy Assistance Program | Govt. prescription assistance program | 1-502-564-8966, extension 4216 |
| Louisiana | E | Louisiana SeniorRx Program | Govt. prescription assistance program | 1-877-340-9100 |
| Maine | E, D, or M | Maine Low Cost Drugs for the Elderly & Disabled Program | Govt. prescription assistance program; will wrap around Medicare Part D | 1-866-796-2463 |
| Maine | L | Maine Rx Plus | Govt. prescription discount program | 1-866-796-2463 |
| Maryland | L | Maryland Medbank Program | Nonprofit prescription assistance program | 1-877-435-7755 |
| Maryland | D, M | Senior Prescription Drug Assistance Program | Govt. prescription assistance program; will wrap around Medicare Part D | 1-800-551-5995 |
| Massachusetts | E, D, or M | The Prescription Advantage Program | Govt. prescription assistance program; will wrap around Medicare Part D | 1-866-633-1617 |
| Massachusetts | L | Mass MedLine | Nonprofit prescription assistance program | 1-866-633-1617 |
| Michigan | L | MiRx Prescription Saving Program | Govt. prescription assistance program | 1-866-755-6479 |
| Minnesota | L | RxConnect/Senior Link Age Line | Govt. prescription assistance program | 1-800-333-2433 |

| State | Population Served: E=Elderly* D=Disabled L-Low income M=Medicare | Name of Program | Program Type | Contact Information |
|---|---|---|---|---|
| Mississippi | | No program | | |
| Missouri | M, Medicaid | Missouri Rx Plan | Govt. prescription assistance program | 1-800-375-1406 |
| Montana | M | Big Sky Rx Program | Govt. prescription assistance program only for Medicare Part D wraparound | 1-866-369-1233 |
| Nebraska | | No program | | |
| Nevada | E and M | Senior Rx | Govt. prescription assistance program; will wrap around Medicare Part D | 1-866-303-6323 or 687-4210 X244 |
| Nevada | D | Nevada Disability Rx | Govt. pharmacy assistance program; will wrap around Medicare Part D | 1-866-303-6323 |
| New Hampshire | L | NH Medication Bridge Program | Nonprofit prescription assistance program | 1-603-225-0900 |
| New Jersey | E, D, or M | Pharmaceutical Assistance for the Aged and Disable (PAAD) | Govt. prescription assistance program; will wrap around Medicare Part D | 1-800-792-9745 |
| New Jersey | E | Senior Gold Program | Govt. prescription assistance program; will wrap around Part D | 609-588-7048 800-792-9745 |
| New Mexico | L | Discount Prescription Drug Program | Govt. prescription assistance program | 1-800-233-2576 |
| New Mexico | L | New Mexico MedBANK | Nonprofit prescription assistance program | 1-866-451-2901 |
| New York | E, M (65+ only) | Elderly Pharmaceuticals Insurance Coverage (EPIC) Program | Govt. prescription assistance program; will wrap around Medicare part D; EPIC considered creditable coverage by Medicare | 1-800-332-3742 |
| North Carolina | M (65+) | NCRx | Govt. prescription assistance program; will wrap around Medicare Part D | 1-888-488-6279 |
| North Dakota | L | Prescription Connection for North Dakota | Govt. prescription assistance program | 1-888-575-6611 |
| Ohio | E, M, or L | Ohio's Best Rx | Govt. drug discount card program | 1-866-923-7879 |
| Oklahoma | L | Rx for Oklahoma | Govt. prescription assistance program | 1-877-RX4 OKLA |
| Oregon | All | Oregon Prescription Drug Program | Govt. drug discount card | 1-800-913-4146 |
| Pennsylvania | E, M | Pharmaceutical Assistance Contract for the Elderly (PACE) & PACE Needs Enhancement Tier (PACENET) | Govt. prescription assistance program; will wrap around Medicare Part D PACE/ PACENET considered cred-itable coverage by Medicare | 1-800-225-7223 |

*(table continues)*

*(table continued)*

| State | Population Served: E=Elderly* D=Disabled L-Low income M=Medicare | Name of Program | Program Type | Contact Information |
|-------|------------------|-----------------|--------------|-------------------|
| Rhode Island | E, D (55+), M | Rhode Island Pharmaceutical Assistance for the Elderly (RIPAE) | Govt. prescription assistance program, will wrap around Medicare Part D | Dept of Elderly Affairs 401-462-3000 |
| Rhode Island | L | Prescription Drug Discount Card | Govt. drug discount card | 1-800-752-8088 |
| South Carolina | M (65+ only) | Gap Assistance Prescription Program for Seniors (GAPS) | Govt. pharmacy assistance program only for Medicare Part D wraparound | 888-549-0820 |
| South Carolina | L | Welvista | Nonprofit prescription assistance program | 1-803-933-9183 |
| South Dakota | | No program | | |
| Tennessee | L | Cover Rx | Govt. prescription assistance program | 1-866-CoverTN |
| Texas | – | No program | | |
| Utah | – | No program | | |
| Vermont | M | VPharm | Govt. prescription assistance program; will wrap around Medicare Part D | 1-800-250-8427 |
| Vermont | E, D | VHAP-Pharmacy, Vscript | Govt. prescription assistance program; will wrap around Medicare Part D | 1-800-250-8427 |
| Vermont | L | Healthy Vermonters | Govt. prescription drug program | 1-800-250-8427 |
| Virginia | L | RxRelief Virginia | Nonprofit grantsmaking program | 1-804-828-5804 or 1-434-361-0331 |
| Washington | All | Washington Prescription Drug Program Govt. drug discount card | | 1-800-913-4311 |
| West Virginia | E, L | West Virginia Rx Program | Govt. prescription assistance program | 1-877-388-9879 |
| Wisconsin | E, M | Senior Care Rx | Govt. prescription assistance program; will wrap around medicare Part D | 1-800-657-2038 |
| Wisconsin | No Rx coverage | Badger Rx Gold | Govt. drug discount program | 1-866-809-9382 |
| Wyoming | L | Prescription Drug Assistance Program | Govt. prescription assistance program | 1-800-438-5785 |

*States define *elderly* differently, and this term could refer to anyone age 55 and older. Source: RxAssist Patient Assistance Program Center. "Statewide Drug Assistance Programs." October 21, 2009. Available online http://www.rxassist.org/patients/res-state-progrms.cfm. Accessed February 26, 2011. Permission from the RxAssist Patient Assistance Program was received to reprint this table. For more information, contact RxAssist at www.rxassist.org.

# GLOSSARY

This glossary provides commonly used terms related to kidney disease and is offered as a brief explanation of such terms. Many of these terms are used throughout the book and some are described in depth in their own entries, as with *dialysis* and *kidney transplantation.*

**albumin**   One of the proteins that can be found in the urine. When this protein is identified, the condition is known as albuminuria. When the relative levels of albumin in the urine are low (between 30 and 300 mg/gm creatinine but above normal), this is termed microalbuminuria. If the levels are higher, or greater than 300 mg/gm creatinine, the condition is called macroalbuminuria. This indicates the presence of serious kidney disease.

**aldosterone**   A hormone produced by the adrenal glands that increases kidneys' retention of sodium and secretion of potassium into the urine and causes blood pressure to be increased.

**alkalemia**   A condition in which the fluids in the body are excessively alkaline. Common causes are persistent vomiting, the use or abuse of diuretics, chronic liver disease, and either primary or secondary hyperaldosteronism.

**amyloidosis**   A rare disorder in which amyloid, a protein-like matter, masses in one or more major organs of the body, such as the kidneys, heart, brain, gastrointestinal tract, or the skin.

**anuria**   The failure to produce any urine. This can become a life-threatening condition.

**autoimmune disorder**   A disorder in which the body's immune system attacks itself; for example, as with lupus nephritis and many other disorders.

**blood urea nitrogen (BUN)**   A waste product produced from the body's normal handling of proteins that is filtered by the kidneys and, if elevated, can be an indicator of kidney disease. The blood urea nitrogen level's rising typically indicates decreasing kidney function. Some conditions can also increase the blood urea nitrogen, including hypotension, dehydration, and intestinal bleeding.

**chronic kidney disease (CKD)**   The presence of impaired kidney disease that lasts for three or more months and is associated with either a decreased glomerular filtration rate (GFR) *or* the leakage of blood proteins through the kidneys into the urine. CKD progresses from Stage 1, a very mild form of kidney disease, and Stage 2, also a mild stage, to the moderate and increasingly severe phases of Stages 3–5. At Stage 5, the patient is usually receiving dialysis or will need to receive dialysis soon or will imminently receive a kidney transplant.

**congenital nephrotic syndrome**   A kidney disease that is inherited and develops either before birth or within the first few months of the infant's life. The child with congenital nephrotic syndrome will usually develop kidney failure (see end-stage renal disease) by age two or three and will need either dialysis or a kidney transplantation.

**corticosteroids**   Medications that suppress the immune system and are often used to control inflammatory conditions, such as glomerulonephritis and allergic interstitial nephritis. Although very effective, corticosteroids have a number of long-term side effects, which increase in likelihood and severity with the amount of corticosteroids that are used. These side effects can include cataracts, mood changes, weight gain, and osteoporosis and other bone diseases.

**creatinine**  A compound produced naturally by skeletal muscle cells and excreted by the kidneys. If the kidneys are not working well, creatinine can build up in the blood. A test for creatinine clearance shows how well the kidneys removed creatinine from the blood. A low level of creatinine clearance indicates that kidney function is impaired. The estimated glomerular filtration rate (eGFR) calculation takes into account the serum creatinine along with age, race, and sex to provide a relatively accurate estimate of actual renal function.

**cystitis**  Infection in the bladder. If untreated, it can develop into a kidney infection (pyelonephritis).

**diabetes mellitus**  A condition in which the pancreas produces no insulin (Type 1 diabetes) or the body cannot use the insulin that is produced because of an insulin resistance (Type 2 diabetes). Diabetes is a leading cause of kidney disease.

**dialysis**  The cleansing of the bloodstream through artificial means after the kidneys have failed, including the use of either hemodialysis or peritoneal dialysis.

**donor kidney**  The kidney that is provided to be transplanted into a person whose kidneys have failed. Most donor kidneys come from deceased individuals, but can also come either from living related donors or from living and unrelated donors.

**edema**  Swelling in the body caused by excessive fluid retention by the kidneys.

**end-stage renal disease (ESRD3)**  Essentially, complete failure of the kidneys. The person with ESRD needs either dialysis or a kidney transplant.

**glomerulonephritis**  Inflammation of the glomeruli of the kidney. This may be caused by an autoimmune reaction or by the body's response to chronic infection.

**glomerulus**  A tiny set of looping blood vessels located in the kidney. The glomeruli (plural of glomerulus) filter the blood. There are approximately one million glomeruli in each kidney in the normal adult.

**hematuria**  Blood in the urine. This indicates a possible infection, kidney stone, the presence of glomerulonephritis, or other medical problem.

**human immunodeficiency virus associated nephropathy (HIVAN)**  Kidney disease that is caused by or associated with the human immunodeficiency virus (HIV).

**hyperkalemia**  Excessively high levels of potassium in the bloodstream.

**hypernatremia**  Excessively high levels of sodium in the bloodstream.

**hypokalemia**  Excessively low levels of potassium in the bloodstream.

**hyponatremia**  Excessively low levels of sodium in the bloodstream.

**immunosuppressive drugs**  Medications that suppress the immune system that are frequently given either to patients with glomerulonephritis, to suppress the abnormal immune system response causing the kidney disease, or to patients with a kidney transplant so that the transplanted kidney will not be rejected.

**kidney biopsy**  A procedure in which tissue from the kidneys is removed to determine the presence of many renal diseases. A kidney biopsy is usually *not* used to detect cancer, because of the risk of leakage of cancer cells from the biopsy site and of the development of metastatic kidney cancer that can sometimes occur.

**kidney transplantation**  The removal of a kidney from a deceased or live donor and its placement into a person whose kidneys have failed.

**nephrectomy**  The surgical removal of a kidney.

**nephrolithias**  The presence of kidney stones.

**nephrologist**  Physician who specializes in treating diseases and disorders of the kidneys.

**nephron**  A very small part of the kidney, which is comprised of an estimated 1 million nephron. Nephrons take the fluid that is built at the glomeruli, and then either reabsorb or secrete compounds into this fluid in order to maintain normal amounts of appropriate fluid and electrolytes in the body and blood.

**nephrotoxicity**  Harm caused to the kidneys. This term is usually used in reference to medications or other substances that can damage the kidneys.

**orthostatic proteinuria** A condition in which the individual has proteinuria only when standing and not while lying down. This condition has no associated long-term risk.

**oxalate** A substance that can combine with calcium in the urine to form kidney stones known as calcium oxalate stones. These are the most common form of kidney stones.

**pH** Refers to the alkalinity or acidity of body fluids, such as the blood and urine.

**polyuria** Excretion of abnormally large amounts of urine.

**proteinuria** The presence of abnormal amounts of protein in the urine, which is an indicator of kidney disease.

**pyelonephritis** Kidney infection.

**renal** Related to the kidneys.

**renal insufficiency** Another term for decreased kidney function. It may refer either to acute kidney injury or to chronic kidney disease.

**renin** A hormone that the kidneys make, which controls the fluid volume within the body as well as the blood pressure.

# BIBLIOGRAPHY

Abdel-Kader, Khaled, Marl L. Unruh, and Steven D. Weisbord. "Symptom Burden, Depression, and Quality of Life in Chronic and End-Stage Kidney Disease." *Clinical Journal of the American Society of Nephrology* 4 (2009): 1,057–1,064.

Adler, A. I., R. J. Stevens, S. E. Manley, et al. "Development and Progression of Nephropathy in Type 2 Diabetes: The United Kingdom Prospective Diabetes Study (UKPDS 64)." *Kidney International* 63 (2003): 225–232.

Adrogué, Horacio, M.D., and Nicolaos E. Madias, M.D. "Sodium and Potassium in the Pathogenesis of Hypertension." *New England Journal of Medicine* 356, no. 19 (May 10, 2007): 1,966–1,978.

Agency for Healthcare Research and Quality. *Comparing Two Kinds of Blood Pressure Pills: ACEIs and ARBs: A Guide for Adults.* October 2007. Available online. URL: http://www.effectivehealthcare.ahrq.gov/ehc/products/12/31/ACEI-ARBConsumer.pdf. Accessed February 15, 2010.

Agoda, L. Y., et al. "Effect of Ramipril vs. Amlodipine on Renal Outcomes in Hypertensive Nephrosclerosis: A Randomized Controlled Trial." *Journal of the American Medical Association* 285, no. 21 (2001): 2,719–2,728.

Akbari, Ayub, M.D., et al. "Detection of Chronic Kidney Disease with Laboratory Reporting of Estimated Glomerular Filtration Rate and an Educational Program." *Archives of Internal Medicine* 164 (2004): 1,788–1,792.

Alper, A. Brent, Jr., M.D., Rajesh G. Shenava, M.D., and Bessie A. Young, M.D. "Uremia." Available online to subscribers at eMedicine Nephrology. URL: http://emedicine.medscape.com/article/245926-overview. Accessed March 18, 2010.

Alpern, Robert J., and Steven C. Hebert. *Seldin and Giebisch's The Kidney: Physiology and Pathophysiology.* Vol. 1. Burlington, Mass.: Academic Press, 2008.

Alsaad, K. O., and A. M. Herzenberg. "Distinguishing Diabetic Nephropathy from Other Causes of Glomerulosclerosis: An Update." *Journal of Clinical Pathology* 2006. Available online. URL: http://jcp.bmj.com/content/60/1/18.full.pdf. Accessed April 8, 2010.

Appel, Lawrence J., M.D., et al. "Long-term Effects of Renin-Angiotensin System–Blocking Therapy and a Low Blood Pressure Goal on Progression of Hypertensive Chronic Kidney Disease in African Americans." *Archives of Internal Medicine* 168, no. 8 (April 28, 2008): 832–839.

Aradhye, Sheeram, et al. *Medicines for Keeping Your New Kidney Healthy.* Mount Laurel, N.J.: American Society of Transplantation, 2006.

Aronson, Jeff. "Dropsy." *British Medical Journal* 326, no. 7387 (2003): 491.

Bahal O'Mara, Neeta. "Anemia in Patients with Chronic Kidney Disease." *Diabetes Spectrum* 21, no. 1 (2008): 12–18.

Ballinger, Susan, M.D. "Henoch-Schönlein Purpura." *Current Opinion in Rheumatology* 15 (2003): 591–594.

Bang, Heejung, et al. "SCreening for Occult Renal Disease (SCORED): A Simple Prediction Model for Chronic Kidney Disease." *Archives of Internal Medicine* 167 (February 26, 2007): 374–381.

Bash, Lori D., et al. "Poor Glycemic Control in Diabetes and the Risk of Incident Chronic Kidney Disease Even in the Absence of Albuminuria and Retinopathy: Atherosclerosis Risk in Communities (ARIC) Study." *Archives of Internal Medicine* 168, no. 22 (December 8/22, 2008): 2,440–2,447.

Beaser, Richard S., M.D., and the Staff of Joslin Diabetes Center. *Joslin's Diabetes Deskbook: A Guide for Primary Care Providers.* 2nd ed. Boston, Mass.: Joslin Diabetes Center, 2007.

Bellando Randone, Silvia, Serena Guiducci, and Marco Matucci Cerinic. "Systemic Sclerosis and Infections." *Autoimmunity Reviews* 8, no. 1 (2008): 36–40.

Bergs, Laura. "Goodpasture Syndrome." *Critical Care Nurse* 25, no. 5 (October 2005): 5–58. Available online.

URL: http://ccn.aacnjournals.org/cgi/contend/full/ 25/5/50. Downloaded May 11, 2007.

Bichet, Daniel G. "Polyuria and Diabetes Insipidus." In *Seldin and Giebisch's The Kidney: Physiology and Pathophysiology.* Vol. 1, edited by Robert J. Alpern and Steven C. Hebert, 1,225–1,247. Burlington, Mass.: Academic Press, 2008.

Blix, Hege Salvesen, et al. "Use of Renal Risk Drugs in Hospitalized Patients with Impaired Renal Function—An Underestimated Problem?" *Nephrology Dialysis Transplantation* 21 (2006): 3,164–3,171.

Bloembergen, W. E., F. K. Port, E. A. Mauger, R. A. Wolfe. "A Comparison of Mortality between Patients Treated with Hemodialysis and Peritoneal Dialysis." *Journal of the American Society of Nephrology* 6 (1995): 177–183.

Bostwick, John Michael, M.D., and Lewis M. Cohen, M.D. "Differentiating Suicide from Life-Ending Acts and End-of-Life Decisions: A Model Based on Chronic Kidney Disease and Dialysis." *Psychosomatics* 50, no. 1 (2009): 1–7.

Brugts, Jasper L., et al. "Renal Function and Risk of Myocardial Infarction in an Elderly Population: The Rotterdam Study." *Archives of Internal Medicine* 165 (2005): 2,659–2,665.

Cameron, J. S. "Bright's Disease Today: The Pathogenesis and Treatment of Glomerulonephritis-I." *British Medical Journal* 4 (1972): 87–90.

Cassell, Dana K., and Cynthia A. Sanoski. *The Encyclopedia of Pharmaceutical Drugs.* 2nd ed. New York: Facts on File, 2011.

Centers for Disease Control and Prevention. *Cholesterol Fact Sheet.* Atlanta: Centers for Disease Control and Prevention, 2009.

Centers for Disease Control and Prevention, National Center for Chronic Disease Prevention and Health Promotion, Division for Heart Disease and Stroke Prevention. "Sodium: The Facts." November 2009.

Centers for Medicare & Medicaid Services. *Medicare Coverage of Kidney Dialysis and Kidney Transplant Services.* Baltimore, Md.: Centers for Medicare and Medicaid Services, 2007.

Centers for Medicare & Medicaid Services. *You Can Live: Your Guide for Living with Kidney Failure.* Baltimore, Md.: Centers for Medicare & Medicaid Services, 2007.

Cerdá, Jorge, et al. "The Contrasting Characteristics of Acute Kidney Injury in Developed and Developing Countries." *Nature Clinical Practice Nephrology* 4, no. 3 (2008): 138–153.

Chadha, Vimal, and Bradley A. Warady. "Epidemiology of Pediatric Chronic Kidney Disease." *Advances in Chronic Kidney Disease* 12, no. 4 (2005): 345–352.

Champagne, Catherine M. "Magnesium in Hypertension, Cardiovascular Disease, Metabolic Syndrome, and Other Conditions: A Review." *Nutrition in Clinical Practice* 23, no. 2 (2008): 142–151.

Che, Qi, Martin J. Schreiber, Jr., M.D., and Mohammed A. Rafey, M.D. "Beta-Blockers for Hypertension: Are They Going Out of Style?" *Cleveland Clinic Journal of Medicine* 76, no. 9 (2009): 533–542.

Chifflot, Hélène, et al. "Incidence and Prevalence of Systemic Sclerosis: A Systematic Literature Review." *Seminars in Arthritis and Rheumatism* 37 (2008): 223–235.

Chu, Hung-Yi, M.D., Ming-Tso Yan, M.D., and Shih-Hua Lin, M.D. "The Clinical Picture: Recurrent Pyelonephritis as a Sign of 'Sponge Kidney.'" *Cleveland Clinic Journal of Medicine* 76, no. 8 (2009): 479–480.

Cibulka, R., and J. Racek. "Metabolic Disorders in Patients with Chronic Kidney Failure." *Physiological Research* 56 (2007): 697–705.

Cochat, Pierre, et al. "Nephrolithiasis Related to Inborn Metabolic Diseases." *Pediatric Nephrology* 25 (2010): 415–424.

Consumers Union. *Treating High Blood Pressure and Heart Disease: The Beta-Blockers. Comparing Effectiveness, Safety, and Price.* June 2009. Available online. URL: http://www.consumerreports.org/health/resources/ pdf/best-buy-drugs/CU-Betablockers-FIN060109. pdf. Accessed February 15, 2010.

Coresh, Josef, M.D., et al. "Prevalence of Chronic Kidney Disease in the United States." *Journal of the American Medical Association* 298, no. 17 (2007): 2,038–2,047.

Corruble, E., et al. "Progressive Increase of Anxiety and Depression in Patients Waiting for a Kidney Transplantation." *Behavioral Medicine* 36, no. 1 (2010): 32–36.

Corsonello, A., et al. "Concealed Renal Insufficiency and Adverse Drug Reactions in Elderly Hospitalized Patients." *Archives of Internal Medicine* 165 (2005): 790–795.

Crumbley, Paul. "Emily Dickinson's Life." *Modern American Poetry.* Available online. URL: http:// www.english.uiuc.edu/maps/poets/a_f/dickinson/ bio.htm. Accessed January 13, 2009.

Cukor, Daniel, et al. "Depression and Anxiety in Urban Hemodialysis Patients." *Clinical Journal of the American Society of Nephrology* 2 (2007): 484–490.

Cukor, Daniel, et al. "Depression Is an Important Contributor to Low Medication Adherence in Hemodialized Patients and Transplant Recipients." *Kidney International* 75 (2009): 1,223–1,229.

Dale, Erin E., and Nicholas G. Popovich. "Sjögren's Syndrome." *U.S. Pharmacist* 32, no. 3 (2007): 72–81.

Daugirdas, John T., Peter G. Blake, and Todd S. Ing. *Handbook of Dialysis.* 4th ed. Philadelphia, Pa.: Lippincott Williams & Wilkins, 2007.

Davison, Sara N., M.D. "Chronic Kidney Disease: Psychosocial Impact of Chronic Pain." *Geriatrics* 62, no. 2 (February 2007): 17–23.

Dember, L. M., P. N. Hawkins, B. P. C. Hazenberg, et al. "Eprosidate for the Treatment of Renal Disease in AA Amyloidosis." *New England Journal of Medicine* 356 (2007): 2,349–2,360.

*Diabetes Mellitus: A Guide to Patient Care.* Ambler, Pa.: Lippincott Williams & Wilkins, 2007.

Diefenhaeler, Edgar C., et al. "Is Depression a Risk Factor for Mortality in Chronic Hemodialysis Patients?" *Revista Brasileira de Psiquiatria* 30, no. 2 (2008): 99–103.

Dimkovic, Nada, and Dimitrios G. Oreopoulos. "Substitutive Treatments of End-Stage Renal Diseases in the Elderly: Dialysis." In *The Aging Kidney in Health and Disease,* edited by Juan-Florencio Macías Núñez, M.D., J. Stewart Cameron, M.D., and Dimitrios G. Oreopoulos, M.D., 443–463. New York: Springer Science+Business Media, 2008.

Diniz, D. H. M. P., S. L. Blay, and N. Schor. "Anxiety and Depression Symptoms in Recurrent Painful Renal Lithiasis Colic." *Brazilian Journal of Medical and Biological Research* 40 (2007): 949–955.

Dionne, Janis M., Margaret M. Turik, and Robert M. Hurley. "Blood Pressure Abnormalities in Children with Chronic Kidney Disease." *Blood Pressure Monitoring* 13 (2008): 205–209.

Divers, J., and B. I. Freedman. "Susceptibility Genes in Common Complex Kidney Disease." *Current Opinion Nephrology Hypertension* 19, no. 1 (2010): 79–84.

Durie, Brian G. M., M.D. *Multiple Myeloma: Cancer of the Bone Marrow. Patient Handbook.* North Hollywood, Calif.: International Myeloma Foundation, 2009.

Edwards, N. Lawrence, M.D. "The Role of Hyperuricemia and Gout in Kidney and Cardiovascular Disease." *Cleveland Clinic Journal of Medicine* 75, Supp. 5 (2008): S13–S16.

Einhorn, Lisa M., et al. "The Frequency of Hyperkalemia and Its Significance in Chronic Kidney Disease." *Archives of Internal Medicine* 169, no. 12 (2009): 1,156–1,162.

Elsayed, Essam F., M.D., et al. "Cardiovascular Disease and Subsequent Kidney Disease." *Archives of Internal Medicine* 167 (2007): 1,130–1,136.

Ernst, Michael E., and Marvin Moser, M.D. "Use of Diuretics in Patients with Hypertension." *New England Journal of Medicine* 361 (2009): 2,153–2,164.

Fadrowski, Jeffrey J., M.D., et al. "Blood Lead Level and Kidney Function in US Adolescents: The Third National Health and Nutrition Examination Study." *Archives of Internal Medicine* 170, no. 1 (2010): 75–82.

Feder, Barnaby J. "A Nazi Past Casts a Pall on Name of a Disease." *New York Times.* January 22, 2008. Available online. URL: http://www.nytimes.com/2008/01/22/health/22dise.html?_r=3&oref=slogin&pagewanted=print. Accessed February 21, 2010.

Feig, Daniel I., M.D., Duk-Hee Kang, M.D., and Richard J. Johnson, M.D. "Uric Acid and Cardiovascular Disease." *New England Journal of Medicine* 359 (2008): 1,811–1,821.

Ferri, C. V., and R. A. Pruchno. "Quality of Life in End-Stage Renal Disease Patients: Differences in Patient and Spouse Perceptions." *Aging Mental Health* 13, no. 5 (2009): 708–714.

Fine, Adrian, et al. "Patients with Chronic Kidney Disease Stages 3 and 4 Demand Survival Information on Dialysis." *Peritoneal Dialysis International* 27, no. 5 (2007): 589–591.

Fine, Derek M., M.D. "Pharmacological Therapy of Lupus Nephritis." *Journal of the American Medical Association* 293, no. 24 (2005): 3,053–3,060.

Flynn, Joseph T., et al. "Blood Pressure in Children with Chronic Kidney Disease: A Report from the Chronic Kidney Disease in Children Study." *Hypertension* 52 (2008): 631–637.

Food and Drug Administration. "High Blood Pressure—Medicines to Help You." February 2009. Available online. URL: http://www.fda.gov/ForConsumers/ByAudience/ForWomen/ucm118594.htm. Accessed Febuary 9, 2010.

Food and Drug Administration Office of Women's Health. *Medicines to Help You: Cholesterol.* August 2009.

Food and Drug Administration Office of Women's Health. Medicines to Help You: High Blood Pressure. 2007. Available online. URL: http://www.fda.gov/womens/medicinecharts/highbloodpressure.html. Downloaded May 20, 2007.

Food and Drug Administration. Public Health Advisory: Non-Steroidal Anti-Inflammatory Drug Products (NSAIDS). Available online. URL: http://www.fda.gov/cder/drug/advisory/nsaids.htm. Accessed May 24, 2009.

Fraser, Sheila M., et al. "Acceptable Outcome After Kidney Transplantation Using 'Expanded Criteria Donor' Grafts." *Transplantation* 89, no. 1 (2010): 88–96.

Frassetto, Lynda A., M.D. "Bartter Syndrome." eMedicine, May 16, 2008. Available online. URL: http://www.emedicine.com/MED/topic213.htm. Downloaded May 24, 2008.

Fulop, Milford, M.D., and Meggan Mackay, M.D. "Renal Tubular Acidosis, Sjögren Syndrome, and Bone Disease." *Archives of Internal Medicine* 164 (2004): 905–909.

Gabrielli, Armando, M.D., Enrico V. Avvedimento, M.D., and Thomas Krieg, M.D. "Scleroderma." *New England Journal of Medicine* 360, no. 19 (May 7, 2009): 1,989–2,003.

Garg, Amit X., M.D., et al. "Long-term Renal Prognosis of Diarrhea-Associated Hemolytic Uremic Syndrome: A Systematic Review, Meta-analysis, and Meta-regression." *Journal of the American Medical Association* 290, no. 10 (September 10, 2003): 1,360–1,370.

Gassman, Jennifer, et al. "Design and Statistical Aspects of the African American Study of Kidney Disease and Hypertension (AASK)." *Journal of the American Society of Nephrology* 14 (2003): S154-S165.

Geiss, L. S. "Diabetes Risk Reduction Behaviors among US Adults with Prediabetes." *American Journal of Preventive Medicine* 38, no. 4 (2010): 403–409.

Gill, Jagbir, et al. "Outcomes of Kidney Transplantation from Older Living Donors to Older Recipients." *American Journal of Kidney Disease* 52, no. 3 (2008): 541–552.

Greenbaum, Larry A., M.D., Bradley A. Warady, M.D., and Susan L. Furth, M.D. "Current Advances in Chronic Kidney Disease in Children: Growth, Cardiovascular, and Neurocognitive Risk Factors." *Seminars in Nephrology* 29, no. 4 (2009): 425–434.

Greenberg, Arthur, M.D., ed. *Primer on Kidney Diseases.* 4th ed. Philadelphia: National Kidney Foundation, 2005.

Griebling, Tomas L., M.D. "Urinary Tract Infection in Men." In *Urologic Diseases in America,* edited by Litwin M. S. and C. S. Saigal, 587–620. Bethesda, Md.: National Institute of Diabetes and Digestive and Kidney Diseases, 2007.

———. "Urinary Tract Infection in Women." In *Urologic Diseases in America,* edited by M. S. Litwin and C. S. Saigal, 587–620. Bethesda, Md.: National Institute of Diabetes and Digestive and Kidney Diseases, 2007.

Gwinnell, Esther, M.D., and Christine Adamec. *The Encyclopedia of Drug Abuse.* New York: Facts On File, 2008.

Hallan, Stein, M.D., et al. "Association of Kidney Function and Albuminuria with Cardiovascular Mortality in Older vs Younger Individuals: The HUNT II Study." *Archives of Internal Medicine* 22 (2007): 2,490–2,496.

Haroun, Melanie, et al. "Risk Factors for Chronic Kidney Disease: A Prospective Study of 23,534 Men and Women in Washington County, Maryland." *Journal of the American Society of Nephrology* 14 (2003): 2,934–2,941.

Harris, Peter C., and Vicente E. Torres. "Polycystic Kidney Disease." *Annual Review of Medicine* 60 (2009): 321–337.

Harwood, Lori. "Stressors and Coping in Individuals with Chronic Kidney Disease." *Nephrology Nursing Journal* 36, no. 3 (2009): 265–277.

Hedayati, S. Susan, M.D. "Prevalence of Major Depressive Episode in CKD." *American Journal of Kidney Diseases* 54, no. 3 (2009): 424–432.

Hellmark, Thomas, Harald Burkhardt, and Jorgen Wieslander. "Goodpasture Disease." *The Journal of Biological Chemistry* 274, no. 36 (September 3, 1999): 25,862–25,868.

Helmick, Charles G., et al. "Estimates of the Prevalence of Arthritis and Other Rheumatic Conditions in the United States. Part I." *Arthritis & Rheumatism* 58, no. 1 (January 2008): 15–25.

Hemmelgarn, Brenda R., et al. "Relation Between Kidney Function, Proteinuria, and Adverse Outcomes." *Journal of the American Medical Association* 303, no. 5 (2010): 423–429.

Heran, Bairaj S., Brandon P. Galm, and James M. Wright. "Blood Pressure Lowering Efficacy of Alpha Blockers for Primary Hypertension." *Cochrane Database of Systematic Reviews* 4 (2009). Available online. URL: http://mrw.interscience.wiley.com/cochrane/clsystev/articles/CD00464. Accessed February 13, 2010.

Heron, Melonie, et al. "Deaths: Final Data for 2006." *National Vital Statistics Report* 57, no. 14 (April 17, 2009): 43.

Hinchcliff, Monique, M.D., and John Varga, M.D. "Systemic Sclerosis/Scleroderma: A Treatable Multisystem Disease." *American Family Physician* 78, no. 8 (2008): 961–968.

Hochman, M. E., et al. "The Prevalence and Incidence of End-Stage Renal Disease in Native American Adults on the Navajo Reservation." *Kidney International* 71 (2007): 931–937.

Hoth, Karin F., et al. "A Longitudinal Examination of Social Support, Agreeableness and Depressive Symptoms in Chronic Kidney Disease." *Journal of Behavioral Medicine* 30, no. 1 (2007): 69–76.

Houssiau, Frédéric A. "Management of Lupus Nephritis: An Update." *Journal of the American Society of Nephrology* 15 (2004): 2,694–2,704.

How, Priscilla P., Darius L. Mason, and Alan H. Lau. "Current Approaches in the Treatment of Chronic Kidney Disease Mineral and Bone Disorder." *Journal of Pharmacy Practice* 21, no. 3 (2008): 196–213.

Hruska, Keith A., M.D., et al. "Hyperphosphatemia of Chronic Kidney Disease." *Kidney International* 74, no. 2 (2008): 148–157.

Hsu, Chi-yuan, M.D., et al. "Body Mass Index and Risk for End-Stage Renal Disease." *Annals of Internal Medicine* 144 (2006): 21–28.

Hsu, Chi-yuan, M.D., et al. "Risk Factors for End-Stage Renal Disease." *Archives of Internal Medicine* 169, no. 4 (2009): 342–350.

Hudson, Billy G., et al. "Alport's Syndrome, Goodpasture's Syndrome, and Type IV Collagen." *New England Journal of Medicine* 348, no. 25 (June 19, 2003): 2,543–2,556.

Ibrahim, Hassan N., M.D., et al. "Long-Term Consequences of Kidney Donation." *New England Journal of Medicine* 360, no. 5 (2009): 459–469.

Isbel, Nicole M. "Glomerulonephritis: Management in General Practice." *Australian Family Physician* 34, no. 11 (2005): 907–913.

John, R., and A. M. Herzenberg. "Renal Toxicity of Therapeutic Drugs." *Journal of Clinical Pathology* 62 (2009): 505–515.

Johnson, Susan L., M.D., et al. "Who Is Tested for Diabetic Kidney Disease and Who Initiates Treatment." *Diabetes Care* 29, no. 8 (August 2006): 1,733–1,738.

Johnston, Valerie L., M.D. "Growth Failure in Children with Chronic Kidney Disease." *aakpRENAL LIFE* 26, no. 5 (2010). Available online. URL: https://www.aakp.org/aakp-library/Growth-Failure-Children/. Accessed November 4, 2010.

Kandel, Joseph, M.D., and Christine Adamec. *The Encyclopedia of Elder Care.* New York: Facts On File, 2008.

Kassan, Stuart S., M.D., and Haralampois M. Moutsopoulos, M.D. "Clinical Manifestations and Early Diagnosis of Sjögren Syndrome." *Archives of Internal Medicine* 164 (2004): 1,275–1,284.

Keith, Douglas S., M.D., et al. "Longitudinal Follow-up and Outcomes among a Population with Chronic Kidney Disease in a Large Managed Care Organization." *Archives of Internal Medicine* 164 (March 22, 2004): 659–663.

Khan, Samina, M.D. "Vitamin D Deficiency and Secondary Hyperparathyroidism among Patients with Chronic Kidney Disease." *American Journal of the Medical Sciences* 333, no. 4 (2007): 201–207.

Kidney Disease Improving Global Outcomes (KDIGO). *Best Practices in CKD-MBD: A Focus on Phosphorus.* 2009. Available online. URL: http://www.kidney.org/professionals/tools/pdf/BestPracticesInCKD_MBD.pdf. Accessed February 13, 2010.

Kimmel, Paul L., and Rolf A. Peterson. "Depression in Patients with End-Stage Renal Disease Treated with Dialysis: Has the Time to Treat Arrived?" *Clinical Journal of the American Society of Nephrology* 1 (2006): 349–352.

Kimmel, Paul L., Karen Weihs, and Rolf A. Peterson. "Survival in Hemodialysis Patients: The Role of Depression." *Journal of the American Society of Nephrology* 4, no. 1 (1993): 12–27.

Kiryluk, Krzysztok, Jerimiah Martino, and Ali G. Gharavi. "Genetic Susceptibility, HIV Infection, and the Kidney." *Clinical Journal of the American Society of Nephrology* 2 (2007): S25–S35.

Klinger, Alan, M.D., American Association of Kidney Patients. "What Are the Symptoms of Uremic Poisoning?" Tampa, Fla. 2004. Available online. URL: http://www.aakp.org/aakp-library/symptoms-of-uremic poisoning. Accessed March 18, 2010.

Konety, Adrinath R., M.D., Geoffrey F. Joyce, and Matthew Wise. "Bladder and Upper Tract Urothelial Cancer." In *Urologic Diseases in America,* edited by Litwin, M. S. and C. S. Saigal, 223–280. Bethesda, Md.: National Institute of Diabetes and Digestive and Kidney Diseases, 2007.

Kovesdy, Scaba P., M.D., et al. "Association of Activated Vitamin D Treatment and Mortality in

Chronic Kidney Disease." *Archives of Internal Medicine* 168, no. 4 (February 25, 2008): 397–403.

Kramer, J. H., et al. "The Association between Gout and Nepholithiasis in Men: The Health Professionals' Follow-up Study." *Kidney International* 64 (2003): 1,022–1,026.

Kurella, Manjula, M.D., et al. "Octogenarians and Nonagenarians Starting Dialysis in the United States." *Annals of Internal Medicine* 146 (2007): 177–183.

Kurella, Manjula, et al. "Suicide in the United States End-Stage Renal Disease Program." *Journal of the American Society of Nephrology* 16 (2005): 774–781.

Kutner, Nancy G., et al. "Association of Sleep Difficulty with Kidney Disease Quality of Life Cognitive Function Score Reported by Patients Who Recently Started Dialysis." *Clinical Journal of the American Society of Nephrology* 2 (2007): 284–289.

Kutzing, Melinda K., and Bonnie L. Firestein. "Altered Uric Acid Levels and Disease States." *Journal of Pharmacology and Experimental Therapies* 324, no. 1 (2008): 1–7.

Lanzkron, Sophie, M.D., et al. "Systematic Review: Hydroxyurea for the Treatment of Adults with Sickle Cell Disease." *Annals of Internal Medicine* 148 (2008): 939–955.

Lapp, Julia L. "Vitamin D: Bone Health and Beyond." *American Journal of Lifestyle Medicine* 3 (2009): 386–393.

LaVeist, Thomas A., et al. "Environmental and Socio-Economic Factors as Contributors to Racial Disparities in Diabetes Prevalence." *Journal of General Internal Medicine* 24, no. 10 (2009): 1,144–1,148.

Lea, Janice, M.D., et al. "The Relationship between Magnitude of Proteinuria Reduction and Risk of End-stage Renal Disease: Results of the African American Study of Kidney Disease and Hypertension." *Archives of Internal Medicine* 165 (April 25, 2005): 947–953.

Lee, Dong-Gi, et al. "Acute Pyelonephritis: Clinical Characteristics and the Role of Surgical Treatment." *Journal of Korean Medical Science* 24 (2009): 296–301.

Lemann, J. Jr. "Composition of the Diet and Calcium Kidney Stones." *New England Journal of Medicine* 328 (1993): 880–882.

Levin, Adeera, M.D., et al. "Guidelines for the Management of Chronic Kidney Disease." *Canadian Medical Association Journal* 179, no. 11 (November 18, 2008): 1,154–1,162.

Life Options Rehabilitation Program. Employment: A Kidney Patient's Guide to Working & Paying for Treatment. 2003: 43. Available online. URL: http://www.lifeoptions.org/catalog/pdfs/booklets/employment.pdf.

Litwin, M. S., and C. S. Saigal, eds. *Urologic Diseases in America.* Bethesda, Md.: National Institute of Diabetes and Digestive and Kidney Diseases, 2007.

Llach, Francisco, and Elvira Fernández. "Overview of Renal Bone Disease: Causes of Treatment Failure, Clinical Observations, the Changing Pattern of Bone Lesions, and Future Therapeutic Approach." *Kidney International* 64, Supp. 87 (2003): S113–S119.

Lund, Richard J., et al. "New Discoveries in the Pathogenesis of Renal Osteodystrophy." *Journal of Bone Mineral Metabolism* 24 (2006): 169–171.

Macanovic, Momir, and Peter Mathieson. *Manual of Nephrology: Drug Therapy and Therapeutic Protocols in Renal Diseases.* Boca Raton, Fla.: Universal Publishers, 2005.

Macías Núñez, Juan-Florencia, et al. "Biology of the Aging Process and Its Clinical Consequences." In *The Aging Kidney in Health and Disease,* edited by Juan-Florencio Macías Núñez, M.D., J. Stewart Cameron, M.D., and Dimitrios G. Oreopoulos, M.D., 55–91. New York: Springer Science+Business Media, 2008.

Macías Núñez, Juan F., M.D., J. Stewart Cameron, M.D., and Dimitrios G. Oreopoulos, M.D., eds. *The Aging Kidney in Health and Disease.* New York: Springer Science+Business Media, 2008.

Maeda, Shiro. "Review: Genetics of Diabetic Nephropathy." *Therapeutic Advances in Cardiovascular Disease* 2 (2008): 363–371.

Mansur, Abeera, M.D., Florin Georgescu, M.D., and Susie Lew, M.D. "Minimal-Change Disease." eMedicine Nephrology. June 11, 2007. Available online. URL: http://emedicine.medscape.com/article/243348-overview. Accessed September 14, 2009.

Markowitz, Glen S., et al. "Lithium Nephrotoxicity: A Progressive Combined Glomerula and Tubulointerstitial Nephropathy." *Journal of the American Society of Nephrology* 11 (2000): 1,439–1,448.

Marshall, S. M. "Review. Recent Advances in Diabetic Nephropathy." *Postgraduate Medical Journal* 80 (2004): 624–633.

Martin, Kevin J., and Esther A. Gonzalez. "Metabolic Bone Disease in Chronic Kidney Disease." *Jour-*

nal of the American Society of Nephrology 18 (2007): 875–885.

Marx, Stephen J., M.D. "Hyperparathyroid and Hypoparathyroid Disorders." New England Journal of Medicine 343, no. 25 (2000): 1,863–1,875.

Mazer, M., and J. Perrone. "Acetaminophen-Induced Nephrotoxicity: Pathophysiology, Clinical Manifestations, and Management." Journal of Medical Toxicity 4, no. 1 (2008): 2–6.

McClellan, William M., M.D., Anton C. Schoolwerth, M.D., and Todd Gehr, M.D. Clinical Management of Chronic Kidney Disease. West Islip, N.Y.: Professional Communications, 2006.

McCullough, K. P., et al. "Kidney and Pancreas Transplantation in the United States, 1998–2007: Access for Patients with Diabetes and End-Stage Renal Disease." American Journal of Transplantation 9, Part 2 (2009): 894–906.

McGregor, Jessica C., George P. Allen, and David T. Bearden. "Levofloxacin in the Treatment of Complicated Urinary Tract Infections and Acute Pyelonephritis." Therapeutics and Clinical Risk Management 4, no. 5 (2008): 843–853.

McNaughton-Collins, Mary, M.D., Geoffrey F. Joyce, Matthew Wise, and Michael A. Pontari, M.D. "Prostatitis." In Urologic Diseases in America, edited by M. S. Litwin and C. S. Saigal, 9–42. Bethesda, Md.: National Institute of Diabetes and Digestive and Kidney Diseases, 2007.

Minocha, Anil, M.D., and Christine Adamec. The Encyclopedia of Digestion and Digestive Disorders. 2nd ed. New York: Facts On File, 2010.

Moe, Sharon M., and Tilman Drueke. "Improving Global Outcomes in Mineral and Bone Disorders." Clinical Journal of the American Society of Nephrology 3 (2008): S127–S130.

Mogensen, C. E. "Microalbuminuria in Prediction and Prevention of Diabetic Nephropathy in Insulin-Dependent Diabetes Mellitus Patients." Journal of Diabetes Complications 9 (1995): 337–349.

Montalescot, G., and J. P. Collet. "Preserving Cardiac Function in the Hypertensive Patient: Why Renal Parameters Hold the Key." European Heart Journal 26 (2005): 2,616–2,622.

Morelon, Emmanuel, et al. "Partners' Concerns, Needs and Expectations in ESRD: Results of the CODIT Study." Nephrology Dialysis Transplantation 20 (2005): 1,670–1,675.

Mujais, Salim K., and Adrian I. Katz. "Potassium Deficiency." In Seldin and Giebisch's The Kidney: Physiol-

ogy and Pathophysiology. Vol. 1, edited by Robert J. Alpern and Steven C. Hebert, 1,349–1,385. Burlington, Mass.: Academic Press, 2008.

National Cancer Institute. What You Need to Know about Multiple Myeloma. National Institutes of Health. September 2008.

National Center for Health Statistics. Health, United States, 2007 with Chartbook on Trends in the Health of Americans. Hyattsville, Md., 2007.

National Institute of Arthritis and Musculoskeletal and Skin Diseases (NIAMS). Questions and Answers about Sjögren's Syndrome. Bethesda, Md.: National Institutes of Health, December 2006.

National Institute of Dental and Craniofacial Research. Dental Management of the Organ Transplant Patient. National Institutes of Health. October 2009. Available online. URL: http://www.nidcr.nih.gov/NR/rdonlyres/078CDF81-2632-463E-A6AE-2B773BF3EAEF/0/OrganTransplantProf.pdf. Accessed November 4, 2010.

National Institute of Diabetes and Digestive and Kidney Diseases. Kidney Failure: Choosing a Treatment That's Right for You. Bethesda, Md.: NIDDK, 2007.

National Kidney and Urologic Diseases Information Clearinghouse. "Growth Failure in Children with Kidney Disease." Washington, D.C.: National Institute of Diabetes and Digestive and Kidney Diseases, 2009.

National Kidney and Urologic Diseases Information Clearinghouse. Prostate Enlargement: Benign Prostatic Hyperplasia. Bethesda, Md.: National Institutes of Health, June 2006. Available online. URL: http://kidney.niddk.nih.gov/kudiseases/pubs/prosteenlargement/. Downloaded May 8, 2008.

National Kidney and Urologic Diseases Information Clearinghouse. Prostatitis: Disorders of the Prostate. National Institutes of Health, January 2008. Available online. URL: http://kidney.niddk.nih.gov/kudiseases/pubs/prostateenlargement. Downloaded May 8, 2008.

National Kidney and Urologic Diseases Information Clearinghouse. Treatment Methods for Kidney Transplantation. Bethesda, Md.: National Institutes for Health, 2006.

National Kidney Foundation. "25 Facts About Organ Donation and Transplantation." Available online. URL: http://www.kidney.or/news/newsroom/fs_new/25fatsorgdon&trans.cfm. 2010. Accessed March 22, 2010.

Naughton, Cynthia A. "Drug-Induced Nephrotoxicity." *American Family Physician* 78, no. 6 (2008): 743–750.

New, J. P., et al. "Assessing the Prevalence, Monitoring and Management of Chronic Kidney Disease in Patients with Diabetes Compared with Those Without Diabetes in General Practice." *Diabetic Medicine* 24 (2007): 364–369.

Niaudet, Patrick. "Denys-Drash Syndrome." *Orphanet*. March 2004. Available online. URL: www.orpha.net/data/patho/GB/uk-Drash.pdf. Accessed February 15, 2010.

Odden, Michelle C., Mary A. Whooley, and Michael G. Shlipak. "Depression, Stress, and Quality of Life in Persons with Chronic Kidney Disease: The Heart and Soul Study." *Nephron Clinical Practice* 103 (2006): c–c7.

Office of Dietary Supplements. Dietary Supplement Fact Sheet: Calcium. National Institutes of Health. Updated October 7, 2009. Available online. URL: http://ods.nih.gov/factsheets/Calcium_pf.asp. Accessed December 29, 2009.

Office of Dietary Supplements. "Dietary Supplement Fact Sheet: Magnesium." National Institutes of Health. Available online. URL: http://ods.od.nih/gov/factsheets/Magnesium_pf.asp. Accessed December 30, 2009.

Ojo, A. O. "Expanded Criteria Donors: Process and Outcomes." *Seminars in Dialysis* 18, no. 6 (2005): 463–468.

Ojo, A. O., T. C. Govaerts, R. L. Schmouder, and A. B. Leichtman. "Renal Transplantation in End-Stage Sickle Cell Nephropathy." *Transplantation* 67 (1999): 291–295.

Online Mendelian Inheritance in Man (OMIM). "Denys-Drash Syndrome." Available online. URL: http://www.ncbi.nlm.nih.gov/entrez/dispomim.cgi?id=194080. Accessed February 15, 2010.

Palevesky, Paul. "Hypernatremia." In *Primer on Kidney Diseases, 4th ed.*, edited by Arthur Greenberg, M.D., 66–73. Philadelphia, Pa.: Saunders, 2005.

Parikh, Nisha I., M.D., et al. "Cardiovascular Disease Risk Factors in Chronic Kidney Disease: Overall Burden and Rates of Treatment and Control." *Archives of Internal Medicine* 166 (2006): 1,884–1,891.

Patzer, Ludwig. "Nephrotoxicity as a Cause of Acute Kidney Injury in Children." *Pediatric Nephrology* 23 (2008): 2,159–2,173.

Pearle, Margaret S., M.D., Elizabeth A. Calhoun, and Gary C. Curhan, M.D. "Urolithiasis." In *Urologic Diseases in America*, edited by M. S. Litwin, and C. S. Saigal, 281–320. Bethesda, Md.: National Institute of Diabetes and Digestive and Kidney Diseases, 2007.

Peitzman, Steven J. *Dropsy, Dialysis, Transplant: A Short History of Failing Kidneys.* Baltimore, Md.: Johns Hopkins University Press, 2007.

Penn, H., et al. "Scleroderma Renal Crisis: Patient Characteristics and Long-Term Outcomes." *QJM: An International Journal of Medicine* 100, no. 8 (August 2007): 485–494. Available online. URL: http://qjmed.oxfordjournals.org/content/100/8/485.full. Accessed December 9, 2010.

Penson, David F., M.D., and Jane M. Chan. "Prostate Cancer." In *Urologic Diseases in America*, edited by M. S. Litwin and C. S. Saigal, 71–122. Bethesda, Md.: National Institute of Diabetes and Digestive and Kidney Diseases, 2007.

Perazella, Mark A., and Glen S. Markowitz. "Bisphosphonate Nephrotoxity." *Kidney International* 74 (2008): 1,385–1,393.

Perez, Gutthann S., L. A. Garcia Rodriguez, D. S. Raiford, Oliart A. Duque, and Romeu J. Ris. "Nonsteroidal Anti-inflammatory Drugs and the Risk of Hospitalization for Acute Renal Failure." *Archives of Internal Medicine* 156 (1996): 2,433–2,439.

Petit, William A., Jr., M.D., and Christine Adamec. *The Encyclopedia of Diabetes.* New York: Facts On File, 2002.

———. *The Encyclopedia of Endocrine Diseases and Disorders.* New York: Facts On File, 2005.

Phillips Andreoli, Sharon. "Acute Kidney Injury in Children." *Pediatric Nephrology* 24 (2009): 253–263.

Plantinga, Laura C., et al. "Patient Awareness of Chronic Kidney Disease: Trends and Predictors." *Archives of Internal Medicine* 168, no. 20 (2008): 2,268–2,275.

Plantinga, Laura C., et al. "Prevalence of Chronic Kidney Disease in US Adults with Undiagnosed Diabetes or Prediabetes." *Clinical Journal of the American Society of Nephrology* 5 (2010): 673–682.

Platt, Orah S., M.D. "Hydroxyurea for the Treatment of Sickle Cell Anemia." *New England Journal of Medicine* 358, no. 13 (2008): 1,362–1,369.

Pleis, J. R. and M. Lethbridge-Çejku. "Frequencies of Selected Diseases and Conditions among Persons 18 Years of Age and Over, by Selected Characteristics, United States, 2006." *Summary Health Statistics for U.S. Adults: National Health Interview Survey, 2006.* December 2007.

Radbill, B., B. Murphy, and D. LeRoith. "Rationale and Strategies for Early Detection and Management of Diabetic Kidney Disease." *Mayo Clinic Proceedings* 83, no. 12 (2008): 1,373–1,381.

Rajagopalan, P. R., M.D., Mark Baillie, Osemwegie E. Emovon, M.D., and Kenneth D. Chavin, M.D. "Results of the African-American Study of Kidney Disease and Hypertension (AASK) Trial." Continuing Medical Education (CME). 2002. Available online to subscribers. URL: http://www.medscape.com/viewarticle/445259. Accessed December 29, 2008.

Rand Corporation. *Hold the Salt: Lowering Sodium Intake Would Improve Health and Save Money.* Santa Monica, Calif.: Rand Corporation. Available online. URL: http://www.rc.rand.org/pubs/research_briefs/2009/RAND_RB9479.pdf. Accessed March 17, 2010.

Rangel, Erika B., et al. "Kidney Transplant in Diabetic Patients: Modalities, Indications and Results." *Diabetology & Metabolic Syndrome* 1, no. 2 (2009). Available online. URL: http://www.dmsjournal.com/content/1/1/2. Accessed February 5, 2010.

Ray, Patricio E. "Taking a Hard Look at the Pathogenesis of Childhood HIV-Associated Nephropathy." *Pediatric Nephrology* 24, no. 11 (2009): 2,109–2,119.

Reamy, Brian V., Pamela M. Williams, and Tammy J. Lindsay. "Henoch-Schönlein Purpura." *American Family Physician* 80, no. 7 (2009): 697–704.

Reilly, Robert F., Jr., and Mark A. Perazella. *Nephrology in 30 Days.* New York: McGraw-Hill, 2005.

Rifken, Dena E., M.D., et al. "Rapid Kidney Function Decline and Mortality Risk in Older Adults." *Archives of Internal Medicine* 168, no. 20 (November 10, 2008): 2,212–2,218.

Rios Burrows, Nilka, Yanfeng Li, and Desmond E. Williams. "Racial and Ethnic Differences in Trends of End-Stage Renal Disease: United States, 1995–2005." *Advances in Chronic Kidney Disease* 15, no. 2 (2008): 147–152.

Rivard, Christopher J., and Laurence Chan. "Hypernatremic States." In *Seldin and Giebisch's The Kidney: Physiology and Pathophysiology.* Vol. 1. edited by Robert J. Alpern and Steven C. Hebert, 1,203–1,224. Burlington, Mass.: Academic Press, 2008.

Robinson, B., et al. "Prevalence of Anemia in the Nursing Home: Contribution of Chronic Kidney Disease." *Journal of the American Geriatric Society* 55, no. 10 (2007): 1,566–1,570.

Rodman, John S., M.D., et al. *No More Kidney Stones: The Experts Tell You All You Need to Know about Prevention and Treatment.* New York: John Wiley & Sons, 2007.

Rodriguez-Iturbe, Bernardo, and James M. Musser. "The Current State of Poststreptococcal Glomerulonephritis." *Journal of the American Society of Nephrology* 19 (2008): 1,855–1,864.

The Royal College of General Practitioners Effective Clinical Practice Unit. Guideline entitled 'Diabetic renal disease: prevention and early management.' 2002. Available online. URL: http://www.nice.org.uk/page.aspx?o=39385. Accessed on October 1, 2008.

Ruggenenti, P., A. Fassi, A. P. Ilieva, et al. "Preventing Microalbuminuria in Type 2 Diabetes." *New England Journal of Medicine* 351 (2004): 1,941–1,951.

Saliba, Wissam, M.D., and Boutros El-Haddad, M.D. "Secondary Hyperparathyroidism: Pathophysiology and Treatment." *Journal of the American Board of Family Medicine* 22 (2009): 574–581.

Salifu, Moro, M.D., Sidhartha Pani, M.D., and Nilanjana Misra, M.D. "HIV Nephropathy." eMedicine. Available online. URL: www.http://emedicine.medscape.com/article/246031-print. Last updated February 4, 2009. Accessed December 22, 2009.

Saydah, S., et al. "Prevalence of Chronic Kidney Disease and Associated Risk Factors—United States, 1999–2004." *Morbidity & Mortality Weekly Report* 56 (2007): 161–165.

Schmucher, H. Ralph, Jr., M.D., and Lan X. Chen, M.D. "The Practical Management of Gout." *Cleveland Journal of Medicine* 75, Supp. 5 (2008): S22–S25.

Schoolwerth, Anton C., M.D., et al. "Chronic Kidney Disease: A Public Health Problem that Needs a Public Health Action Plan." *Preventing Chronic Disease* 3, no. 2 (April 2006): 1–6.

Segev, Dorry L., M.D., et al. "Perioperative Mortality and Long-term Survival Following Live Kidney Donation." *Journal of the American Medical Association* 303, no. 10 (2010): 959–966.

Sesso, Ricardo, and Sergio Wyton L. Pinto. "Five-Year Follow-up of Patients with Epidemic Glomerulonephritis due to *Streptococcus zooepidemicus.*" *Nephrology Dialysis Transplantation* 20 (2005): 1,808–1,812.

Shankar, Anoop, Ronald Klein, and Barbara E. K. Klein. "The Association among Smoking, Heavy Drinking, and Chronic Kidney Disease." *American Journal of Epidemiology* 164, no. 3 (2006): 263–271.

Shoback, Dolores, M.D. "Hypoparathyroidism." *New England Journal of Medicine* 359, no. 4 (2008): 391–403.

Shu-Chuan, Jennifer Ye, and Hsueh-Chih Chou. "Coping Strategies and Stressors in Patients with Hemodialysis." *Psychosomatic Medicine* 69 (2007): 182–190.

Siedner, M. J., et al. "Diagnostic Accuracy Study of Urine Dipstick in Relation to 24-Hour Measurement as a Screening Tool for Proteinuria in Lupus Nephritis." *Journal of Rheumatology* 35, no. 1 (January 2008): 84–90.

Singh, Ajay K., et al. "Correction of Anemia with Epoetin Alfa in Chronic Kidney Disease." *New England Journal of Medicine* 355, no. 20 (November 16, 2006): 2,085–2,098.

Singh, Gurmeet R. "Glomerulonephritis and Managing the Risks of Chronic Renal Disease." *Pediatric Clinics of North America* 56 (2009): 1,363–1,382.

Stanton, M. C., and J. D. Tange. "Goodpasture's Syndrome." *Australian Annals of Medicine* 7 (1958): 132–144.

Staples, A. O., et al. "Anemia and Risk of Hospitalization in Pediatric Chronic Kidney Disease." *Clinical Journal of the American Society of Nephrology* 4 (2009): 48–56.

Steer, Andrew C., Margaret H. Danchin, and Jonathan R. Carapetis. "Group A Streptococcal Infections in Children." *Journal of Paediatrics and Child Health* 43 (2007): 203–213.

Steinbrook, Robert, M.D. "Medicare and Erythropoietin." *New England Journal of Medicine* 356, no. 1 (January 4, 2007): 4–6.

Stevens, Lesley A., M.D., Josef Coresh, M.D., Tome Greene, and Andrew S. Levey, M.D. "Assessing Kidney Function—Measured and Estimated Glomerular Filtration Rate." *New England Journal of Medicine* 3354, no. 3 (June 8, 2006): 2,473–2,483.

Stinghen, Andréa E. M., et al. "Immune Mechanisms Involved in Cardiovascular Complications of Chronic Kidney Disease." *Blood Purification* 29 (2010): 114–120.

Straub, Deborah A. "Calcium Supplementation in Clinical Practice: A Review of Forms, Doses, and Indications." *Nutrition in Clinical Practice* 22 (2007): 286–296.

Suri, M., et al. "Denys-Drash Syndrome." *Indian Pediatrics* (December 1995): 1,310–1,313.

Szeifert, Lilla, M.D., et al. "Symptoms of Depression in Kidney Transplant Recipients: A Cross-sectional Study." *American Journal of Kidney Diseases* 55, no. 1 (2010): 132–140.

Taber, S. S., and D. A. Pasko. "The Epidemiology of Drug-Induced Disorders: The Kidney." *Expert Opinions on Drug Safety* 7, no. 6 (2008): 679–690.

Thompson, Joanne, et al. "Albuminuria and Renal Function in Homozygous Sickle Cell Disease: Observations from a Cohort Study." *Archives of Internal Medicine* 167 (2007): 701–708.

Tong, Allison, et al. "Experiences of Parents Who Have Children with Chronic Kidney Disease: A Systematic Review of Qualitative Studies." *Pediatrics* 121 (2008): 349–360.

Toussaint, Nigel D., Grahame J. Elder, and Peter G. Kerr. "Bisphosphonates in Chronic Kidney Disease; Balancing Potential Benefits and Adverse Effects on Bone and Soft Tissue." *Clinical Journal of the American Society of Nephrology* 4 (2009): 221–233.

Tryggvason, Karl, M.D., Jaakko Patrakka, M.D., and Jorma Wartiovaara, M.D. "Hereditary Proteinuria Syndromes and Mechanisms of Proteinuria." *New England Journal of Medicine* 354, no. 13 (2006): 1,387–1,401.

Tseng, Chin-Lin, et al. "Survival Benefit of Nephrologic Care in Patients with Diabetes Mellitus and Chronic Kidney Disease." *Archives of Internal Medicine* 168, no. 1 (January 14, 2008): 55–62.

Tsui, Judith I., M.D. "Association of Hepatitis C Seropositivity with Increased Risk for Developing End-stage Renal Disease." *Archives of Internal Medicine* 167 (June 25, 2007): 1,271–1,276.

United States Department of Health and Human Services. *2008 Annual Report of the U.S. Organ Procurement and Transplantation Network and the Scientific Registry of Transplant Recipients: Transplant Data 1998–2007.* Rockville, Md.: Health Resources and Services Administration, Healthcare Systems Bureau, Division of Transplantation, October 2009.

United States Renal Data System. *USRDS 2009 Annual Data Report: Atlas of Chronic Kidney Disease and End-Stage Renal Disease in the United States.* Bethesda, Md.: National Institutes of Health, National Institute of Diabetes and Digestive and Kidney Diseases, 2009.

Vieira, Lisa. "Expanded Criteria Donors Offer Hope for Patients Needing Kidney Transplant." *Journal of the American Association of Physician Assistants* 22, no. 3 (2009): 33–36.

Von Essen, Marina Rode, et al. "Vitamin D Controls T Cell Antigen Receptor Signaling and Activation of Human T Cells." *Nature Immunology* 11, no. 4 (2010): 344–349.

Waikaur, Sushrut S., M.D., and Wolfgang C. Winkelmayer, M.D. "Chronic on Acute Renal Failure:

Long-Term Implications of Severe Acute Kidney Injury." *Journal of the American Medical Association* 302, no. 11 (2009): 1,227–1,228.

Wald, Ron, et al. "Chronic Dialysis and Death among Survivors of Acute Kidney Injury Requiring Dialysis." *Journal of the American Medical Association* 302, no. 11 (2009): 1,179–1,185.

Waldman, M., and G. B. Appel. "Update on the Treatment of Lupus Nephritis." *Kidney International* 70, no. 8 (2006): 1,403–1,412.

Wallen, Eric M., Geoffrey F. Joyce, and Matthew Wise. "Kidney Cancer." In *Urologic Diseases in America,* edited by M. S. Litwin and C. S. Saigal, 335–378. Bethesda, Md.: National Institute of Diabetes and Digestive and Kidney Diseases, 2007.

Walser, Mackenzie, M.D. *Coping with Kidney Disease: A 12-Step Treatment Program to Help You Avoid Dialysis.* Hoboken, N.J.: John Wiley & Sons, 2004.

Warady, Bradley A., and Vimal Chadha. "Chronic Kidney Disease in Children: The Global Perspective." *Pediatric Nephrology* 22 (2007): 1,999–2,009.

Ward, Michael M., M.D. "Laboratory Abnormalities at the Onset of Treatment of End-Stage Renal Disease: Are There Racial or Socioeconomic Disparities in Care?" *Archives of Internal Medicine* 167 (2007): 1,083–1,091.

Waterman, A. D., et al. "Attitudes and Behaviors of African Americans Regarding Early Detection of Kidney Disease." *American Journal of Kidney Disease* 51, no. 4 (2008): 554–562.

Weaver, Arthur L., M.D. "Epidemiology of Gout." *Cleveland Clinic Journal of Medicine* 75, Supp. 5 (2008): S9–S12.

Wei, John T., M.D., Elizabeth A. Calhoun, and Steven J. Jacobsen, M.D. "Benign Prostatic Hyperplasia." In *Urologic Diseases in America,* edited by M. S. Litwin and C. S. Saigal, 43–70. Bethesda, Md.: National Institute of Diabetes and Digestive and Kidney Diseases, 2007.

Weiner, I. David, and Charles S. Wingo. "Hyperkalemia: A Potential Silent Killer." *Journal of the American Society of Nephrology* 9 (1998): 1,535–1,543.

Wild, S., G. Roglic, A. Green, et al. "Global Prevalence of Diabetes. Estimates for the Year 2000 and Projections for 2030." *Diabetes Care* 27 (2004): 1,047–1,053.

Wu, Eric Q., et al. "Disease-Related and All-Cause Health Care Costs of Elderly Patients with Gout." *Journal of Managed Care Pharmacy* 14, no. 2 (2008): 164–175.

Wyatt, Christina M., and Paul E. Klotman. "HIV-1 and HIV-Associated Nephropathy 25 Years Later." *Clinical Journal of the American Society of Nephrology* 2 (2007): S20-S24.

Wyatt, Christina M., et al. "The Spectrum of Kidney Disease in Patients with AIDS in the Era of Antiretroviral Therapy." *Kidney International* 75, no. 4 (2009): 428–434.

Zappitelli, Michael, M.D. "Epidemiology and Diagnosis of Acute Kidney Injury." *Seminars in Nephrology* 28, no. 5 (2008): 436–446.

Zhou, Xin J., Zoltan G. Laszik, and Fred G. Silva. "Anatomical Changes in the Aging Kidney." In *The Aging Kidney in Health and Disease,* edited by Juan F. Macías Núñez, M.D., J. Stewart Cameron, M.D., and Dimitrios G. Oreopoulos, M.D., 39–54. New York: Springer Science+Business Media, 2008.

# INDEX

Page numbers in **boldface** indicate major treatment of a topic. Page numbers followed by *t* indicate tables.